Meeting Challenges

By Doug Perry

Meeting Challenges is a comical story of adventure, lust, love and life's experiences. It intergrates racial, political, and ethical questions to provoke the reader's imagination to stretch and allows for various viewpoints to be contemplated. Meeting Challenges the second in the series is a sequel to The Gain. While the story can be enjoyed alone there is a depth that can be gained from reading them in sequence.

Thank you to all of the good people and events that have inspired me to write this novel. I am glad to be able to do this work and enjoy it deeply. The beings and places may only exist in my mind, but in there, they seem vivid and exciting. I hope you enjoy my writings as much as I do. Blessing to all of you.

Table of content

4
Going Fishing

Stepping out of the washroom Jay looks around the coffee shop. He sees the staff behind the counter hurrying to supply the line of patrons with the beverages that they want. He sees the crowded room filled with those who are alone and those conversing with each other. He sees the stresses on the faces of most of them. Hearing the background music muffling the many conversations as the barista shout their orders at each other. Turning to Heather Jay tries to remember the details of the few days before he had dinner with Reggie. Knowing that they would be fresh in her mind; He stands there for a few slow deep breaths to calm him self, and to recall the events of those few days. Putting them into sequence Jay gains perspective on what would be relevant topics for him in the coming evenings conversations. Then he starts thinking about going back to work in a few days, going fishing in the morning, and going home with his beloved tonight.

"Ok, I can do this" Jay says to himself under his breath as he lifts his foot to step toward Heather. Seeing her looking at the other washroom as he steps back toward his seat Jay spins his head and looks at that closed door. 'Two washrooms, oh fffrigg' he thinks as he steps into her view. "Ready to go?" offering her a hand to hold as she stands up beside him.

"Oh, I thought I saw you go into the other toilet just a few seconds ago, I thought maybe the first one you went in didn't work or something." Heather says looking at Jay with a perplexed expression.

"No." Jay smiles into her eyes, "everything worked in there as well as can be expected. Does this me look as good as the one you watched going into the other washroom, or do you want to wait and take that one to the movie?" Jay smiles hard with a bit of a laugh escaping his lips and a sparkle in his eye. Taking a last glance around the room as he starts walking with Heather toward the side door that faces the cinema.

She smiles at him, holding his hand, "Jay I was impressed with your answers to all of Reggie's questions. What was the look on his face?" Heather looks up at Jay for a second as they walk toward the cinema door.

"He looked a little surprised. He is an odd duck but polite and seems to be smart, I think I'll call him in the morning and see if he wants to come fishing with us too." Jay replies as he pulls the door to the cinema open and steps aside for Heather to enter first. Jay stepping inside takes her hand again and leads to the line-up to buy tickets. "It starts in twelve minutes."

"Oh, Jay I got the tickets already, before the coffee. Lets go get seats." She says as she searches her purse for them. Pulling them out as they walk toward the escalators and handing them to him. "There was no line when I came by so I thought it best to get them first."

Riding up the escalator with his arm around her Jay notices that he is still feeling the effects of the vercset. Searching deep within himself he feels it exploring his senses and reaches through it to see if he can find Trentia's feelings from there. He can't, at least he can't be sure if he can feel her still through the vercset. He can feel the vercset in him though and now that he is still he can feel its' lingering effects of extending his senses within his body and mind. Feeling Heather beside him he feels how he is emotionally connected and the depth of his feelings toward her. He notices the warm glow in and around his heart. The content feeling of safety and joy and companionship and affection, the openness and sharing and security all percussing through him from skin to skin. Delving deeply into these feelings Jay watches his memories of their interactions and feels a calm filling him as they reach the top of the escalator. With his arm around her and a smile on his face Jay takes the few steps to the attendant and hands her the tickets.

The attendant looks at them, the tickets, and back at them while reaching to grab some 3-D glasses. "Here Sir, Mam, theatre 6, over there then left".

"Thank you" Heather says, taking her glasses and holding Jay's arm as they walk as directed. "I hope it is a good movie, I could use some excitement" as she smiles at Jay.

Smiling back and looking into her eyes, "Yeah, excitement is good, I'm sure James Bond won't let us down." Feeling his body reacting to the decrease of adrenaline from the situation of his morning, "it will be good to watch some excitement". His sensations made more noticeable by the lingering vercset's effects Jay thinks to him self 'it will be nice to watch some excitement without being involved in the outcomes'.

They find some seats about a third the way back almost in the middle. Jay offers to go get snacks but Heather says she is still full from dinner. Jay concurs. After a moment of comfortable silence they start joking about the last James Bond movie they watched and comparing notes of the few released before that. After the previews, as the movie is starting, Heather pulls some truffles and a vitamin drink out of her purse. Jay is surprised and remembers how thoughtful she always is. These are what he would have gotten himself if they had been available at the concession. It brought tears to his eyes as he put on the glasses. He had done all that he had done on Ramga thinking that he would not be back for such a long time, if ever, and now has to face himself about it all. But just now he will focus and simply enjoy the movie.

After the movie and the long drive home Jay takes a shower manually and scrubs himself dry with the towel. Realizing that his body hair is not fully grown back he puts on his robe and finds some pajamas while Heather readies herself for sleeping. When she gets into bed she asks if he plugged his phone in to charge. Jay gets up and does it, gets himself a glass of water and takes his regular before bed herbal supplements. He looks at his phone, turns it on, and fills the water filter. Jay goes back to his phone and opens the text function to contact Reggie.

"I'll send Reggie a text now so that he can have a chance to get it in time to come fishing." Jay says to Heather. He texts (Reggie, I enjoyed the interview etcetera. I am going fishing in the morning with friends. It would be great if you could join us. It will give me a chance to thank you for the thought provoking experience, and maybe get you some more subjects. Meet me at Granville Hotel Marina before 8am today. Jay).

"Do you think it is OK to text him so late?" Heather asks with her head sunken into the pillow.

"It is a text, he won't answer if he is busy or asleep." Jay says as he looks at her head sticking out from the covers. He makes his way to his side of the bed and climbs in. Jay searches his feeling for a second then cuddles up to her and gives her a kiss. "Good night" he whispers into her ear. Feeling the emotional comfort of being home after a long adventure Jay listens to the sounds of the room. Feeling the familiarity of his old bed and Heather beside him he smiles and takes a deep breath. The familiar smells of earth fill his nostrils and bring his mind to the life he lives here, the shops near by, the beach walks, the sunsets and the farm not too far away. The window is open a little and he can hear the birds in the trees outside. He can also hear the music from one of the neighbours' patio, and smell the fresh soil on the garden across the fence. Taking another deep breath Jay focuses on how his body feels as he relaxes more into the pillow and mattress. Stopping his thoughts and only paying attention to the sensations of his body as he relaxes more with the next slow deep breath; focusing to relax where he finds tension in his muscles and joints. With the next inhale Jay fades into dreams of James Bond and the Gowrlacks, riding Brebails and eating strange foods. Jay hears an odd sound and feels a bump against his ribs.

Heather roles toward him, "Jay that is your alarm, you got fishing this morning, I'm not getting up."

Disoriented Jay looks around the room. Remembering the short day before and then remembering his fishing plans with Gary. "Oh", Jay sits up on the side of the bed and looks in the direction of the sound. He can't see the phone but gets up and takes the few short steps to the kitchen to slide his finger across the screen and bring the room back to silence. Feeling himself he notices that he feels strong and clear minded, but still disoriented from the end of his adventure on Ramga. He looks at the time on his phone and thinks about what he needs to do. He puts some water in the kettle. Then looks at the espresso machine. His eyebrows go up, he fills it with water and turns it on, checks the grounds funnel/holder, warms it with hot water from the sink and fills it with fine ground French roast beans. Looks in the fridge and pulls out the milk and places it on the counter. Looks back in the fridge and takes out the bread, butter and peanut butter, then with a smile on his face turns and pulls the honey from a cupboard and places it with the other items. Still smiling he walks to the washroom, removes his pajamas and gets into the shower. After toweling himself off Jay walks naked back to the kitchen and steams his milk, drips his espresso (missing the first few drops, and then running it short), and pours it into his slightly frothy milk. Taking a tiny sip, closing his eyes and smiling as he takes a deep breath. 'You can't get that on Ramga!' he thinks to himself and puts down the cup. Looking at Heather as he slips past to get his clothes, being as quiet as possible so she can sleep easily.

Once fully dressed for his day of fishing he returns to the kitchen and his coffee. Jay makes his two peanut butter and honey sandwiches with lots of butter and packs them in a bag with a banana and two cans of coconut juice for his lunch. He checks the time and then his pockets before putting his jacket on. Checking his texts to see if Reggie replied then grabbing a toque for his head. Jay walks back and gives Heather a kiss on her cheek and says "see you for dinner" before slipping into his shoes and locking the door behind himself.

After starting the van Jay sits and looks at the street. It is quiet, only a few birds, one lady walking a dog near the park and the city bus pulling up to the bus stop a few blocks away. He thinks about the situation that brought him home early the day before and remembered what Herfermks said about him getting placed on the Gyrekian moon if there was any trouble. Taking out his phone he dials Reggie's number, after a few rings he hears a sleepy and confuses voice.

"uchn, Hello?" Reggie asks.

"Hi, Reggie, did you get my text last night?" Jay quarries with a familiarity like they are close friends.

"Who are you?" Reggie asks.

Jay remembers that Reggie may not feel that close or recognize his voice. "It is Jay, from dinner last night. Something happened and I am back early. It is important that I talk with you. Can you meet me at Granville Hotel Marine before 8 AM? If you like you can come fishing on a charter boat with me, and two of my friends. The experience could help with your public relations work."

Reggie thinks about Jay's words, he is suspicious of why Jay would be back early but to him it is the next day and he has no way of knowing how long Jay was gone. Pondering this for a few seconds as he wakes up a bit more his curiosity gets him, he looks at the time, "That gives me an hour to get there, I live near the restaurant we met at last night, how long will it take me to get to that marina Jay?"

"About 5 minutes, 10 if you walk. There will be beer but bring a snack for lunch, we will be back in time for the evening meal" Jay says. He thinks for a second, "I'm driving in, from home. I can pick you up at your place if you like, in about 40 minutes?"

Reggie thinks about what his interactions with Jay were. "Ok, in front of the restaurant?"

"Ya, that's perfect, do you want me to stop and pick you up a mrruk on the way?"

"Mrruk? How," Reggie asks.

"hahaha, well, a good coffee, made right can taste about the same, see you in forty minutes Reggie!" Jay taps the red spot to end the call, puts the phone down and starts driving. Enjoying the familiar views on the way, liking how the rising sun sparkles off of so many things, the river, the jets, and the buildings. Then close to the restaurant Jay stops at a small cafe that makes a good latte and asks for a restratto latte and an americano with three short shots in it to go. He adds a dash of cinnamon and a half spoon of dark sugar, gives it a good stir then a shake of coco powder on top and another stir, and puts on the lids. With the coffees in the cup holders in his dash Jay drives to Gabe's Souvlaki, parks and looks around for Reggie. Seeing Reggie walking toward him from behind Jay reaches across the van and pops opens the door.

Arriving at the van Reggie pulls the door wide and looks in at Jay, after a pause, "good morning".

"There is your coffee, it should taste like a mrruk, get in" Jay smiles to him.

Reggie hesitates as he examines Jay's expression, then as he starts climbing into the seat of the van "so how long were you there, and what happened?"

Jay smiles at him. " It was only about four months, maybe five, of earth time. I did some off world work with Herfermks and visited Akwerts with Trentia. There were some planetary security issues. I think due to my being selected as a top story for social media, after having the first tour with the birds for a very long time, I was to be investigated. A non member of our team sent me back and said he would meet me last night to retrieve me but he did not show up." Looking at the surprised expression on Reggie's face, "try the coffee, I think you will like it!"

Reggie hesitates continuing to look at Jay, then looks at the coffee and reaches for it. He slowly takes off the lid and smells it. Looks at Jay with wide eyes, "It smells ok" stairs out the window for a few seconds and then takes a drink. "uum, yeah, it's not bad." Takes another drink and turns to look at Jay again. "So what do you want from me?".

Jay looks at him and takes a drink of his own coffee. "Well Reggie. I realize that my 10 years is not up yet. But I understand that my time with the team may be over. I only have you as a contact and am willing to do whatever the team needs of me. So if you could ask Herfermks if I am getting sent to the Gyrekian's moon now, or what? Reggie, I had an earlier conversation with the ryberrian who sent me back and talked to Herfermks about it. Herfermks told me not to converse with that ryberrian directly but to go through him only. At the time when other ryberrian wanted to send me back, all the data on his tablet make it seem too important for me to do as I was asked. According to Trentia it was accurate, but as he did not show up when he said he would, I suspect something is not as it should be."

Reggie looks at Jay and takes another drink of the coffee. He looks around on the street and in the back of the van. Then he takes another drink. "So are we actually going fishing today, tell me about that".

Jay smiles. "before leaving after dinner last night I had a busy life. I had plans to go fishing today with a friend from work and his brother in law from out of town. So that is what was on my social calendar for today, here on earth. There is room on the boat for more than are going and I can afford to pay for your spot on the fishing charter. After working on your world and starting to get comfortable with your culture I realized how odd it must seem for you to have to live here. Reggie I would feel honored if you would join us for a day of fishing. We will probably talk about sports, and politics, and women, and family, and work, and enjoy jokes about our world and each other. You will likely catch a fish; they are delicious, and nutritious. If you have other commitments or don't trust me enough I understand."

Reggie looks at Jay trying to read his expressions. "So, you want me to communicate with Herfermks for you, and separate from that you are inviting me to come spend the day on a sea vessel to catch some fish with your friends?"

"Yip" Jay replies.

"Ok, I'll go fishing. I'll send a message to Herfermks that he will understand while you drive us to the marina. I can't say when we will get a reply." Reggie pulls out his tablet and looks at Jay as he starts the van and pulls out into the sparse traffic. Reggie works his tablet's screen while they drive. "Jay, what is the last event you can mention that Herfermks would remember or know about before you were sent back to here.

Jay looks at him then back at the street. "The second morning after visiting Trentia's family in Akwerts."

After a few more blocks Reggie says "You know Jay, I understand that you probably have been told not to say anything about what Herfermks does with you. When I left there was some time after you arrived. I remember when Trentia left our organization, I think less than a year after your arrival there. I remember little about you, we never actually met, but I did hear you worked hard and that you were a successful recruit of mine. I worked from another city so that it would be impossible for us to meet. I sent a message to Herfermks saying that you returned here the next morning after visiting with Trentia's family in Akwerts. I said that you are well and that you would like to hear from him sooner than latter." Reggie looks at Jay. I also told him that you are taking me fishing with friends in a boat on the water, and that you made my coffee taste like mrruk. I am leaving my tablet open for his scans to work through. But I have no way of knowing when you will be contacted."

"Thank you Reggie. We will park here. It is a few blocks to the marina but the van will be safe here and this parking is free. Did you bring a snack?" Jay looks across the van at Reggie as he opens his door to step out.

"I brought a tomato and some cookies." Reggie smiles and finishes his coffee.

"Well, I've got two sandwiches, a banana and two coconut drinks. If you like the peanut butter and honey I'll swap you one for some cookies. You are welcome to have one of the coconut drinks." Jay says with a smile.

"Thanks Jay, but can't I drink the water that the boat floats on?" Reggie asks.

"You can, but it has a lot of salt in it, hehehe" Jay snickers. "We can't drink it, it makes us more thirsty and dehydrated."

"Oh. What is the beer like Jay, I haven't tried it. You said there would be beer to drink." Reggie inquires.

"It is stronger than the beer that the birds like to drink on Ramga, it is bubbly and served cold. It thins the blood and dulls the mind, but brings a feeling of happiness and willingness to share information" Jay looks at his phone to see the time. "We have a few moments, they are probably some snack machines at the marina. I'll get something incase you don't want too much beer."

"Thanks" Reggie looks at Jay with curiousness for a few seconds. "Jay, did you like the beings you met on Ramga?"

Jay turns his head and stops walking. "Yeah I did actually. It was scary at first. I hoped that they wouldn't catch me. You know being a human. But I was having a great time there and making friends everywhere I went. I liked my job too."

"is that why you are treating me like an old friend?" Reggie looks into his eyes watching his response.

"In my life you are, kind of, you gave me the greatest gift that I have ever heard of; and after living in your culture briefly I feel I can trust you more than most of the humans that I have known." Jay looks at him, "It is strange." Pointing to the side of the marina building "the vending machines are around there," Jay looks around "Gary's car is over there if you want to go down onto the dock and see if you can see three guys in a charter boat I'll catch up with whatever I can get from the machines." Jay starts walking.

"I'll go with you Jay" and Reggie follows Jay toward the corner, then to the vending machines. "This one has snacks," Reggie says "the mixed nuts and fruit bits looks good."

Jay puts in a $ 5 note and pushes the buttons to make them come out. Then steps to the other machine, "water, pop, coconut water, or fruit juice?"

"What is the difference between water and coconut water?" Reggie asks.

"Water is like from the tap, coconuts grow on trees and are filled with very health fluid that taste like slightly sweet water. They grow in the warmer parts of this planet." Jay says, can you check its' biocompatibility with your tablet?"

Reggie looks at him, "get me one I'll do that, thanks Jay."

Jay looks at his money and gets a can and hands it to
Reggie. Then gets two more as Reggie is scanning the can and
working on his tablet. Jay looks at Reggie in time to see him
nod with a smile and starts walking ahead toward the ramp
down to the docks. The gate is tied open so they go through.
Half way down the ramp Jay can see Gary and his brother in
law talking to a guy and loading their stuff onto his boat.
"that's them there" Jay says as he points.

"Ok," Reggie replies "it looks like a good vessel. But it doesn't
look like it can go under the water."

"No, if it goes under the water we will be in great danger,
hahaha" Jay laughs until a tear comes out. "No Reggie our
fishing boats stay on top of the water, it makes it more
challenging this way. It is safe though."

A few steps behind Reggie, Jay waves to Gary and calls out to
him. "Gary, I brought a friend, I just realized last night that he
might like to join us but didn't know if he could make it until
this morning."

"Great," Gary replies reaching out a hand to shake with
Reggie. "My name is Gary and this is my brother in law Ted
and our captain Jody."

Reggie shakes Gary's hand then Ted's, then Jody's. "I've never fished from a boat before."

"Isn't it exciting," Ted says, "I've never seen the ocean before today."

"Well the weather is good, 5 km wind from the south west, nothing more expected. The fish are biting in the straights off the mouth of the river, near Point Grey, and near Roberts creek." Jody says.

"Permission to come aboard" Jay asks as he puts out his hand to shake with Jody.

"Welcome aboard, you too Reggie. Do you prefer Reggie or Reg?" Jody asks him.

"Reggie please" Reggie says as he steps aboard. "Where should I put my lunch?"

"Inside, down there in the fridge if you can find room. I brought food for six just in case, but you are welcome to do as you please." Looking at Jay's hand, you brought food too." then looking at Gary, "We agreed on lunch didn't we."

Gary looks at Jay, then at Jody, "Yip, lunch provided, and guaranteed fish or the next trip for half price." Gary looks at Reggie going into the cabin and then at Jay again, "you forgot? It was last night. haha, so you had a long night ahy?"

"Well," Jay scratches his head and smiles, "you did say lunch included, and beer. There better be beer. It seems like a long time ago now, my bad. Should we get the money dealt with before we leave the dock?" as he pulls out his wallet.

Gary pulls his out too. "I'm paying for Ted too." and hands some bank notes to Jody.

Jay looks at the notes and pulls what he thinks is the same amount. "I am paying for Reggie, is this the correct amount?" and hands the money to the captain.

Jody counts the money, "you having a rough day Jay," and hands back a five."

"Not yet" taking back the note and smiling at Jody, "Got coffee?"

"Can you make it Jay? I want to get under way, It is in the galley." as he turns to the stairs. He hurries to the top, sits checks his instruments and starts the motor.

Jay goes inside and starts looking around the cabin. Sees the coffee maker, a drip machine. Looks in the cupboards until he finds the filter and grounds. Fills the machine with water and grounds and sets the thing to do what it can. Checks the fridge and sees lots of beer and food and milk and cream. Looks to the left and sees some bottles of scotch, rum, vodka and liqueurs. He smiles to himself and goes out then onto the dock. "Captain, Want me to get the lines?"

Jody looks at him, looks around the entire boat, then at the path between the other boats that they will be leaving through. "Yeah, just untie them and get aboard, don't push us off yet."

Jay does. Gary and Ted are sitting in the deck chairs and Reggie is standing looking around at the stern of the boat. Jay goes beside Reggie and says softly "there are no stabilizing mechanisms so best to sit or hold something before we start moving."

Reggie looks at Jay with a questioning matter of fact expression for a second then looks at the deck chairs smiles back at Jay and sits down in one. They hear the change of the engine sound and feel the pulse as the captain puts it into gear. They start to move, slowly out of the slip, turning, and between the other boats toward the far side of the inlet. As they approach the middle they turn and head west into the bay. Reggie and Ted both seem taken by the view. The morning sun is brightly sparkling off of the buildings, boats, and the water behind the boat.

Jay thinks about the sunrise he enjoyed at the sea two days earlier before going swimming for the day. He compares the brilliance of this one to the magical dazzle of the one at the sea. Smiling to himself and enjoying the birds he asks in a loud voice "who wants a coffee and how do you like it?"

Gary looks at him, "black"

Ted smiles, "white and sweet"

Reggie turns his head to Jay and smiles, "same as this morning if you can"

Jay looks up to the dodger and steps half way up the ladder. "Captain, your coffee sir, how do you want it?"

"haha, Well if you are gonna call me sir, I'll take it with a tiny shot of granny mate"

Jay goes and makes the coffees, by the time he has them on a tray the boat is under the bridges and passing the buoy at the inlets entrance. As he picks up the tray he feels the boat softly lunge with acceleration and hears the hum of the engines increase. Serving his fishing mates first then putting his own coffee down Jay climbs to give Jody his drink. Placing it beside him and looking at the controls he can see that the boat is only at half throttle. "Fast boat?"

"Yeah, it will do 45 mph but it is best if keep it under 30. It handles better and the fuel consumption is bad at top speed." Jody Takes his cup and has a sip, turns one eye toward Jay and gives him a nod. "Perfect." Jody makes an adjustment on the radio and turns to Jay for a second, "get out on the water much?"

"Yeah, I got a sail boat, in the marina under the bridge. I'm not much of a fisherman though, I'm hoping that all changes today." Jay smirks.

Jody looks at his expression then back at the water. "You will catch something even if I have to get into the water and put it on the hook myself there is no way I'm gonna take you out for free!." Then he looks at Jay with the most stern and serious look on his face.

Jay looks back at him and they both start to laugh. "Where we gonna fish?" Jay asks.

"I'll call around and see where it is best. I'll know in about ten minutes." Jody says.

Jay goes back down stairs and gets his coffee and sits on the icebox facing the three men in chairs. Reggie is listening to Ted talk about life back in Montana. Jay sips his coffee and thinks how much better it would taste with a little granny in it. Gary asks Reggie where he grew up. Jay turns to Reggie to hear his response and hears silence.

"Reggie, was it a city or town, I remember you mentioned it being by the sea, or was it a lake?" Jay asks.

"Actually a farm town, near a small city on the sea side." Reggie replies.

"So you were a farmer like Ted? What did you grow?" Gary asks.

"Actually my parents worked for the government in administrative capacity in the farm town. We didn't grow anything. The farms in the area mostly grew fruit. Some meat animals were also produced but we didn't participate in any way. As soon as I was old enough I left for the city to further my education." Reggie replies and takes a big drink of his coffee.

"I was raised on a farm, and still do some farming" Ted says. "There is no lake or sea near where I come from. Some ponds and creeks, But this ocean is really something. How deep is it?"

"Well" Jay says, "here it is only about a hundred feet but if we go that way it is several hundreds feet and it we go between those two islands it is hundreds of feet deep there too."

"Where is he taking us to fish?" Gary asks.

"He wasn't sure. He said he was gona check, I guess he is gona radio his friends and see where the fish are." Jay says. "We are turning south so I suspect we are going to the mouth of the river. I heard that there are still salmon coming up the river."

"I hope so." Reggie says.

"Do you like salmon Reggie?" Ted asks.

"Yeah, I have it in restaurants often. Sushi, baked, barbequed, pickled, I like it all." Reggie says.

Jay looks at Ted, "what kind of fishing do you do in Montana?"

Ted shakes his head, "not much, there is fishing there, bass, trout, but I don't do it. I went out about five years ago with some friends and shot a deer. That was something." shakes his head some more. "Won't do that again."

Gary looks at him, "why not?"

Ted looks at each of them. "One of my friends almost shot another friend by accident. His gun went off when he didn't think it was loaded. We slept in the forest and in the morning realized that we were in a cow pasture with trees. The farmer told us not to come back. When we did kill the thing it wasn't with the first shot. My friend wounded it, then it ran about 300 yards before it fell down. When we got there it was hiding under some bushes bleeding from the guts. Clearly it was suffering. I wanted to shoot it in the head but my friend insisted in shooting it in the heart. It took him two shots to kill it. Then we had to cut the guts out and bring it back to the car.

It was about a mile to the car. Hahaha. That thing was heavy after the first hundred yards. My two friends where arguing about who should carry it next most of the way back. All three of us were covered in blood and because we killed it so slow the meat was tough as hell. Because we didn't bleed it properly it was messy for the butcher and he charged us extra. Because my friends are assholes we argued about who should get what parts until the last peace was eaten a year later. In the end it would have been cheaper to take my wife out to a fancy restaurant 30 times than the full expense of the 3 days of hunting. There was the license, the gun registration, the gear to camp, the first night in a hotel, the booze. Nope did that once, once is enough."

"Well" Reggie says, "I hope fishing works out better for us than your hunting experience"

Gary and Jay both start laughing, after a second Ted starts laughing to. Reggie looks at them and although he isn't sure what was the funny part of Ted's story he starts laughing a bit too.

The intercom comes on and they hear the Jody say "I heard that several boats have caught salmon in the straight this morning so we will start there. Will one of you like to steer so I can get the gear ready?"

Gary looks at Jay then Reggie, Ted looks at Reggie then at Jay; Reggie looks at Jay then at Gary and Ted.

"It is easy," Jay says. "He will probably have it on auto pilot anyways, There just needs to be someone there incase we want to stop, or have to turn to miss another boat." He looks at them "Reggie you and Ted should do it, it will be fun. Go for it Ted, you will have a better time than you did hunting for sure."

Ted looks at Reggie, "lets give it a try"

Reggie gets up looks at the ladder going to the upper deck where Jody is, then looks at the others. "Ok Ted lets do this." he turns and goes to the ladder climbing to be greeted by Jody looking back at him when he steps onto the top deck.

"Reggie right?" Jody asks. Seeing the nod "well it is easy, just go straight that way. See here the number on the compass, keep this line on that number." he turns the wheel a little one way turning the boat, "see the numbers move," then turns it the other way until the number moves back. "It is that easy." Jody looks at Reggie's eyes, "have you controlled a vessel before?"

"Something similar yes" Reggie says.

"I'll be back up in 5 minutes if you have a question push the intercom button here and ask." Jody says. "Are you ready?"

Reggie looks at the controls, he sees the throttle the radio, the chart plotter, the fish finder and the various gauges indicating how the motor is doing. "Ok, should I grab the wheel?"

Jody nods, "yeah, if anything happens pull back the throttle slowly and I'll be back up here." He steps out of the seat and lets Reggie sit down before letting go of the wheel. "Hay Reggie, looks like Ted is coming up to sit with you." He goes down the ladder as soon as he can get past Ted.

Ted nods at Jody as they pass each other. "Reggie, you got balls man. I wouldn't want to be driving. I thought they were joking about us driving this boat." Ted stands and looks at him for a moment then sits in the seat beside him. "It is great out here huh!"

Reggie looks at him and smiles. "yeah, I never thought I would do anything like this, it is great." Steering the boat is not that hard. Later you should do it, get Jody to show you how." Reggie looks at the gauges then the compass. It has moved off the number a bit so he moves the wheel a little. He sees that the compass went the wrong way so he moves the wheel a bit the other way. After a few seconds the compass comes back.

"Apparently we are going right over there. In the middle I think." Reggie looks at Ted, "he said about five minutes."

"Wow, this is a fast boat" Ted says as he looks back at where they came from. "It looks like we are half way to that island over there."

Reggie looks at the chart plotter and then at the island, then back at where they came from. "Yeah, almost. See it here. We are this dot here." pointing at the chart plotter on the dash between them.

"That's handy," then Ted looks at the fish finder and points, "what's that one do?"

Reggie looks at the compass for a split second then at the fish finder. He looks at the display then pushes the buttons changing the screen several times. "It shows what is under the water and how deep things below the boat are, it also indicates traveling speed and water temperature." with wide eyes looking into Ted's, "an impressive technology."

"I'll say, what are those dots?" Ted says pointing at some small shapes on the screen.

Reggie looks at them for a second then at the water in front of the boat then at the compass then back at the screen. He pokes the buttons on the fish finder changing the screen several times, Looks at the water and compass again and corrects the wheel a little then pokes the buttons some more. "I think it is some things moving in the water below us, Lots of things." Reggie smiles at Ted "maybe those are the fish."

Ted looks at the screen and starts smiling too "I hope so."

Jody coming back up the ladder, "Hay boys, we are there, Reggie, ease back on the throttle."

Reggie looks at Jody then at the water in front of the boat then at the throttle and slides it slowly back. He feels the boat slowing and hears the motor quieting down. He continues to bring it slowly back until Jody is standing between him and Ted and the lever is at the neutral position. He looks at Jody and stands up. "Here you go captain, Thank you it was interesting to drive, nice vessel."

Jody smiles as he opens a panel and flicks some switches. "I'm changing the controls so that I can steer from below and coach you all on fishing on the lower deck." flicking more switches the chart plotter and fish finder go off. "Go on down you two, I'll be right behind you." Jody opens a panel and pulls out a camera and mounts it on the visor above the middle of the dash. He checks the wires flicks some switches in the panel and on the camera, checks the LEDs are on and adjusts the position of the camera, "that should do it" he says to himself as he turns and notices he is alone. Taking a deep breath he starts down the stairs. At the bottom he waits as the others are chatting and fondling the fishing gear. "Ok Boys, you each get a rod, but before you pick it up think about where you are going to be when you are fishing. We are gona be traveling slowly and your lines must not get crossed with each other's. One on each side and two off the back, OK" he looks at them all looking a little puzzled. "Put a chair where you are gona fish from so that you can sit until you catch a fish. Get your beer in place beside the chair or your coffee, and then take a rod and sit in your chair pointing off the edge of the boat."

Jay laughs, smiles at Jody and says, "yeah I think I'll get a beer, anyone else want one?" as he steps toward the cabin.

Gary and Ted both concur asking for one. Reggie moves a chair to one side of the back deck and picks up the rod closest to him, then looks at Jay opening the fridge inside and asks for one too. Gary and Ted set up their chairs at the stern (back) of the boat and each take up a rod. Jay returns with five open beer, passing one off to Jody then one to each of the others before putting his down on the gunnel so that he can put his chair in place and get his rod ready. Jody takes a big slug of his then wipes his mouth with his sleeve. He looks at the situation of the gear on the rods and the positioning of the chairs. Then slides out a cooler from the corner and opens it.

"Ok boys here is the bate." as he hands each of them a five inch long shiny dead fish. "Put one of these little fish on your hook so that it will stay on. Push the hook through the eyes and catch it in the gills or something similar to that. You see the flashers at the tip of your rods, once you get the fish on the hooks, you are gona let the hook into the water then let about 10 feet of line loose so that the flasher goes into the water. About then I'll pass you a weight to clip onto your lines. When the fish pulls the hook hard the weight will slide down to the flasher. Any questions?"

The three men are busy with their bate.

Reggie having done as Jody said, as fast as he said it is busy with his beer. He tastes it, smells it, gets out his tablet and scans it and works his screen a little before putting it away. "Tell me Jody, is the beer always served cold at sea?"

Jody looks at him with wide eyes, "not always, do you want a warm one?" Watching Reggie with his beer, sipping it, looking in the can, "if you like I have other brands."

"Oh no, this is good" Reggie smiles at him and notices Jay trying his best not to laugh as he is turning his face away from the others. "Lets get my weight on the line Jody. How does it work, the line, it goes through here, and there right?"

Jody points at the one end of the weight, "yeah, then it goes between the metal coils, and the grip will hold it, until the fish pulls hard."

"Oh, good idea, then it slides to the flasher?" Reggie squeezes the line between the wire loops and his rod slides across the deck, as he works the line to finally get it clamped between the wire loops on the lead weight.

Jody picks up the rod and sets the handle into the holder on the gunnel of the boat in front of Reggie. "Grab it when you are ready and let the line out for about 60 feet, there is a black mark on the line at every twenty feet so let it out until you see the third black mark on the line pass the end of the rod"

Reggie and the others are all getting their gear into the water Jody turns on the flat screen hooked to the camera on the dodger and sets up the view screen so he can see what's in front of the boat on it. He sets up his fish finder to see what is under them and adjusts the sensitivity to show details so that he can determine if there are fish under them. He puts the boat in gear and they start moving again. This time slower, about 6 km/hr. Then slows a little. He fiddles with the controls on the fish finder to widen the viewing area under them and slowly turns the boat a little.

"Ok" Gary says and turns to Jody, "my beer is empty I need another."

"They are in the fridge Gary put your rod in the holder and get some." Jody looks at him.

Ted looks at Gary too, checks his own beer and it is still full, looks at the floor then at Gary as Gary is getting up. "Did you use that beer for bait, where did it go?'

Gary puts the rod in the holder and turns to Ted. "The first thing you have to learn about beer in Canada is the faster you finish one the sooner you can start the next. It might be different where you come from in Montana, but here we know where to put the beer" smiling at Ted and giving a big nod, "I'll bring one for you incase you figure it out. If you don't Reggie can have it when it gets warm." Then turning to Jay, ready for the next Jay?"

Jay smiles at Ted and looks at Reggie to see if he is getting the humor. "Sure Gary, its good to be ready, right? Can you get me a bud light this time." looking at Gary heading for the fridge.

"There is an odd sensation on my rod" Reggie says as he stands holding it awkwardly as it bends and line is being pulled off the spool.

Jody stops the boats motor and says, "pull your lines in Ted, Jay, I'll get Gary's" as he quickly steps over and grabs it form the holder. "We gotta get the lines out of the way so the fish won't tangle them. Just reel it up, till the weight is at the tip of the rod. Reggie keep your line taught, reel it in slowly when there is pressure then fast when the pressure decreases."

"Ok," doing his best to follow the instructions, "It is a fish isn't it?" Reggie's arms being pulled to move by the tension on the line, "I can't believe how hard it pulls. What kind of fish is it?"

"Tasty I hope" Ted says as he pulls in his line.

"Probably a salmon, right Jody" Jay interjects.

Jody looks at how the rod is bending and tells Reggie, "Don't pull too hard it could break the line. Let the tension off a little on your reel."

Reggie obviously enthralled with the experience, "what?"

Jay having pulled his line in places his rod in the holder and steps past Gary with his hands filled with beers to adjust the tension controller on Reggie's rod. Hearing it clicking madly as line is slowly release even though Reggie continues to wind it in. "does that look better Jody?"

"Good save Jay" taking a beer from Gary and smiling, "looks like we will have an good day today, the sun will be hot in an hour or two and the fish are biting."

Gary hands beers to Ted and Jay then places one beside Reggie and looks at him, "first time you caught a fish Reggie?"

Taking his eyes off his rod to look at Gary for only a split second, then in the water, then at the fish finder, then back at the rod, "can you see it on the device?" looking at Jody, "the depth fish screen thing, can you see what kind of thing I caught, it pulls so hard, maybe it is something else."

Jody looks at Gary and Jay smirking and starts to laugh, "well whatever you caught counts, my guarantee is that you will catch something, as long as it isn't the bottom I'm licensed for you to pull it up. When we see it, if it is not a salmon we can through it back."

Jay sees the worried look coming onto Reggie's face and curtails his snickering to say, "the fish finder is not that sophisticated as to determine what kind of fish, and it has a limited field of scanning, it likely won't show your fish, don't worry there is nothing else in these waters that would bite the bate."

Watching Reggie continue to wind the reel Jody sees that he is making some progress. "It's coming up" as he steps to a panel and opens it to pull out a big net on a hoop with a handle that he extends like a telescope. "When it comes to the surface, see how the line is pointing away from the boat, you might have to move to the other side if it come this way, we don't want it under the boat. You three stay out of his way" as Jody looks at the others. "Get it beside the boat and I'll scoop it into the net. So we can pick it up"

Ted stepping back from the edge incase Reggie has to follow the fish around the stern, "why don't we want it under the boat, it can't damage the boat can it?"

Gary looks at him, "the prop, it can cut the line or get tangled. Then we lose the fish."

Reggie takes a few small quick steps to the stern as the fish swims behind the boat, then back toward his side stopping in the corner while he continues to wind the rod. They all see the flasher reflecting the sun a few times about 20 feet from the boat then as Reggie continues to wind on the reel finally they see the fish surface for a second. "woe, there it is Reggie" Reggie's face bursts with relief and joy seeing it coming closer to the boat.

"Lift the rod and keep reeling it in" Jody says as he stands behind Reggie, "When it is closer I will step out beside you and scoop it with the net" Jody opens the door to step out onto the swim grid at the stern. Then looks to see the fish is going toward the bow, and the flasher is out of the water, almost at the rod. He steps beside Reggie toward the bow and readies the net with both hands leaning over the edge of the boat. "Someone hold my legs, keep reeling, lift that rod, YA" and stuffs the nets hoop between the boat and the fish then twisting and pulling it around the fish and lifting it in one slick motion, "IT'S IN THE NET" he yells. Then spins the net and grabs the web with one hand "pull me up, it is a good one."

Reggie stops reeling and looks to see Jay and Gary grab Jody's belt and pull him a little as he straitens up and pulls the netted fish into the boat. Smiling hard and looking at the three men, and then at the fish squirming in the net. "Wow shiny and big, it smells good, what do we do with it now?" Reggie watches as Jody, without hesitation, opens a compartment in the floor and dumps the fish out of the net into the ice and water in it.

"That is what happens, that way if you decide not to kill it, it will be easier to get the hook out with out damaging the fish." Jody looks at Reggie then the rest of them. "Is it a keeper?" Looking at their smiles "are you taking them home for food or letting them go?"

Jay looks at Reggie and can tell he is unsure what to say. "Yeah we like that one Jody. Reggie if you don't know how to cook it

I can show you" Jay turns to Jody, "Do we kill it first or take the hook out first?"

Jody gets gloves, puts them on and picks up a bat. "I'll bonk it and pull the hook out." He grabs the salmons back sliding his left fore finger and thumb into its gills, pulls it out of the icy water and onto the deck. Then one good bat on the head and it stops moving. Squeezing into the gills with his grip the mouth opens and he looks in, the line is going into its' stomach. "He swallowed it" then with several hard tugs, the hook and some intestines come out from the fishes mouth. Jody hands the hook back to Reggie "put new bait on this and put it back in the water, don't forget to reset the weight."

Ted asks, "How do you know it was a he?"

Jody looks at him, turns the fish over, "Oh, my bad, She. See these little fin things here, the male is more pointy, and the size of the fish, this is pretty big for a female." he looks up at Ted, "we will see the eggs when we clean it after, but now get your gear back in the water and maybe you will get the next one." Jody stands up and goes back to the controls. He looks at the screen showing in front of the boat and at the fish finder and the chart plotter and then at the four men holding their rods. "Ok let them out to the same length, 60 feet, the third black mark on the line." Jody looks at the view screen again and puts it into gear and pushes the throttle until the fish finder says 6 km per hour.

A few minutes pass with the four watching their lines and sipping their beers. Jody slows the boat a little and tells them to let out another ten feet of line.

Gary asks, "Can you see some fish under us?"

The others all look at Jody as he nods and smiles. Looking at the screen then the fish finder again Jody says to them, maybe another ten, so the fourth black mark should be at the end of your rods." and he turns the wheel slightly to give a wide space between them and another boat near by. "Music? Do you guys want to hear anything special?" He takes out his Ipod and starts turning it on.

Ted says, "Actually I'm enjoying the sounds of the boat and the birds."

Gary finishes his beer and asks, "are you offering to sing to us Jody?" as he sticks his rod in the rod holder, "I'm not gona pay extra, but if you want to sing to us I don't mind" As he walks to the fridge and gets his third beer.

As Gary has his face in the fridge choosing his next beer the reel on his fishing rod starts to let out line and makes a sound of fast clicking, his rods' tip bends towards the water. The other three men look at it and with out a word they start reeling in their lines, Jody turns the motor off and steps over to grab Gary's rod. Jody looks at Gary standing up by the fridge with a surprised look on his face.

"Did I catch one?" as he hurries out to the deck and puts down the opened beer. "I'll take that" as he reaches for the rod.

"Got a hold of it?" Jody asks before letting go. "It pulls hard but keep reeling it in, keep tension on it." Jody sees Gary nodding and turning the handle on the reel. He looks around and gets the net, then looks to see that the others have reeled in their lines. They have and are watching him, "who wants to net this one?" He looks at them all with questioning expressions but not saying anything. "Reggie, you saw what I did last time, it's like that, just scoop it around the fish fast and then lift right away. You do it" and holds the net out towards him.

Reggie's eyes get big as he starts to smile and puts his rod in the holder. "Ok Gary, I'm going to net your fish."

Ted's expression changes to relief and Jay smiles ear to ear. Both of them holding their rods and moving as far out of the way of Gary as possible. The fish swims one way then another as Gary is pulling it up. It first surfaces about twenty feet behind the boat, then down and up again with a little jump about ten feet off the port stern. As it gets closer Gary has his rod at the center of the back of the boat and the fish is near the surface just behind the boat. Reggie climbs out onto the swim grid with net in hand and gets down on his knees with the net in both hands ready to dip for the fish.

"Easy now Reggie, keep the tension steady Gary, wait until it comes closer Reggie" Jody coaches with his beer in hand. He turns giving a cheers motion with his beer to Jay and Ted. Leaning over the back of the boat to watch Reggie's and Gary's teamwork with the catch.

"Now" says Gary.

Reggie thrusting the net, sweeping and twisting it around the fish, "Yeah, got it!" as he lifts the fish in the net almost tipping off into the water with it. Feeling Gary's hand on his shoulder pulling him back, "Whow, thanks Gary" Turning with a smile and holding the net with the struggling salmon in it "It's a good one"

Gary smiling at the fish "Yeah" he picks up his beer and downs it. "I'm gona have another beer."

"OK" Jody says reaching for the net, "lets get that one on ice and catch some more." He takes the net, opens the hold with the first fish in it and dumps the new fish from the net into the ice filled water. He puts his gloved hand on it's back as it squirms and slides his fingers into the gills to grip it and bonks it with his bat. This time the hook is in its mouth so with a push, twist and pull he gets the hook out of the fish. As he is closing the door to the hold Jody says "check your bate and get those lines back in the water" He looks at the four men and goes to the controls. Jody starts the motor and looks at the flat screen, the fish finder, and the chart plotter. He turns the wheel a little and puts it into gear. The boat starts to move and he adjusts the throttle a bit. Jody looks back to see all four men sitting in chairs each with a beer in one hand and the rods in their other hands. "Ha ha." The sun is starting to feel warm on the side of his face as he checks the fish finder and adjusts the wheel a little then speeds up so slightly. "Are you ready?"

Reggie turns to Jody, "you didn't say, so we went to 80 feet of line again." Then he looks back at the others to listen to the conversation.

"The first time I went fishing I was five years old" Gary says. "My mom told my dad that he had me for the weekend because she was helping her sister with her wedding. He got me dressed for the woods and took me out with his friends to go up some creek past Whistler. They were not too impressed with me coming along. But I caught the most fish."

Ted says, "I heard you caught some little trout and a bull head"

Gary laughs and looks at him "those four trout were longer than from my elbow to my finger tips, and the catfish was bigger than my hand." Gary smiles "I was only five years old and so excited that I practically pissed myself when I got the first one."

"hahaha" Jay laughs "Yeah, the same thing is happening to you today, you are catching fish and getting pissed!"

Ted laughs, Reggie looks at Jay with a worried expression.

Gary picks up his beer for a drink and notices that it is empty, "I need another beer" and stands up. As he reaches down to put the rod into the rod holder it bends and the reel starts clicking fast to release line. "Hey, I got another one," Gary grabs the reel and starts fumbling to grip the handle, he looks at Ted, "Ted grab it for me would you, could you reel it in for me" Gary holds it closer to Ted.

Ted quickly puts his rod in the rod holder and takes Gary's pole, lifting it to keep tension until he gets a good grip on the reel's handle. Ted starts winding and turns to ask "Gary, who is going to reel in my line?"

"fuck" Jays rod bends and his reel starts releasing line. "I got one now too"

Jody had already turned off the motor and starts reeling in Ted's line. Reggie is finishing reeling in his line and is holding the loose line between the flasher and hook to control it from bouncing too much. Jay kicks the chair he was sitting on across the deck a little to give himself a little more room to maneuver. Ted is reeling on Gary's fish as it is pulling very hard and going around towards Reggie's side of the boat. Jody ducks under Ted's arms as Ted holds the Rod high to keep the line from crossing his own.

"Thanks Jody" Ted says as he frantically reels in the line now that the fish is giving him some slack.

"Mine isn't pulling that hard" Jay says while he reels it in seemingly with ease. Then his rod bends hard and the line is pulled out a bit, it changes angle to behind the boat, "it's starting to fight now"

Jody hands Reggie the rod. He grabs the net and gets out on the swim grid watching Ted bringing the fish to the surface, "It looks like a big one Ted, see if you can get it over this way somehow."

Ted looks at Jody, then Reggie as he is putting away his rod and line. Then back at Jody. "How?" he asks, as he is reeling and the fish changes direction again and again.

Reggie starts softly laughing. He looks at Jay working his rod and reel trying to control the fish. With a big smile he watches Jody again readying the net as Ted tries to lead the fish by moving his rod. Reggie looks for Gary and sees him standing inside the cabin looking out at them.

Gary sees Reggie look at him, winks, smiles and without a word turns and steps toward the fridge.

Ted watching the fish near the surface working it's mouth trying to let go of the hook. He keeps reeling and keeping tension, and trying to get the fish pulled to where Jody can net it. "I think it is gona be coming your way it seems to follow a bit" stepping to the corner and leaning over a bit "here it comes Jody"

Jody is focusing on the fish and as it swims closer he thrusts his net into the water in beside it, scooping under the fish and pulling up all in one motion. "Ah ha, Got ya." In one swift motion Jody lifts turns and dumps the fish on the deck and then moves with the net to where Jay is working to get his fish up. "OK Jay, I'm ready for you, bring it as close as possible"

Gary is back with his beer and looking down at the fish flapping on the deck. "Looks like a barbeque fish to me" having a sip and looking at Ted and Reggie, "who wants to whack it?"

Ted looks at Reggie. Reggie responds by putting the rod into the holders and getting the bat. He changes it from one hand to the other then back. Then he gets down on his knees and grabs the salmons back like Jody did, sort of, without putting fingers into the gills. Reggie tries to hit its' head. The fish moves and Reggie almost lost it and missed it. Hitting the deck instead. Jody looks over his shoulder for a second then back as Jay's fish is starting to surface a few feet from the boat. Reggie laughs and swings the bat again bonking the salmon hard right on the top of the head. It starts to quiver.

"That's it," Gary says "that's just the nerves Reggie you got it good that time." Gary takes another drink of his beer. "How is your fish doing Jay, you want me to ask Ted to get it up for you, he did a great job with mine?"

Jay laughs, "I got it Gary but thanks for the offer"

Jody sees his chance and juts the net into the water and under the fish, twists and lifts "he hay, Yeah Jay. This is a nice one too." Jody stands to look at the quivering fish and some blood and the gear on the deck as he holds the netted fish up with both hands. "Reggie could you open the lid to the ice where the other fish are please"

Reggie gets up, steps and does it. He watches Jody dump the fish out of the net into the icy water "want me to bat it for you?"

"Sure Reggie", Jody smiles and goes to put his net away.

Reggie quickly grabs and bonks Jay's fish, correctly this time, it stops moving with the first hit.

Jody has an impressed expression on his face." here, I'll get the hooks out, it can be tricky." Jody puts on his glove and grabs Ted's fish that was quivering and bleeding on the deck from its' gills and looks into its' mouth. He reaches into his back pocket and take out his needle nose pliers. "This one is really stuck" Jody reaches the tip or the pliers deep into the fish's mouth and grips the line end of the hook. He pushes and twists and torques and out it comes. He slides the fish into the icy water and watches Ted move the line out of his way. Jody grabs Jay's fish from the icy water and with his fingers in the gills looks into its' mouth. "It is in the gills Jay, that is probably why it didn't fight at first." He grabs the hook with his pliers and jiggles it until it comes out.

"What about his slippery stuff from the fish on the deck?" Reggie asks.

Jody looks at him, "you hit the fish here Reggie, you gotta clean it up!" Seeing his guilty expression Jody starts to laugh, "don't worry, that is part of fishing, I'll get that in a minute." he looks at the four fish and the four men. "Ok guys, we got four fish on ice, We can continue for a while with catch and release or we can go to the cove and have some beers. What do you think?"

Jay's heart is still pounding from reeling in the fish. He looks at the others.

Gary says "either way for me" and moves his chair to sit down.

Ted says, "well, I pulled one in, that is the fun part, except eating it and I'll do that later. Beach?"

Reggie looks at Jay and the fish in the ice water "beach"

"Beach, it is then" Jay says. "What about the lines?"

Jody has a rag in one hand and a hose pumping out water in the other. As he gets down to clean the slime and blood from the deck he says "If you can take the flashers and waits off the lines and hook the line to the poles with a little tension and leave them in the rod holders that would be great. I'll get the hooks in a minute" Jody makes short work of the deck, closes the fish hold and takes the hooks putting them back into his tackle box. He looks around "I'm going back up to steer from there, you four are welcome to do as you please" He flicks some switches at his control station and goes back up the ladder.

Gary is sitting in his chair "Ted have you ever caught a fish that big?"

Ted looks at him, "not quite, it is the hardest I have ever felt one pull that is for sure."

"It was great" Reggie says, "I really liked every part of it, the net, even the feel of it squirming before I hit it."

"I never caught one before either, not in the ocean, I caught a salmon in the river once when I was a kid. It was exciting but this was better." Jay says then lifts his beer toward his lips and notices it is empty. "I need another" and Jay gets up. "Anyone else want another beer?"

"What about lunch?" Reggie asks.

"We can have our snacks but I think lunch won't be until we get to that cove he mentioned" Gary replies "Jay, you can bring me one." Then makes his way through the cabin to the head (toilet).

Ted says "beer me" and looks at Reggie.

"OK, bring me one too Jay" Reggie lifts his beer to his mouth and tips it back, like he had seen Gary do several times, chugging down the last from it.

Jay chuckles as he sees Reggie tilting back the can to get the last from it. Jay gets up thinking to himself, 'I better give him something to eat before he forgets what not to say.' "Reggie, I'll get you a snack to have with that next beer." Jay collects his sandwiches and the coconut drinks and beers from the fridge. Hands a beer to Ted and puts one down by Gary's chair then gives Reggie one; and a sandwich and a coconut drink. He smiles at Reggie and sits down with his own sandwich and opens his coconut drink. Looking at Reggie until he gets eye contact then gestures with the coconut drink and nodes with wide eyes then looks at the beer. He sees Reggie smile and subtly nod back as he opens the coconut water.

Gary comes out, "Ted" and tosses Ted a beer, steps forward looking at the drink in Jay's then Reggie's hands, and hands them both beers. "Coconut water aye? Is that stuff good?"

"Yeah" Jay answers.

Reggie takes a drink of his, "actually it hasn't got much flavor, but it feels good in my mouth."

Ted looks at it then sips his beer. I drank a lot of it when I was in Mexico two years ago. My wife and I went to Merida for my cousin's wedding. He was getting married to a Mexican woman. It was in that city. The hotel had a guy with a cart full of fresh ones out front every afternoon. He chopped the top off and would give us a straw to drink it with. I tried to chop one open." Slowly shaking his head side to side, "I was surprised how much skill the man had. One morning I saw him in the ally beside the hotel trimming the ends of the coconuts, and stacking them in his cart. He took about six or seven strokes at each one shaving the end that he would cut off when you buy it. He would hold it in one hand and chop off the husk with the machete using his other. He turned it by tossing it up and inch or so and catching it as he took the next chop."

Jay says, "They taste better fresh like that but, they can't be grown here so I drink it from the can."

"I've never tried one" Gary says.

Jay moves his arm towards Gary holding the can of coconut water, "here try it."

"No" Gary says, "What if I like it more than beer?"

Ted starts laughing.

Reggie sees the smirk on Jay's his face, "good joke Gary." Reggie didn't see how it was funny but he understood that the others did find it funny. He looked at Jay and notices Jay starting to eat his sandwich. Reggie starts unwrapping his sandwich and takes a bite.

Ted gets up and leans over the side to look in the direction the boat is going. "Are we going to go up that river?"

Jay sees the others look at Ted, "probably just past the breakwater by the beach. On the other side of it is a cove. There is easy anchoring and almost no waves. Perfect place to sit and enjoy the afternoon."

Gary looks at each of them in turn for a second, "You guys want to smoke a do-be?"

Ted looks a little nervous, "Is it safe?"

Jay sees a perplexed look on Reggie's face. "Ted, in this country no one cares if adults out on a boat blaze. If you want to, it is totally safe" Turning toward Reggie, "Most of us in this city smoke marijuana at least once in a while. I seldom do, but others do it every day." Jay sees Reggie look at him and points with his eyes at Reggie's tablet, and gives a nod.

Gary looks at the others. "Should we ask Jody if he wants some?"

Jay looks at Gary, "maybe the next one, just let him steer the boat for now"

Reggie picks up his tablet and starts working his fingers on the screen.

Gary nods, unbuttons his right shirt pocket and pulls out a fatty and a lighter. He licks the outside of it, puts an end in his mouth, and ignites the other with the lighter. After taking a big toke, he passes it to Ted.

Ted looks a little nervous, taking a quick glance at Jay and Reggie as he accepts the reefer from his brother in law. Reggie watches what Ted does with it carefully as he slides his tablet back into his jacket. When Ted has filled his lungs he looks at Reggie and passes it to him. Reggie takes it between the tips of his fore finger and thumb, looks it over pretty good and exhales as he moves it in front of his lips. Taking a long slow inhale as Jay watches the cherry glow and grow until his lungs have fully expanded. Then Reggie reaches toward Jay with the spliff only to see Jay shaking his head and gesture to Gary with a nod of his head.

Gary looks at Jay, "Today, here, and you still won't take a puff?" Gary reaches and takes it smiles and takes another hit then passes it to Ted again.

As ted takes it he looks at Gary, "It's good stuff, I got a buzz already." Ted takes a long toke and passes it to Reggie as he struggles to hold in a couple of little coughs; retaining most of it.

Reggie exhales fully as he accepts what is left of the joint. Takes a full fast breath in,,, then out. Puts it to his lips and sucks it hard again.

"Fuck Reggie, you know what to do with it don't you?" Jay says.

Reggie looks up at Jay with his eyes wide as he finishes his toke and reaches to give it back to Gary. Shrugging and slowly getting a smile across his face Reggie gets a sparkle in his eyes.

"You have good lungs, I can't take a hit like that" Ted says.

Reggie smiles watching as Gary passes the roach to Ted, then slowly exhales." When I was a youth, I spent some time working at a farm, in a warm climate. We had some stuff growing there on the farm that we would smoke. I worked there for a few years so I got accustomed to it. I don't do it here in the city because I have to work and my social world is restrictive." He sees Ted finishing his puff and offering to pass the remaining bit of a roach. Reggie looks at it and gripping carefully it with his finger and thumb nail he holds it in front of his lips sucking air past it as the last of it starts glowing, it's cherry larger on the side being held, then it disappears into his mouth. "hU, cHUhc" Reggie's eyes as big as saucers, "It burnt my throat, hahaha" then coughing.

Jay starts laughing before the others. They feel the boat slowing down and turning. Looking out the sides they realize they are entering the river and turning to go behind the breakwater. Reggie's eyes are watering as he reaches for his coconut water. He guzzles the last of it and takes a deep breath. Then smirks at Jay. Ted stands and looks out the side of the boat looking at some large birds and Gary stands looking back and forth up the river and at the beach.

"That's an eagle!" Ted says "and two more over there."

Jay steps beside him and points at the log boom about a hundred feet beside them, "those are seals on those logs"

Reggie steps beside them, "are they friendly?"

"We don't communicate with them. The won't bother us but if we try to get too close they might bite us." Jay says. "There are lots of eagles here in the river Ted. All the way up to that barge in the distance, they are often sitting on the top of those poles that they tie the log booms to."

Jody checks his chart plotter and pushes the buttons to drop the anchor. He sets the GPS and alarm in case they start to drift and turns the engine off. Stepping toward the ladder and looking down, "Ok guys, you want to barbeque, or go to the beach and buy some burgers?"

"What do you mean?" Ted looks at him.

"For lunch" Jody says, "I can cook, it's included, but at the nude beach they sell food and stuff so if you would rather go there for something to eat, I'll put the dingy in the water and row you to shore instead"

Ted says, "nude beach, really?"

Jay says "the food is good at the beach, but I'm just as happy having beer and barbeque on board."

Gary says "can you see the beach from up top Jody?" then looks at Ted, "go up"

Jody looks around, then at Gary, "Yeah, you can all sit up here if you like"

Reggie looks at Jay and softly asks "nude beach?" with a puzzled look.

Jay looks back at him and softly says "clothing optional, you can walk there from the university."

Gary folds up his chair and passes it up to Jody then moves
to the next one as he notices Ted is climbing up the ladder.
Turning to Jay and Reggie "Are you two going up top?"

"Yeah" Jay smiles at him "barbeque on the top deck is good
with me" then looking at Reggie. "Did you get an answer to
the text yet?"

Reggie smiles at Jay for a second and says, "You want to do
this now or after lunch?"

Jay looks at Reggie and smiles. "Jody, what are you cooking
for us?"

Jody looks down at them "corn on the cob, honey garlic
buffalo wings, kimchi marinated beef skewers, sourdough
buns with butter and cheese, and apple strudel."

"Sounds great" Jay looks back at Reggie, "I'm full from my
sandwich and the beer and coconut drink, I bet it will be best if
I come back hungry to enjoy the rest of the day at the beach
and a great meal."

"hahaha, Ok Jay," taking a quick look around "lets go inside," Reggie gestures with one hand and then follows Jay inside, "Jay I have to urinate, is there a toilet on this vessel."

Jay looks down the corridor toward the bow. "I bet it is the door on the side." Jay walks down to the door and opens it. Then turns around and opens the door on the other side, "That's it." looking in the room and pointing, "the button there above the toilet is the flush, the liquid chemicals will probably be blue. "Jay steps back to let Reggie go in.

Reggie stand still "no Jay you first, when they send you back here you come out and I will go, I can wait.

Jay starts to laugh, "ha-ha, so you can hold it ten years aye, that will be a record for this world!" Jay steps into the bathroom.

Reggie gets the joke and snickers as he works the screen of his tablet. "He says this will do it, don't take any steps until you are there." Reggie reaches in and closes the door. "Ok"

Getting back

Jay sees the room fading to a foggy black and then unfading to a room with a few beings that seem translucent and are moving extremely fast and some equipment, then fading again and unfading to the room where he first met Herfermks Trentia and Sihiryan. As the room un-fades into view Jay sees Herfermks and Sihiryan looking at him. "Hi, is everything OK?" Jay asks.

Herfermks and Sihiryan look at each other and then at Jay as they start to smile and look him up and down. Herfermks scans Jay with his tablet as Sihiryan walks to Jay and embraces him and then stares into his eyes like she is surprised to see him alive. Hands him an audio set and smiles.

"Here Jay, put these on. Then we can talk easier" as she hands the tiny parts to him.

Jay looks at her, takes the electronics and puts them in his ears and mouth and on his neck. He makes a few sounds and pushes the mouthpiece with his tongue until it feel comfortable. "What happened?" Jay asks. "It is good to see you too Sihiryan, Herfermks, good to see you too!"

Herfermks looks up from his tablet to Jay, after a second "Good to see you Jay, It has been a good while since you have been here, things are a little different now."Herfermks steps toward Jay extending his arm and gently holding Jays shoulder. "Trentia has left our organization, Torky has left too and has gone back to his home world. The rest from the team are in other units now. You will be stationed on the Gyrekian's moon. First you will go through a day or two of reorientation with Sihiryan and a short meeting with me off world."

Jay looks at him then at Sihiryan. "How long has it been?"

Sihiryan looks at him with a softhearted smile, "four years Jay" looking at him like an old friend, "sorry we didn't get to go to the forest. It would have been interesting."

Jay looks at her thinking about how four years passed for them and for him it is the next day. "I hope the forest is still there!"

Herfermks looks at Jay with a perplexed expression on his face, then at Sihiryan for a second. Then back at Jay. "Jay everything is Ok here, there where a lot of issues to be dealt with concerning security and politics after you left. Things are back to normal now. The planet, Ramga is ok, this city, Shiyhra has not changed, and everyone you knew is in good health. If you would like to do your orientation in the forest maybe it would be good." Herfermks smiles and looks at Sihiryan and then back at Jay again.

With a surprised expression, Sihiryan looks at Herfermks then at Jay "I guess that could work."

Jay looks at them both, "I still didn't grow back my body hair so I'm ready."

Herfermks looks at Jay and smiles. "We learned a lot from out lax precautions last time Jay. First you will spend a few minutes in the lab. Right after that we all can get something to eat. Then you can go to the forest."

"On the way to the lab we will change your clothes, do you remember where your locker is Jay?" Sihiryan asks.

Jay looks at her, "for me it was yesterday that I last used it, Lets go. "Jay starts walking to the door.

Herfermks and Sihiryan look at each other and start to follow out the door and down the hall. When they get to Jay's locker Jay taps it and looks at them. Herfermks works on his tablet for a few seconds and a different locker opens.

Jay looks at it, then in it. "Ok, my clothes can go in here but what will I wear?" he sees Sihiryan opening a cupboard across the room and he starts getting undressed. Folding his close and putting them in the locker Jay asks, "Herfermks, is there a way that my phone battery can remain charged until I go back to earth."

Herfermks looks at Jay, "interesting, let me see it."

Jay hands him the phone. Herfermks looks at it and works the buttons a little. Then he scans it with his tablet. Herfermks works on his tablet and scans the phone a few times. "Interesting Jay, the only thing I can think of is to put it in a time freeze unit until you take it out of the locker, I don't have one here on Ramga though. Can I take it for now and put it in the locker later when I get one for it?"

Jay looks at him, "of course Sir, thank you, my things are under your control. Do as you please with them."

Herfermks slips the phone into his pocket as Jay is putting on pants and a Kyranin robe. He watches as Sihiryan hands him his footwear and a tablet. Herfermks looks at the tablet, "Jay let me see that tablet for a minute please." He taps it to his and then sits it on top of his and works on the screen until Jay is finished dressing and Sihiryan has adjusted his hair and checked the fit of the clothes. Handing the tablet back to him.

"This time I will know if anyone wants to interfere with your schedule."

Jay looks at Herfermks, "So what happened, was that guy correct to send me back when he did."

Herfermks looks at Jay, "no harm done Jay, he meant well and saved us some meetings but it was not his place to do it." Herfermks looks at Sihiryan then back at Jay, "lets go up top for a meal and some drinks now, you two can go over that too in the forest."

Jay looks at Sihiryan to see her smile a knowing smile at him. "I am hungry, I hope I can get something with sinnt sauce.

"Don't worry Jay we have had time to study all your likes and dislikes and biological functions and the changes that happen with our adjustments. When you get out of the lab this time you will enjoy anything that any other kyranin would like." Sihiryan smiles and touches his arm as she gestures toward the door.

Jay looks at her with a surprised expression. They walk quietly to the elevator and it opens as they approach. A korob steps out and nods at them, then they get in. Herfermks strokes his fingers on the elevators control panel and then on his tablet as it starts to move. It opens and they walk down the hall and go into the lab. Sihiryan gestures at the chair, and Jay sits in it. Herfermks works the controls as Sihiryan watches him. They converse about what he is doing a little. Jay sits quietly in the chair listening to them and noticing what is happening to his body. He starts thinking about his last day there, about Trentia and his time under the sea. He remembered the large portion of vercset that he had eaten and wondered what had happened to Trentia and the large portions that they had brought back from the cave. "What happened to Trentia, where did she go?"

Herfermks looks at Sihiryan and sees her eyes looking back at him. "She is good, shortly after you went back she left this organization and took other work far from here, it allows her to travel and it seems that she likes it as she has not communicated with us since she left." He turns to Jay to see Jay's expression, "I have checked on her and she is happy in her new life, I would not interfere with her there but it is part of my obligation to past team members to check on them to be sure they are safe and happy after they leave their work here." He sees Jays face lighten and the stress release from his eyes. "Lets go eat now" and starts toward the door.

Jay gets up and follows with Sihiryan beside him. "He must be hungry."

"Just before you faded into the transport room he mentioned being in a twenty hour meeting on some planet that I never heard of. I guess they didn't have food he liked" Sihiryan says.

As they get to the elevator Herfermks looks at them and pats and rubs his pockets then pulls out Jay's phone and some other devices. "I left my tablet in the lab, Sihiryan could you please get it for me" He asks as the elevator opens.

She looks at him, "of course, I'll meet you two up top in a few minutes." and she turns, and starts back towards the lab.

Herfermks steps into the elevator and says, "Get in Jay, could I see your tablet please?"

Jay passes it to him as he steps into the elevator.

Once they are both inside and the door starts to close Herfermks starts working the screen of Jay's tablet and the room starts fading to black then to light green that quickly become a forest. "Jay I can't take it anymore, I have to eat something" handing him his tablet, "don't touch the screen Jay." Herfermks takes a look into the forest around them and slowly sniffs the air. "I'll be back in a minute stay here" and he starts running between some trees.

Jay watches thinking it is an odd situation. After only a few seconds Herfermks is out of sight and can't be heard. Then in the distance Jay hears a shrieking squealing noise for a second. Then nothing. After a minute Jay hears some tiny rustling in the trees above him. He looks up to see a bird of some kind eating a small creature. He looks into the forest and can see several odd looking insects eating leaves and something with scales that is about the size of a rabbit licking the nectar from a flower. Jay takes a few deep breaths and likes the way the air feels in his lungs. A minute later Herfermks waves and calls his name as he walks toward him between the trees. He can see Herfermks smiling with a joyful content look.

Herfermks looks at Jay, "Ok Jay. Here look at your tablet. You see this setting here, this is when we went to, this one here is when we left, this one here is where we went, and that one is the elevator. Do you get it?"

"I can see the four... sets of data, but I don't know how to read them."

"Good, so what you do now is switch them back around the other way. So Jay, put two fingers on the two whens, and then move them both at the same time to drag them to the alternate positions, at the same time, like I said. You can't do them one at a time they will disappear. If they disappear you will have to punch them in and that is complicated Jay. You don't want to get into that situation Jay, do you understand?"

Jay looks at him. He holds the tablet with one hand and twisting his hand one way first, puts two fingers on the times. He then turns his hands over sliding his fingers so that the times move to the opposite locations on the screen, "ok"

Herfermks nodding his head and says "good, now do it with the locations the same way."

Jay carefully repeats his action with his hands and fingers on the screen with the two locations. He looks over the screen well to see if he can understand the characters and the format of the information displayed.

Herfermks points with his finger to another position on the screen, "this will tell you when it is ready, once it is ready wait until you are ready and anyone you are taking with you is in physical contact with you. Then when you are certain that you are ready think about where you are going to, and get ready to be there. Once you are ready to be there check that you have everything that you want to bring with you and that it is safe to leave. When you are certain that you are ready to go say the command." He looks at Jay and puts his hand gently on Jays shoulder.

Jay looks back at Herfermks "what is the command?"

Herfermks smiles at him. "Well Jay, I am not aloud to share the command with anyone that is not of the highest security clearance of the Ryberian military science and oversight authority." Looking into Jay's eyes, with a serious look on his face, "if you where to over hear me mention the command you would surely never repeat it to anyone, or alone, incase you were under surveillance would you?"

Jay looks back into Herfermks eyes pondering the words he just heard. "No, I probably wouldn't even know what it was related to, and I would never share anything you said to me unless it was information of a social nature to be shared with our mutual friends."

Herfermks says, "think", then still looking at Jay he raises his eyebrows "complete transfer now." Herfermks keeps looking at Jay, secures his grip on his shoulder and still looking in Jay's eye, nods at him.

Jay thinks 'complete transfer now' and sees the forest fading to black and the elevator appearing around them. He feels the elevator moving and Herfermks releasing his grip on his shoulder. Jay turns toward the door and looks up at Herfermks beside him to see him smiling and nodding his head. The door opens at the roof top restaurant and Jay gestures for Herfermks to step out first. He follows Herfermks to a table near the edge with a view of the sea in the distance between the taller buildings.

Herfermks looks around and makes some hand signals to the server. "Jay take that chair so you can see the sea. I am sure you have some questions. It is best if you save them for another time. I have signalled to the server that you and Sihiryan will have the special and I will have my regular." He looks around the deck to see who is there. "Privacy is not as it once was Jay" moving his chair a little and waving at Sihiryan as she steps out from the elevator Herfermks gives Jay another nod.

Jay looks over to see Sihiryan walking toward them and then back at Herfermks. "I am glad we are able to have time to share a meal. It is an honor to spend time with you sir." As Sihiryan approaches Jay stands to greet her "hello Sihiryan, Herfermks has ordered for you already. Thank you for joining us for breakfast," then looking at the angle of the sun, "or is it a late lunch?"

Sihiryan looks at Jay with a concerned expression on her face and smiles "thank you Jay." Handing the tablet to Herfermks, "Here you are sir. Thanks for ordering, did you get me a mrruk?" looking back at Jay as she sits down.

Herfermks looks at her, "I used the hand signal for two specials and one regular for me, I don't know if it will include your mrruk."

Sihiryan looks at the kitchen, "unless they are new to Ramga I bet they will figure it out."

Jay looks at them, one then the other for several seconds. "It is a beautiful day."

"Yes" Herfermks agrees, I have meetings here for three days and will be busy but I would like to visit the caves with the artifacts in the south before I go back to Ryberia. Would you two like to join me?"

Jay asks, "do you refer to Tewes' archeological find under the sea?"

Sihiryan looks at Jay with a surprised expression. "He does, for a year now it has been on social media a lot" she looks at Herfermks then back at Jay "I am surprised you have been following it Jay"

Jay sees the server walking toward them with a tray holding four cups, "I think he has our mrruk."

The server puts the tray on the table, put two cups in front of Herfermfs and the two mrruks in front of Jay and Sihiryan. "I will return with your meals shortly."

Jay sips his mrruk and looks at the expressions on Herfermks' and Sihiryan's faces. Seeing no tension he says, "When I visited under the sea some years ago I met Tewes at his shop across from Crenshaws in Atwerts. He told us about the finds in the caves and that he hoped to have them researched soon."

Herfermks looked at Jay with interest. Sihiryan looked surprised.

"Herfermks, did Trentia show you the artifact that we found in the caves near Atwerts?" Jay asks.

Herfermks looks at Jay and after a few seconds, "no," He takes a drink from one of the cups. "what was it?"

Jay sees the server coming out of the kitchen, "our food is coming" and he smiles. "We found a heavy carved statue of a three legged being in some old ruins of and amburst city. I thought she might have mentioned it to you. We had talked about bringing it to Tewes' shop to have it analyzed."

Sihiryan looks at Jay then smiles at the server as he places her meal in front of her "thank you," then back at Jay "that sounds interesting."

Herfermks smiles and nods at the server as he puts Jay's meal on the table and a small plate of kreptigs in front of him. Then looking at Jay for some seconds. "She didn't mention anything. It was a time when other concerns were pressing. Tell me about this artifact."

Jay looks at his meal and picks up his fork. "Well, it was about, twice as long as this fork. It was heavy and smooth and had three legs but was shaped like an amburst or kyranin, other than that."

"Was it clear?" Herfermks asks.

Jay takes a bite of his meal and looks into Herfermks eyes, "I didn't get a good look at it in the light. I'm not sure, it may have been."

Sihiryan samples her food and smiles. She looks at the interested look on Herfermks face and asks, "are you an archeologist in your heart Herfermks?"

Herfermks looks at her and smiles. "I did spend some time studying artifacts of various cultures." and takes a drink of one of his cups. If it was interesting enough for Trentia to want to bring it to Tewes it must have been something rare. Trentia did work with him for some years and was respected in that scientific community."

Jay looks at him then her, then he takes more bites of the food. "This is good. Thank you for your efforts to make me comfortable, the last meal I had here was not so enjoyable."

"Would you like a side dish of kreptigs Jay?" Herfermks asks as he raises his hand to signal the server.

"No, no please,,, please no" Jay responds.

Herfermks laughs and looks at Sihiryan, "did you see him eat one before?"

Sihiryan smiles, "he seemed to like them when I was watching, hahaha"

Jay takes a sip of his mrruk and looks at the sea. Then asks, "How is your meal sir?"

Herfermks looks at Jay for a second and realizes it is just a topic change. "Good I prefer the beverages on the Gyrekian moon but this is pleasant." Smiling and looking at Sihiryan then Jay, "I have heard of a great opportunity for you on the moon. They have a career opportunity for you there. I have arranged for you to interview for it in a few days."

Sihiryan looks at Herfermks. "He will have to travel for a few days to get there." Then at Jay and back at Herfermks, "I thought he would be here for two or more days working with me."

Herfermks smiles, "yes, I believe it is next week they expect him, I will be sure to confirm the appointments so that travel time is not too cramped."

A few bites in silence then Jay starts to think about going to the forest and then to go to live on the moon; and start his work there. He looks at Sihiryan. "What kind of camping gear will we need for the forest?"

Sihiryan looks at Jay then at Herfermks and back at Jay. "Camping gear? Don't worry Jay, everything is easy in the forest, you will have a great time there with me."

Herfermks watches Jay's expression and hesitation before having another bite. He has a sip from his other cup and pulls out his tablet and scrolls through several screens and looks at Jay. You will like camping here Jay, it is different but you will like it." Looking over at the view screen, I heard that the Vwortek have designed new suits to use when visiting other worlds, what do you think of them Sihiryan?"

"Well," she takes another bite, gives Herfermks and then Jay a blank stare, "I guess it is an improvement, for,, their,, perceived acceptance by other cultures?" then gives Herfermks a questioning look.

Jay looks over at the view screen and sees a presentation about the suits showing how they adjust to fashions of various worlds. He smiles and nods at her.

Herfermks asks, "what do you think of it Jay?"

Jay takes his last bite from his plate and looks at Herfermks while chewing it. After swallowing "Well, if they feel better wearing those suits I support their efforts. I like them and accept their challenges as, perhaps, greater than mine, to fit in socially. I am glad that they are willing to make efforts to be happier interacting with other species. I suspect it will further their ability to be accepted by many species of the alliance."

Sihiryan looks at Jay then Herfermks. "That is a respectful and serious response Jay. I am impressed and inspired by it. Thank you for presenting the needs of the Vworteks so softly. It gives me the idea to consider their cultural and personal needs rather than the usual Kyranin view of their ways of interacting." She smiles and has the last bite of her food.

Jay takes another bite as he notices Herfermks tablet shift position slightly.

Herfemks looks at Sihiryan then at Jay, then back at Sihiryan. "Sihiryan, do you have all what the two of you will be needing to spend a few days in the forest?" Turning to look at Jay with a questioning expression.

Sihiryan looks at Jay then at Herfemks, "what do you have in mind? We won't need much, the forest has everything that we need."

"Well," Herfermks pauses "Jay hasn't got a room here now, and it is still light, will you take him to the forest this evening or should I arrange for accommodations for him?"

Sihiryan looks at Jay then Herfermks. She takes a sip of her beverage and looks at Jay for a second. "Jay, would you like to stay with me in my room tonight. It is best if we arrive in the forest in the morning. That way we have the day to explore and find a comfortable situation for your first night of camping".

Looking at Sihiryan's calm serious expression "sure, that would be great, I am honored to be your guest." Jay searches his memories of Kyranin etiquette and can't remember anything relating to being invited to stay in a Kyranin friends' home. Then thinks about not having any luggage, not even a toothbrush. "Should I go to the market and purchase a few basic items?"

Sihiryan takes another sip then looks at Herfermks looking back at her and turns to Jay. "No Jay, I'll go to the marker in a few moments and leave you here with Herfermks. You know where my room is, let yourself in when you get there and make yourself at home."

"I wanted to ask you Jay" Herfermks pauses and picks up a kreptig from his plate, "do you think you will be happy on the moon for a few years?"

Jay thinks to himself, 'it could be interesting' and looks around at the few other tables with patrons. "I suppose I will learn to love it" Then looking into Herfermks' eyes "will I have occasions to travel from there?"

Sihiryan interjects with a topic change "Would you like me to pick up any special treats for camping Jay?" Gesturing with her arms and face, "wine, pastries, preserved foods?"

Jay turns and looks at her as his curiosity starts to swell. "I'm not sure, whatever you choose, I trust your judgment. Oh, some fine thread to clean between my teeth would be great."

Sihiryan finishes her drink and stands "It was good to see you Herfermks, Jay I will see you later." She smiles at them both, turns, and walks toward the elevator.

"Would you like my last kreptig Jay? I noticed that there wasn't any in your meal?" Herfermks looks at Jay like he should take it.

Jay thinks it this odd, as he knows that Herfermks should remember that he does not like the kreptigs. Seeing the continuing expression in Herfermks eyes Jay responds "Oh, Thank You so much sir, I was looking at yours and was thinking how I wished that my meal had included some." Giving Herfermks an expression indicating his lack of enthusiasm about eating one as he reaches to pick it up. "You don't mind?"

Herfermks smiles, "no Jay not at all, I am happy to see you enjoying it, I ate earlier and am more interested in my drinks. You have it my old friend." Lifting one of his cups to his mouth and pouring it's contents into his mouth, them watching as Jay slowly bites the kreptig in half.

Jay's eyes open a little wider as he chews. Then the second half goes in his mouth. "mmmm, that is good. I didn't think I,,, It is better than I expected. That's a pleasant surprise"

"Finish your beverage Jay" Herfermks says as he stands up. "I'll walk you to the elevator. I have to go to the lobby down stairs to wait for some diplomats.

Jay looks at his drink and thinks to him self 'I am a little thirsty,' he chugs down the last from his cup and smiles up to Herfermks as he stands. "To the elevator then" smiling and gesturing for Herfermks to walk first, "After you sir."

Herfermks walks to the elevator waving at the server and giving a nod of appreciation to him as he looks out from the kitchen door way. Taking out his tablet before reaching the elevator and starting to work the screen "Jay, do you remember the friends we made on Vwotia?"

Smiling as he walks Jay recalls the little Pixies. "How are they doing?"

Reaching the elevator Herfermks Smiles. "They sure liked your Jay, They always ask how you are doing." He gestures for Jay to enter first and follows him inside handing him the tablet. "Jay" as the elevator door closes, "do you see where to activate the screen?"

Jay notices Herfermks hand grasp his shoulder as he looks at the screen of the tablet and feels his heart speeding up. "The time is that code and place is that code. This indicates that it is ready, Are we ready?"

Herfermks nods his dead as Jay looks up at him.

Jay thinks 'complete transfer now' and the elevator starts to fade to black then to another room. As the room appears Jay notices that it is a very old structure with walls made of stone, and a dilapidated door. The ceiling is wooden beams with stones on top and cracks showing sunlight coming through. There are large insect like looking things in the corners and in the cracks between the stones. The floor is thickly covered with dust. "Where are we?"

Herfermks asks is a soft voice, "remember how to set the path back?" and points at the tablet.

Jay looks at the screen and holds his fingers above the two sets of symbols indicating the times and looks at Herfermks. Seeing him nod Jay touches the screen with his two fingers and switches the positions. Jay takes a good look at the two sets of symbols. Then he puts his fingers above the two sets of symbols indicating the locations and sees Herfermks nod again. Putting his fingers on the spots and switching the positions then looking at the four sets of data he notices that one of the times has changed. "Herfermks, the time changed here!"

In a soft voice Herfermks responds "quietly Jay. That is the present time here, now, so it changes." Herfermks opens his hand for Jay to put the tablet into it. "OK Jay, take out your tablet. Then set the return times to the same as on mine, to the elevator and when we left."

Jay takes a look at the symbols on Herfermks tablet then opens his own tablet. He looks at the screen and scrolls through several menus but can't find the right icon.

Pointing his finger at Jay's tablet screen, Herfermks leans close to Jay and whispers "these three icons, or any three icons in the same alignment, touch them and ask with thought to open time share six. The words to think are, "time share six open"

Jay puts his three fingers on the icons on his screen and thinks the words. Nothing happens.

Herfermks sees the surprised worried expression on Jay's face. "Think the words as a fraise, as a complete thought, the meaning of the words together as one."

Jay tries it and it works. He has the screen open and looks at it to see if he can find a keypad or something to get the symbols from.

Herfermks whispers into his ear tap your tablet gently on mine and think "read open time share six specifics."

Jay thinks about the words for a second then thinks it again as he taps the tablet to the other one. He looks at his screen and sees that the symbols are now matching what he read on Herfermks tablet. Showing the screen to Herfermks Jay sees him smile and put his tablet into his pocket Jay does the same.

Herfermks looks out the cracks in the door, opens the door, listens and looks carefully from every angle. Then sneaks his head out a little to see down the wall in either direction. Jay sees past him and determines that they are in an old abandoned town or city. Herfermks steps outside, still examining his view then around the corner of the structure and looks back at Jay sticking his head out. He points in the other direction with a gesture indicating that Jay should check the other side. Jay's heart speeds up as he carefully walks through the rubble to the far corner of the building they arrived in. Peaking his eyes around the corner, then his head, Jay sees that they are on a small hill at the edge of the ruins of a castle. He looks at the terrain of the slope and landscape beyond it. He sees weeds and shrubs and bushes and something similar to grass. There are trees a short distance away that are the edge of a forest that fills the distance to the horizon. The trees are of three types. The tallest have leaves on the clumps of branches and brightly colored flowers near the tops. Jay sees some small furry creatures peaking out from behind a bush at him, some tiny movements in the upper branches of a few trees and a large flock of birds far away over the forest. Jay then looks back at the ruins. He notices small grey fuzzy creatures in some of the cracks in the walls, and some large insect looking things on the ground and on the walls. Finally he looks back at Herfermks who is looking at him. He walks back to him.

Jay asks in a soft voice "what was I looking for?".

Herfermks smiles, "what did you see?"

Jay describes the tall trees and the shorter ones with the broad leaves and bright plumes in the middle, the shrubs that look like they are full of berries, the various creatures that he saw and the bugs. Then He adds, "these ruins look like they were abandoned after some great battle, but not too long ago because nothing grows between the rocks."

Herfermks looks at him for a few seconds. "I was here ten years ago, in this time, and it was a peaceful community. The creatures that lived here are more like me than you Jay." He looks in the doorway that they came out of, that was my home here. I have been visiting here for hundreds of years then a few years ago I came back at this time and this is what I found. No crops, no shops, no families, no friends." He looks around, turns to look up the corridor between the buildings near by, "Would you like to investigate it with me?"

Jay thinks about what he has been asked. "What do you mean?"

Herfermks is looking at the forest in the distance. "There are other cities and other tribes and other species on this planet. There is little technology here though, not for thousands of years. This particular species does not exist in that time. These rock structures took generations to build for these beings. The rocks were shaped with only other rocks for tools. The wooden beams for the roofs were carved from the trees with tools made of sharp rocks. These beings were mostly artists, they sang, danced, painted images, told stories and loved their children enough that four or five generations would live together in harmony." looking into Jay's eyes, "I miss them Jay, I just want to know what happened to them, would you like to go back and watch with me?"

Seeing the emotion in Herfermks' eyes Jay realizes that this is a personal issue for Herfermks and suspects that is why he is asking rather than just telling him what to do next. "Sure, I would be glad to be with you to do this, anything that I can do to help I will."

"Thank you Jay" Herfermks looks around. "That door was like a common meeting room, similar to a pub, but like a home, not a business." The fields around the village and the rooftops all had crops growing. All of the streets were like a mixture of parks, playgrounds, private patios, side walk cafes and markets." looking at Jay, "Your appearance would likely attract a lot of attention, the other species on this planet did not look much like you do."

"Are you going to change my appearance?"

Herfermks looks him up and down "no." He takes a step toward the view of the forest and looks at it. "I will put you out of faze just enough that they won't be able to see you. It may be odd for you as you might be able to notice their feelings and thoughts more than you can hear their sounds." Turning back to Jay "lets watch from the forest first to choose the time to watch from here" and starts walking. "Common Jay, we will climb one of those tall trees and watch from there. That way we won't cause any random interference."

Jay starts to follow walking as fast as he can following behind Herfermks as they start down the slope toward a knoll at the edge of the forest. About every fifteen steps Jay runs a few strides to catch up again. Contemplating being out of 'faze' gets Jay curiosity going. "What do you mean out of faze is it safe?" A couple of big breaths and a few running strides, "how does out of faze work?"

Herfermks keeps walking, "oh, don't worry Jay it is totally safe." pointing into the forest "that one looks taller than the others lets go up that one." Changing direction a little toward the tree he chose. "The flowers will help hide us, I guess I could go out of faze too, lets do that Jay, that way I will be able to see you better and know that you are ok."

Jay, breathing heavily now trying to keep up, "how do we go out of faze?"

Herfermks says, "we slow the process of tuning into the new time just enough so that we are following it as it passes without actually getting into it. So we will be still slightly in the black zone that you experience as we transfer from one time to the next, the transition process will be slowed to match the rate of actual time passing but following it rather than matching it. We will be nearly in their time, but not quite. We can see into the time we are entering before we appear in it. When we are going backward in time it is the other way, they can see us just before we are there."

Jay is making sense of it logically in his mind when his toe catches the root of a shrub and trips. Falling hard Jay makes a thud sound and exhausts an "uofh," "ooh fuck, that hurts" as he roles over and takes a breath. "Uh, I tore the knee of my pants and my hand is bleeding."

Herfermks stops, turns, and walks back to Jay. Looking down at him, "Jay, I am surprised, you are so brave for such a fragile creature," Reaching down to help Jay up with one hand and taking out his tablet with the other. He scans Jay and fiddles with his screen a little. Then points the tablet at Jays knee "is that helping?"

Jay looks at his knee, "yeah, what are you doing?"

"It is some frequencies to initiate tissue corrections, and some radiation that mimics the natural radiation of your form, and some variation of the restructuring technology to change your form that is specifically useful to correct the damage from the trauma." Herfermks look at his hand and resets the controls on his tablet and points it at Jays bleeding palm. "Tell me Jay, with you life expectancy so short, and your body so fragile, how can you be so willing to take all the risks that you do?"

Jay looks at him "what do you mean, I am carful, I don't take risks" "hahahaha, Ok hahaha, I see why the birds like you Jay" standing straight and putting the tablet away. "It is hard for me to understand your perspective on what is safe I guess. Here grab my arm" as he takes out the tablet again and works the screen "Jay, pay attention" he opens his tablet to the time share six screen and adjusts another area on the screen. "This is for opening the data detail screen." Herfermks looks back at the screen and it changes to a map showing where they are. When he touches it a window opens and shows a configuration of symbols like the ones in the boxes in the time share six screens. He taps a point on the screen and makes a counter clockwise circle and gets a close-up of the area. Then changes the angle of the tablet and the map becomes a 3-D image of the terrain. He taps and makes a clockwise circle and three windows open up. One is a top view with a grid of the close up area, and the others are cross sections one from the front and one from the side. "Watch" He adjusts the dot in each of the three images so that the dot in the 3-D image is just on top of a large branch high up in the tree. "See," then he touches his thumb to the configuration of symbols and slides it off the bottom of the screen. Then lifting his finger and looking at the screen as it changes back to the time share six screen. "Watch this Jay" Herfermks slides his thumb up from the bottom of the screen to the 'to place' position and the new symbols appear there. Looking at Jay, "with me so far?" then taps another area of the screen that opens a window with what looks like a lot of slide controls. He scrolls down the page then puts one finger on the symbol at the start of a slide and uses another finger to adjust the position of the mark on the line. "Both fingers must be in contact to make the adjustment Jay. Don't try this unless you are sure, each line does something different and it matters that they are set correctly" then looks at the tree. "Ok Jay, we are going to go up there, we will stop just out of faze so we can adjust to the branch's location for a few seconds before we solidify. When you get there, step onto the branch a few times, softly, until you feel it under your feet.

Grab a smaller one for balance and gently adjust your grip
on it until it feels like you are holding it." Then looking at Jay,
"does that make sense?"

Jay looks at him and tightens his grip on his arm, "yeah"

"Any questions"

Jay looks at him then the tree and pauses, "mmm, no"

Herfermks checks his screen and then they fade to black. Then
Jay notices that the tree looks a little fuzzy around them. Jay
adjusts his feet to feel the branch beneath them, and grabs
through a branch once before he gets it the second try. He
adjusts his grip and his feet a few times until they feel solid.
Herfermks makes some more adjustments on his tablet. Jay
starts looking around and notices that the daylight is fading
then changing from light to dark faster and faster like a strobe
light from a nightclub in the 80's. He looks at Herfermks' tablet
and then at the ruins of the castle.

"There" Jay exclaims, "I see them"

Herfermks adjusts his tablet's screen controls and the strobing stops and then starts to go slowly again, then slower. "Watch Jay tell me if you see anything odd. Any other species or any violence."

Jay watches as the days show as passing about one a minute. He gets familiar with the patterns of the steaks and spots of color from the movements of the beings and their things. Then some changes start to happen. "What's happening, it's changing now."

Herfermks slows the pace and they watch as the amount of activity in the area changes. They notice that there is a lot more beings than before and that they are building huts in the fields. They slow it down more and see that many of the beings are not lizardish but look more like monkeys. Then a third species arrives in a large number and the monkeys start to flee in small groups. Herfermks slows it down more so that each day takes about ten minuets. They watch as the new species wearing clothing and weapons are interacting with the host species amicably. This continues for many weeks. But once in a while one of the regular movements stops taking place.

Jay comments. "It looks like some of them are going missing or changing their routines."

Herfermks says "Ok Jay we will go back to my place now and walk amongst them and see what is happening."

Jay looks at him as he is adjusting some of the sliding controls in the program. "What are you doing now?"

"We will see a day pass in ten minutes when we get there but they wont see us." Herfermks looks at him, "ready?"

Jay nods. As it starts to fade to black Jay asks, "can they hear us?"

The room is appearing around them and Herfermks is still working his screen. "No, we can talk but try not to get in any ones' way."

The door is closed. Jay notices that there are less cracks in it as he leans toward it to peek through them.

Herfermks says, "If no one is looking open it. Jay it will seem so slow to them that they wont notice."

Jay opens the door and sees the being racing past in various directions and hears constant whizzing and softly screeching

tones and what seems like the hum of a badly tunes engine.
" I guess we can hear them"

"Watch the interactions Jay I'll slow it down more. "Herfermks
says as he adjusts some of the slide controls. "Lets go into their
social room Jay" as he stats walking while working the tablet.

Jay sees the pace reduce until he can see individual faces on
the beings as they hurry around. He notices that the lizard
looking ones give the others a wide birth and wait for them to
get out of their way rather than crowding them.

Jay turns to Herfermks and sees that he has gone.
Remembering the door that He had pointed to earlier Jay
follows and enters the room. He sees Herfermks sitting in the
corned with some old lizard like beings. Looking around the
rest of the room he sees only a few groups sitting and
conversing. He walks to Herfermks and asks what is going on.
Jay watches as Herfermks adjusts the slides on his tablet some
more, and the being there start to interact at normal speed.

Herfermks looks at Jay and says, "lets listen Jay, your
translator may take a few moments to adjust to the sounds
from the time distortion but you should be able to understand
them soon." Herfermks looks across the room then back at Jay,
"no females in here or children playing." then looks back at
the old ones talking.

Jay listens too. First just mumbling and static then he can hear them complaining about their guests. They are talking about friends missing and killings after altercations. Then he hears one of them suggest that they have a great feast and eat all of the other beings. The others nod and agree it would be a good idea. Then after a moment of thought one of them says to the others it would take all of us to hunt to be able to get them all and that it would have to be done all at the same time. One of the others says that he has heard others talk about this same idea and some of them have disappeared. Jay looks at Herfermks "can we help them?"

Herfermks looks at Jay "maybe but it is not going to be easy to get permission. We have no authority here and what happened is between indigenous species. More important is that it happened some years ago so the time distortion could cause problems planet wide."

Jay looks at Herfermks as he listens to the old being talking about the friends and family members that are missing. He feels angry and looks at Herfermks again then around the room. With a solumn scowel "Lets go see what these others are like", and starts walking towards the door.

Herfermks watches him take a few steps and gets up and follows. Out side the door he sees one of the other species children talking with an adult lizard.

The child asks, "How do you get the rocks to be the right shape to stay in the walls?"

The adult lizard looks at the child and answers, "it is easy Grulit, we brake the sides of the rocks so that they are flat and won't roll off of each other. Then when we stack them they won't move."

Grulit asks, "but Derasto do the rocks mind when you break them, can they feel the pain, do they cry?" and picks up a rock and taps it on another rock.

Derasto has a perplexed look on his face. "I have never heard a rock complain." He looks at the child and at the rock in its' hand. "Can you hear what the rock says?"

Grulit says, "It makes a sound when I hit it to another rock but I can't understand what it is saying."

Derasto says, "that is interesting, I never thought that the rocks might be trying to communicate when we hit them together. I don't believe the rocks have feelings Grulit." He looks around at the rock walls and the rocks on the ground. "Is there anything else that makes you think that they might be trying to say something?"

"My mother told that all things have life in them and all things are filled with love. She says that some things force others to do what they want then to and every thing needs to eat." Grulit looks at Derasto's face, then deeply into his eyes, "Derasto, if the rock didn't like being broken to make houses for you to live in and you found out would you stop breaking rock?"

Derasto looks into Grulit's eyes, "I don't know. I never thought about it. We have always broken rocks and cut wood to make homes. I guess we could stop making them if the rocks didn't like it. But the rocks have never complained. When they roll down a hill they make the same sounds."

Grulit looks into Derasto's eyes again "when you eat the plants do they cry and try to get away?"

Derasto smiles, "No" smiling at the child, "the plants seem to be happy"

Grulit asks, "Can you teach me how to eat the plants?"

Jay turns to Herfermks standing a few feet away, "lets go back and see why the monkeys left."

Herfermks looks at him, "come to the market and the pool first," and starts walking up the path between the homes. Jay, each structure houses a family. When a family gets to big for the structure they trade with a smaller family with a bigger structure. The men all spend a few hour each week building new structures and the rest of the time they work the fields and collect food and socialize." Then turns to Jay, "when it is the season they all work diligently to make the beer and the wine"

Jay looks at the walls of the structures. There are elaborate murals paintings on most of them. He can hear singing coming out from several homes, and drumming from others. There are children playing here and there, children of both species. He stops walking and watches as a lizard being is teaching one of the others how to brake and stack the stones to make the walls. "Herfermks, you will want to see this."

Herfermks walks back and watches and listens as the skills are being taught. It is clear that they are getting along quite well and enjoying each other's company. "Interesting Jay" he turns and starts walking again. "The market and pool are just up here, common."

Jay follows seeing similar situations as he walks past
several structures before getting to the market. At the entrance
to the market there is a structure with a sloped wall of various
sized rocks, Herfermks climbs it and looks into the market. Jay
follows climbing up and standing beside his friend. They look
across the market and the pool. The two species are
communicating and interacting in a friendly manner. Then at
the edge of the pool a woman of the new species steps
backward out of the water on the foot of child lizard. The
woman stumbles and turns around and kicks the child hard
and accuses it of attempting to trip her. An adult lizard quickly
picks up the child and suggests that she stepped backward
onto the child in defense of the child. Several of the other
species walk over and surround the three. They shove and hit
the woman holding the injured child until she escapes the
group. One of the group nods to an onlooker who follows the
woman out of the market.

Herfermks looks at Jay. "They are far more aggressive but less
industrious." shaking his head "It is obvious why the monkeys
left." There is nothing we can do Jay. I can go back and visit
them before this time. I can enjoy their culture before they
become extinct. But there is nothing we can do to help them
change the way they are. They won't all agree to eject the
others before there numbers are too small."

Jay feels his heart drop realizing that Herfermks is right. "It is
sad, the more aggressive are going to destroy the others. But I
can see what you mean, we can't help" he turns to Herfermks
"even if we went back and taught them to keep the strangers
out of their village a time would come when they would be
over run by the more aggressive."

Herfermks says, "Ok Jay" and grabs his arm, "think the command to your tablet and we can go back, I'm ready."

Jay remembers the tablet and the elevator and that he is going to Sihiryan's then camping in the morning. He thinks about the conversations at the roof top cafeteria and that he enjoyed the kreptig. Then he thinks 'complete transfer now' and nothing happens. "Nothing happened."

Herfermks turns to look at Jay, "Is our hand on the tablet?"

Jay smiles and puts his hand into his pocket touching the tablet and thinks the command again, and the market starts fading to black. The elevator is around them in a few seconds and Jay sees Herfermks taking out his tablet. Jay looks up at his face.

Herfermks looks down at Jay with a solemn look. "Well Jay. Thank you. It was hard for me to go and watch that, I am glad that you came with me." He works on his tablet a little. "I am going to spend some time with my family. I will make travel arrangements for you to arrive on the Gyrekian moon and I will meet you when you arrive."

Jay gives Herfermks a hug.

Herfermks looks at him with a questioning expression. "You are not coming with me Jay, and a simple touch is enough for that."

Jay pulls back from the hug. "An earth tradition when you say by to a good friend, especially after and emotional experience. I am happy I was there with you to witness that with you sir. Thank you, I will see you in a few days."

Herfermks disappears and a second later the elevator door opens at Sihiryan's floor. Jay steps out and takes a slow deep breath, and thinking about the experience on that world and starts walking toward Sihiyan's room. When he gets there he announces his arrival to the door and it opens and the room welcomes him, suggests a beverage, and offers him a shower and tells him where the robes are. Jay looks around, it is almost the same as Trentia's room, the decorations are different, and the bed is higher. He notices a particularly bright piece of art on the wall between the door and the kitchen. Standing back to take a good long look at it he decides to have a shower before the beverage. He looks around and walks to the shower area and undresses. He folds his cloths and puts them on a basket that is there. He looks at the controls for the shower and asks the room if it can set the shower to wash him the same way that Sihiryan likes it. The water and fluids start coming out and Jay steps into them. He likes the warmth and is surprised at the jets from the panel that come up from the floor. It takes great care and efforts to clean the bottom of him while the jets from the two sides and the top massage and wash the rest of him. Then it blow dries him and he gets a robe from the closet and goes to the kitchen. Looking in the fridge Jay finds some juice that is familiar. He pours himself a glass and sits in the chair facing the wall screen.

Jay sips his drink and says "room, display the social media main events of the last three days." As he watches the stories about celebrities and the Vworktek suits and political views about things like Tewes' caves, he starts to think about his friends still waiting for him to come out of the bathroom on the boat and starts laughing. "Room, turn off the view screen please." Jay finishes his drink and washes the glass. He gets under the covers of Sihiryan's bed. As he feels the comfort of the pillow under his head he falls asleep.

Sihiryan found mouth-washing gear for Jay at the amenities shop a block down the street from the building. She checked the weather predictions for the next few days on her tablet and started back toward the entrance of the building. Putting Jay's oral hygiene tools in her pouch with her tablet, she looks up she and notices two of her work colleagues from the building. Seeing that they have noticed her too she nods and smiles.

"Sihiryan, How are you doing?" the amburst male says to her.

She stops walking "good Trecbeth, how are you? Shrehanker, good to see you, was it a good day in your department?"

Trecbeth smiles as he extends his hands to greet Sihiryan. Shrehanker puts an arm around Sihiryan's shoulders and leads her to turn directions, "yeah, a good day, lets go for a drink at Delcomkis. If you are hungry the pastries are fresh there at this hour." Seeing that Sihiryan is hesitant by the look on her face and the hesitation to reciprocate the embrace. "If you can't come we can do something another time."

Sihiryan smiles at her and lifts one arm around Shrehanker and grasps Trecbeth's hand with her other. "I was going to have an early night, but I can do that later, hahaha, yeah lets go for a drink or two."

"Great" Trecbeth says, "It was an exciting time in out department with the racial factions and their alarmist concerns about the Vworktek's new suit technology."

"Yeah" Shrehanker adds, "It is astounding how some worry about issues that actually don't effect them." Looking at Trecbeth "we will have to visit three worlds in the next 20 days to hear the concerns of various inter species relations committees." Then looking at Sihiryan, "and the Vworktek don't go to any of those three planets unless invited."

Sihiryan looks at her then him. "Sounds like you need some drinks." Then at him, "what are we going to have?

He looks at both females and smiles. "I have three days off so it is grandillia-sours for me, if they can make them."

Shrehanker laughs, "not for me, I'm going to have wine and zrectas seeds"

Sihiryan thinks for a moment then as they enter the establishment "I have never had a grandillia-sour or zrectas seeds, what are they like."

Delcomkis has a wide sidewalk cafe style entrance with a musician singing and playing soft music on a string instrument in it. The ceiling is about 40 feet high and draped with brightly colored fabrics. The walls are fashioned to look like the bark of a huge tree. There is what looks like huge branches with little gazebos hanging from them on rustic looking ropes. Each gazebo has three small cozy double chairs facing the small table between them and an umbrella like top. The room is about 70 feet wide and 60 feet long. The floor is glass with water running under it. There are 7 of the gazebos. The rest of the room is filled with couches in front of coffee tables and small round tables with bar stools around them. The room is only about 1/4 full of patrons, mostly kyranins, and one a group of birds that have moved some of the round tables together to stand around. The back of the room opens to the restaurant area with only about twenty tables, a bar on one side and the kitchen on the other. The corridor through the middle of the room is like a cross connecting the bar to the kitchen and the entrance room to the entrance of the party room down the stairs at the back. The opening to the party room is only about 10 feet wide and 12 feet tall. The carpeted stairs are round, fanning out to the whole room; about 3 feet long each and there are five of them. There are gaming tables in the near corners, and walls dropping from the ceiling that look like drapes to help decrease the sound from the band in the far end from disrupting the games. The band is on a sloped stage so that from anywhere in the room you can see them like they are beneath you, while they are actually above you. There are tables with chairs on both sides of the room and doorways leading to a spa on the left side and theatre like lounge on the right side. There are hygiene rooms in each corner. The band is playing, the restaurant is about 1/2 full, the gaming areas are well attended and the dance floor is hopping.

Shrehanker looks at her with wide eyes "Well, the grandillia-sour will not please your pallet as a kyranin, but it will be the start of an exciting evening. The seeds will be something that you won't want to forget. They are safe but you will see things differently after a few bites. If you want an early night best stick to the wine."

As they enter the restaurant section Sihiryan asks "are we going to sit in here?"

"No" Trecbeth says. "Through to the theatre, Provok, one of the Korobs we work with is doing some poetry and comedy there. His performance starts in a few moments."

Sihiryan smiles, "the Korob that was with you last month at the lake watching the game when I saw you?"

Shrehanker gently puts a hand on her side and gives her a gentle shake "you think he's cute don't you Sihiryan?"

Trecbeth laughs "You did smile at him a lot at the game Sihiryan. Are you open to that inter species marriage movement?"

"No, but I do think he is cute" Sihiryan says, "he had a lot to say that day and he seems smart."

As they enter the lounge Trecbeth points to a table with four chairs near the front, "lets sit there". Then as they walk toward it making their way between the tables and sofas he waives at a server, "Sir, please, some kreptigs and hot wine for us. We will sit there." pointing to the table again.

Choosing the middle chair facing the stage Sihiryan sits
first. She takes out her tablet and checks grandillia-sours and
zrectas seeds. After seeing the toxicity levels very low on both
she says, "I'll have one of each"

"Each of what?" Shrehanker asks.

"You are brave" Trecbeth submits as he sits down, "but you
can't buy zrectas seeds in here"

"Is that what you mean you are having a sour and some seeds,
I'll give you some seed, I have them baked into these biscuits"
as she pulls out a few cookies from her satchel.

Sihiryan smiles as the waiter walks up.

He puts the three cups of hot wine on the table and the bowl of
kreptigs between them. "Is there anything else? The
performance will start in a few minutes and I won't take any
orders until he is finished"

Sihiryan looks in the young ambursts eyes for a second then
says "Please, three Grandillia-sours sir." Taking a sip of the

wine "mmm, this is perfect, it warms the mouth and grows a froth at the same rate, thank you."

The server smiles stepping backwards and nods before turning away to get the drinks.

Shrehanker asks, "Trecbeth, would you like a biscuit as well?"

Trecbeth looks at her, "oh, please yes, do you have a good supply? It will be fun to share it with Provok after his show."

"hahaha, do you think it is a good idea?, He is going to have to do another show latter too." Shrehanker asks.

Sihiryan looks at her then at Trecbeth, "maybe I should just have a half biscuit."

Taking a drink of the wine and nodding, "mmm. This is perfect, I have a good supply, the biscuits are not that strong," She takes a napkin and puts several more biscuits from her satchel onto it. "Do you like the sound from the band in the party room, I am new to their style of presenting?" she picks up one of the biscuits and pops it into her mouth glancing her eyes to them both.

Sihiryan looks at Trecbeth as he listens to the band's music coming from the next room. He gets a serious look and nods. "They have a style of their own but I like it"

Sihiryan takes another drink of her wine and nods too. "I have heard them before on the social media broadcasts, late at night, on the education institute's programs." Picking up one of the biscuits and taking a small bite. "It is an interesting sound." Then taking a kreptig and chomping it down in hast, "the flavor of the biscuit is new to me."

Trecbeth moves his chair to face the two women better. "They raise the rhythm with the strings while bobbing the mood of the music with the drums and contrast it with the strength and tone of the lyrics. The words are interesting."

"mmm" Sihiryan nods, "strong statements about their emotions and desires for freedom from family expectations." turning her head to look back and forth at them, I didn't look at them when we walked through, where are they from?"

The others both shake their heads as the server steps up and puts three glasses of grandillia-sour on the table. "The biscuit looks good, what is it?"

Shrehanker looks at him and hesitates, "I brought them from my home world, I'm a Kuroberote. You are welcome to try one but I must warn you they do have a kick!"

He smiles at her, "I have a break when the performance starts, could I join your table and try one."

She sees the sparkle in his eyes and feels her heart thump. "Well" shifting in her seat and looking into his eyes, "I would feel my heart warmed by your company at our table young sir." Continuing to look into his eyes as he nods and steps back before turning to go back to the bar.

Sihiryan nudges her with her arm, "he is young." then winks at her, "but he is hansom too. Hahahah."

Trecbeth smiles at her and winks "do you think he has any idea what he just did?"

"hahahaha" Shrehanker looks at him then Sihiryan "I bet is innocent, there are so few of us here that he likely never have met a woman from my world before".

Sihiryan thinks about their short interactions, "I don't understand, maybe he flirted a little but what are you saying he is innocent of?"

Trecbeth sees Shrehanker's wide eyes looking at Sihiryan. "In her culture a male being so forward in their first conversation is almost equivalent to a proposal for marriage in yours." He looks at Shrehanker's eyes then back at Sihiryan's "their mating is only for a period long enough to raise a family but that is usually about 40 years in their culture. On the Kuroberote home world if a male approaches a female in that manner and fails to follow through it is a disgrace for his entire family."

Sihiryan looks at Shrehanker and into her eyes for a second, "In our culture and from what I know of Amburst his behaviour was simply a friendly flirt indicating that he finds you attractive"

Shrehanker smiles back at her "I understand, I find the young male attractive too, I have lived on many planets and am open to any situation, but it still got my heart pounding to be treated that way, I love it here on Ramga!" Lifting her grandillia-sour, nodding at Sihiryan and shifting her gaze toward Trecbeth with a smile "a toast to cultural exchanges here on Ramga and around the Galaxy" waiting for the others to put their glasses to their lips, then she downs the drink. "I love how they make me feel but the flavor is not my favorite"

Sihiryan nods in agreement and takes another nibble of her biscuit. "So you are not offended that the server has no intention of anything serious?"

As the lights dim they notice the server picking up a tray of glasses from the bar and starting to walk in their direction, Shrehanker leans to Sihiryan's ear. "I know he just wants to fuck me, and I like the idea that we can do that together. But, every girl where I come from likes to feel the rush of hearing a proposal; even if we would never accept it" and gives her a wink as she sits back into her chair.

As Provok is entering the stage from the side, the server sets the four glasses from the tray on the table, moves the fourth chair to beside Shrehanker and puts the empty tray under it. He leans to her ear, "my name is Srenkita" as he gracefully strokes her shoulder with his hand, sliding it down her back, around her side and comfortably resting it on her thigh.

Provok stops at the front centre of the stage and clears his throat, fidgets and stutters "ii I aaaa a'm rr ready to start," then clears his throat. "Well, as you can imagine it it's a little awkward for me to be up here, all alone, with nobody to bump and nudge as I am talking." he looks around the audience, "You all know how we are, this is it folks, this is the one and only time, ever, that you will see one of my kind alone, standing alone" lifting his arms up into the air just higher than his shoulders, "It's ok, I understand, take some pictures, send them to your friends. It's not funny for me though I'll tell you that," Clearing his throat again, and loosening his collar. "I'm going to go straight into the poetry now" he reaches into his pocket and pulls out a tablet and works the screen for a second, "Ok, here it is" he looks back at the screen like he is reading it then up at the audience. "What are the looks about?" you want me to say the poems without reading them?" His posture slouches a little, as he looks one-way at the crowd then the other. Then puts the tablet away in his pocket as he gets a sad look on his face. "They told me it was a tough audience here, I was going to do a classic to get things started but I can see you want something new" He strokes his hair back and takes a deep breath. "Shallow skies, the rumble of glowing tall-broad ships sifting the clouds, straining to stop, to hover, bursting the calm to shimmer their light through the trees onto the night's sweet ground. Creatures so scared, the billowing air giving no heed, nor a single care. With opening hulls and greetings of cones, colored light searching for bones and the flesh that makes them grow. Then arrows and hooks with lines,,, lifting what's on the hooks. To study for books, to show, the creatures ask why, these things in the sky take their families and friends away, to see and record without asking a word. They cannot learn what they loved, or did for play. They look up with disgust at the tall-broad ship, shaking their heads and holding their hips. Then say Go back through the sky,,, so our loved ones won't die to be taken for waist, and your pride. As whatever you find you could not understand. Our freedom so grand as to live here, so close to the land."

A few seconds of silence followed by smiles and nods.

"Thank you, I think, I can't tell if you liked it, If you were all Korobs like me I would have been bumped hit and kicked a thousand times if you liked it." Provok sees and hears some laughing. "About the poem, it was inspired by a conversation I had with three birds that I shared some beer with at the beach, well they shared it and I was there. I wanted some." He looks around the room, and sees they are all looking at him. "They told me how happy they are that we have such great technologies, not that they need any of it, but as we have such great technology we can produce beer and good beer according to them, in such quantities that we never run out." Looks both ways. "You know when I first got here to Ramga I went into a bar and saw that there was buckets of beer. I got one. I like beer I thought, and so I got one to take home. So I stepped outside the bar and bumped into the first bird I ever saw. He looked down at me and saw that I splashed out some of my beer from the bucket when I walked into him. He said to me "Leave that beer for me and go get yourself a new one." I was so scared that I offered him my tablet too. He laughed so hard that he fell over and rolled over onto the street. I took my opportunity and went back inside and told the bartender about how I was robbed. The bartender told me since I gave my beer to the bird my next one was free. I thought he was scared of them too." Provok could see some laughing and others waving at him. He put his arms up nodded his head and said "blessings to the birds." Stepping down off of the stage as the lights came back up and the doors to the party room opened. Provok walks up to Sihiryan's table and smiles at her then greets his workmates.

Srenkita with his hand still on Shrehanker's thigh smiles at her and finishes his drink then says what time he finishes his shift.

Shrehanker looks at him for a few seconds as she starts to smile "If I'm in the other room come and find me"

Srenkita leans forward and kisses her on the cheek then takes his tray, puts the empties on it and goes back toward the bar.

Provok takes the chair and moves it to the other side of the table to face them. "What do you think," patting Shrehanker on the knee with one hand and Trecbeth on the shoulder with the other while bumping his foot against Sihiryan's feet then sides of her legs.

The other two nod, and Sihiryan says, "I heard several Kyranins laughing a few times, and I liked the poem a lot. Is it your own poem?"

"Yes" as he looks at the server who just put a drink in front of him. "Thank you" patting her on the leg as he turns back to Sihiryan. "We met at the park once some weeks ago correct?" as he bumps her ankle with his foot again.

Sihiryan smiles and nods thinking that she is going to trap his foot with hers if he kicks her again. "Have you been doing this kind of thing long?"

"No this is my third show." Provok smiles as he pats Trecbeth on the shoulder, I have to thank Trecbeth for setting them up for me"

As his foot touches her ankle he feels Sihiryan lifts her foot under his as her other foot slaps the top of his. 'She caught it' he thinks. His gaze stops roaming and fixes on her eyes as he sees her body stop moving from the action of catching his foot. He feels the grip on his foot from hers' through his shoe and has a shocked look on his face. Still looking into her eyes and speechless he swallows. He has no idea what it means to be grabbed by a kyranin woman. To be grabbed by her feet must mean something but what? The pause goes unnoticed by the others and he notices Sihiryan's eyes opening wider and her face smiling at him. He feels his heart starting to speed up and the rush of fear and excitement filling his organs and flesh. Still without words he reaches for his drink, continues to look into her eyes, and starts to smile back at her. Not that he has thought what to do next but he is smiling back at her because he sees her still smiling, with more intensity, at him. Thinking that it looks like a friendly smile the excitement grows faster than the fear in him. Not knowing what the grip on his foot means, "did you like my show?"

As Sihiryan forces his foot to the floor, slide out from under it and holds it down with both feet she nods keeping eye contact.

Provok takes a drink and looks down at his glass then back up at Sihiryan. He feels her pressure and massage on his foot and examines her smile. "I live near here, are you familiar with the area?" He sees her eyes still fixed on his, "I have a view of the mountains form our place, it has the sea in the background. Do you live in the city?"

Trecbeth asks, "What is in your drink, it is an odd color Provok?"

Turning to him then looking back at Sihiryan and Shrehanker for a split second each "It is a mixed drink from Korob, I am surprised to get it here. It is a mixture of juice from three sedative plants and the juice from a stimulant berry and the extract from a root that dulls pain that is preserved in alcohol. A sharp flavor, slightly sweet and warming to the mouth and chest." He looks at the tree of them each for a second, "It is called a spelunker. Would you like a taste?"

Trecbeth reaches and takes the glass with one hand and slides the grandillia sour to replace it. "Yes, try mine".

Shrehanker smiles at their exchange, "That's called a guardillia sour, I would love to taste your drink, a spelunker you say? Would you like to try a cookie from my world?" as she passes him a cookie.

Sihiryan presses hard into his ankle with a toe, "I will taste it too".

Provok takes the grandillia sour in one hand and picks up the cookie in the other and looks into Sihiryans eyes again. He thinks about her grip on his foot and with one nervous action pops the cookie into his mouth and washes it down with the entire sour. "Humm. That isn't sour at all,,, I like it".

Sihiryan laughs, "Well then you can share mine with me" and slides it to him then reaches for the spelunker from Trecbeth.

Trecbeth hands her the drink and leans forward to be sure his grandillia sour is empty then looks up to see Provok taking a drink from Sihiryans. Starting to smile "so you like them" Raising an arm in the air and waiving at the server, I'll get some more for all of us".

Sihiryan takes a sip of Provok's drink as she looks into his eyes, smiles putting it down on the table and sliding it toward Sherhanker. "It is good, tangy, and leaves my mouth wanting more." looks away from his eyes examining the other features of his face. "How was the cookie?"

Sherhanker laughs, "he washed it down so fast I bet he didn't taste it?"

Provok looks at her thinking about the massage on his foot. "Well actually I could have taken more time to enjoy it but it was good."

Sherhanker passes another one to him. "This time enjoy it and tell me what you think of it, I brought it from my home world" She picks up the spelunker and smells it then takes a sip, then a small drink. "It is good" and raises the glass toward Provok, smiles and nods, then hesitates as if she is waiting for something. As he lifts Sihiryan's grandillia sour and takes a big drink of it she has a sip of his, smiles and passes it to him.

Srenkita arrives at the table, "What could I get for you" as he looks at each of them in turn ending with Sherhanker to whom he gives a wink.

Trecbeth responds, "a grandillia sour for each of us and could we each also have one of these, spelunker, I think they are called?"

Srenkita smiles, "a good choice sir" then he turns toward the bar.

Sihiryan looks at Trecbeth, "I have to work early tomorrow and for the next two days, I was serious about having to leave early"

Provok looks at her with concern as he thinks about the grip she still has on his foot then looks at Trecbeth.

Trecbeth winks at Sherhanker and says "Oh, well the drinks are ordered already, as soon as they are done, we can see that you make it home."

Sihiryan laughs and gives Sherhanker a nudge with her hand, "you are training him I see"

Sherhanker laughs. "You don't have to stay Sihiryan, It is good to see you but if your work needs you we understand."

Shihiryan reaches for her wine glass and looks at Provok's eyes again, "I won't leave just yet" taking a sip then looking at Provok when did you decide to take up performing?" and slides one foot up his shin and past his knee.

Provok takes the last of the glass of sour in a gulp and a deep breath before answering. "I thought about it when I was a child. Of course it wasn't a career choice, it was a dream, but in the past few years here on Ramga I decided to see if I could do it."

"You seemed nervous at the start of the show" Sihiryan asks, "is that part of the act?"

Provok smiles and brings his thoughts above the table, "actually the first time I did it, at the amature preforming association, I was so scared I couldn't tell the jokes. The audience was laughing so hard that I thought it could be part of the act." He looks at her smiling and looking at him talking to her. "I am still a little nervous on the stage but mostly it is part of the act."

Sherhanker looks at them noticing the connection that is starting between them. "I liked the poem"

Trecbeth lifts his glass, and gestures towards the bar "The new drinks are coming, lets finish these" and lifting his glass, "a drink to Provok's performances present and future. May they be uplifting to most and enjoyed by many" then puts his glass to his lips.

The others do the same finishing there drinks as the new ones arrive and are put on the table in front of each of them. Srenkita smiles and winks at Sherhanker again as he takes the empties and near empties away on his tray. Sihiryan looks at the two drinks in front of her and notices how she already feels. She thinks about the cookie she ate and contemplates the added effects it will soon bring. Slouching a little in her chair and thinking about Jay and camping, and Provok's foot under hers, and that she can't go to his place. She takes a deep breath. Looks at her two friends, smiles, and lifts the spelunker "to new beginnings". She waits for the others to lift their glasses and takes a slow big drink as the others follow.

Sherhanker half finishes her glass and notices that the two males did finish theirs and that Sihiryan's still has about two thirds in it. "How about some cookies, to create a thirst for the sours?" and she puts a cookie in front of each of the four of them.

Provok smiles feeling the drink fill his belly and her foot now resting on his thigh, and seeing the cookie in front of him. "Where is your home world"

Sherhanker smiles at him, "not close by, do you like the cookies"

"She is from Kuroberote" Sihiryan says.

"Oh" Provok says as he takes a bite of the cookie and looks around the room. "Kuroberote" then looks at Sherhanker, "I know of that world" and takes a drink of the grandillia sour. Making a silly smile at Sihiryan, "How are you doing?"

Sihiryan takes a nibble of her cookie and a sip of her spelunker and nods, "good, I like to dance, do you ever dance?"

Provok takes a bite of his cookie and then the rest of it, chews swallows and washes it down with the rest of his grandillia sour. "I can dance," Then looks at the glass, "why do they call them sour?"

Sihiryan slides hers' toward him as she sees that Trecbeth notices and how he is starting to laugh, "after our drinks would you dance with me?"

Feeling her feet on his shins he smiles and picks up the glass, "Yes, I would love to dance with you," taking a big drink then asks, "in here or in the party room?"

Sihiryan looks at the others for a second. She takes another drink from her glass and gets up with the glass in her hand, "in there."

Provok stands up and finishes the grandilia sour and starts toward the other room.

Sherhanker looks at them then at Trecbeth. Then at his drinks and says, "We will follow you two in a few moments."

Shiryan reaches and takes her half cookie, smiles, pops it in her mouth and finishes the spelunker and nods at them then follows Provok to the dance floor. To dance with a korob is like doing a jig and swing dancing mixed with a little bit of disco and salsa. Sihiryan catches up with Provok near the middle of the dance floor. The music has a varying rhythm with a slow drum beat, and whining wind instrumental tune that is the foundation for the lyrics. When he stops and turns to see her she steps right into him and slides her arms under his and up his back to grip his shoulders. Being a lot taller than him she slides one leg between his in response to his first step. She feels his arousal on her thigh and smiles down to him. The music slows and softens almost as soon as they start dancing and she leans her head down beside his. "I do have to leave early but I do want to see you again."

Provok looks up into her face and focuses his eyes into hers. "I am Korob, I am attracted to you" with a worried look on his face.

Sihiryan smiles then puts her head down and talks into his ear, "don't tell anyone, none of your friends, not anyone, I will invite you to see me in a few days." and she slides into him in time with the music. Her arms on his back feel the tension in his back increasing as they dance. She feels his arousal changing angles on her thigh as he leads her in the embracive dance movements toward the side of the floor with chairs and tables.

The music starts to change again and he leads her, holding her hand to a table. He pulls out his tablet and hands it to her. With out a word he watches as she taps hers' to his and checks the screens to see that they have each other's contact information. "Sihiryan, you know I can't start anything serious with you, I'm a Korob".

Smiling to him, looking at how cute he looks and liking the way he is looking back at her. "I understand" Then looking around the room and then the tablet, then toward the door. "Will you be Ok alone here now, I do have to go, I do have work for three days starting in the morning".

Provok looks at her and the room flashing and moving behind her, "yeah" looking her all up and down, "yeah, I understand, I'll say nothing, I'll hear form you in some days. And I will be happy when you do contact me" then looks around the room. "I am good here, hahaha, I hope my next performance goes well, those are good cookies." smiles into her eyes and softly grips her hand "Have a good night."

Sihiryan gives him a hungry look and winks as her tablet indicates an incoming communication. Still looking at Provok she lifts the tablet to view it. Starting to turn as she moves her eyes to the tablet she sees it is Sherhanker and Trecbeth from the other room. She sees their images waiving and smiling and talking and the words scrolling like subtitles on a foreign movie read (there is a dance group from Nilbask giving a surprise performance in 5 minutes. Six dancers, and three Krebits with their own musicians; miss a dance and see it with us.) Looking back at Provok, Common it is a special show in the performance lounge" reaching her hand toward him "I'll leave after it".

Provok takes her hand and follows closely back to the table in the other room. Smiling at the others as he arrives, "She dances well"

Sherhanker moves to the chair beside her so that Sihiryan and Provok can sit together facing the stage. "I ordered wine for you both. It is about to begin."

The doors close to the dance room and the lights dim as the server Srenkita arrives with a tray full of drinks and he starts putting them all on the table. "I brought us each a sour as well, I hope it is OK" as he looks for a free chair to get for himself.

Trecbeth smiles looking into his eyes, "thank you".

The others are busy with adjusting their positions and deciding who gets what drink as Srenkita returns putting a chair tightly beside Sherhanker's and sitting in it. The curtains open and the show begins. Four bright blue female dancers glide across the stage from different corners as the music begins. A soothing melody on wind instruments as the girls circle around and slide into a huddle in the middle of the stage. The low tones of an intersecting melody lead out two fat, almost round girls moving so gracefully from the back of the stage toward the first four. Then the chimes of glass bells softly begin to compliment the fluidity of the other sounds, guiding the three Kerbits in movement as they seemingly float down from the ceiling.

"I have never actually seen one before" Trecbeth says.

Sihiryan leans forward focusing her eyes, "are they naked?"

Provok stops moving as he watches them moving to the music "these girls are as small as children, but the way that they move is delightful."

Sherhanker takes a drink of wine, "I checked my tablet, and this group has been performing together for about 30 years. I saw them once on Kuroberote at a special festival. They are all adults and yes they are all naked, and they don't like to interact with other species. But they give a great show."

Provok still keeping very still, "I heard that the Kerbits have wings and fly but I never imagined that they would look like that, how do they move so slowly in the air?" Picking up a glass and taking a big drink, "I have to go up next."

Trecbeth starts laughing softly, "don't worry they won't expect you to take your cloths off"

Sihiryan starts to laugh too and puts her arm around Provok "you are great on stage" hugging him a little so her breast presses into his shoulder a bit then reaching for a glass as well. After a drink of the sour she realizes how intoxicated she is becoming. She thinks about what her friend said about the biscuits and then tried to remember how many she ate. Thinking about the number of drinks she had she has another drink of the sour and looks at Provok beside her. 'He is cute, fuzzy and cute' she thinks and laughs, smiles and shakes her head side to side then her attention is absorbed by the activities on stage. The soothing sounds perfectly in time with the movements of the dance. With it's mingling aerobatic and acrobatic movements holding her attention fully. The brightness of the colors filling her eyes, and a full fuzzy feeling fills her body from the seeds and drinks.

By the end of the performance all of the drinks on the table are all empty. They all stand to wave and cheer and praise the performers. Sihiryan's duty to leave early felt further away from the moment than was normal for her and this brought her to a deeper thinking of the situation. Searching her feelings she realized that her attraction to Provok is real and more than just lust, her desire to spend time with her friends is just that, she had been working a lot lately and the intoxication of her mind, senses and body was justified considering how much they all drank. She assessed the time to be spent debriefing Jay for three days in the forest and decided that she could stay a little longer and not start the debriefing until the next evening. The camping would be more fun if they focused on it first anyway.

Provok slides his hand up her leg and over her hip to hold her back as he turns to look up into her face and eyes, "my show is next, in 15 minutes. I have to go in the back to prepare. I will see you soon" and he turns and walks away.

Srenkita picks up his tray and fills it with the empties, "more drinks?" he asks then slowly turns and smiles at Sherhanker as he stands straight.

"Just wine this time Srenkita" Sihiryan replies as she sees him turn to her and nod before heading to the bar.

Trecbeth asks, "You are not bolting to your early night yet?" and smiles at her.

Sherhanker turns to him then looks at Sihiryan and starts to laugh. "Maybe we should get something to eat?"

With a silly grin on her face, "I don't like eating this late" Sihiryan replies.

Sherhanker puts some more of the biscuits on the table and sees Trecbeth's hand coming for one.

Sihiryan reaches for one too and starts to laugh, "hahaha, what are these seeds that taste so good called again?"

"Careful with those Sihiryan, they will make you see thinks differently" Sherhanker says, "Zrectas seeds have physcobalancing effects. That is to say they can cause you to re think your priorities."

"Is that why I'm still here having a good evening with you two, or is just because I like to have a good evening with friends?" Sihiryan jests and laughs. She reaches to Trecbeth's hand and to Sherhanker's on her other side and smiles at them both. I am glad I came out. I have been putting in a lot of hours lately at work and haven't had much social time. Then turns to Trecbeth, "are you in a committed relationship? I only ask because it seems that we have both had a little romance tonight but you didn't seem to have any interest in anyone at all."

Trecbeth smiles at her. "Actually I do have a relationship with a female under the sea. I will see her in a few months, after our tour of conferences and the many meetings here afterwards. I am not married but my inner demands for intimacy are small outside of my relationship. Why do you ask?"

"I thinks it is the seeds" Sihiryan says. "It has me wanting to know the personal sexual thoughts and choices of who ever I think about" with a perplexed look she turns to Sherhanker.

Sherhanker looks into her eyes. "Hahaha. That is a odd situation Sihiryan, are you asking me what my desires are?"

Sihiryan looks into her eyes and slowly smiles then says, "No, but I am more and more curious about it. I have never had this curiosity before about what others think or desire or lust about. Do you think it is the seeds?"

"I hope not," Shrehanker retorts, "if it is it will be with you for a full day or more. I haven't heard of that reaction before but it does have a kick" reaching for a biscuit for herself, "maybe it was the korob drink you tried?"

"Or the sours" Trecbeth submits. "The sours can have an aphrodisiac effect."

Sihiryan looks at him then her, then him again and thinks about how she feels, "no this is mostly intellectual, I'm interested to know more than wanting to do. It is odd for me to be like this, I usually don't think much about the thoughts of others unless it effects me somehow." then with a perplexed look on her face she thinks, 'I must be pretty loaded', "hahaha, what did you think of Provok's poem?"

Trecbeth looks at her then at Shrehanker.

Shrehanker nods "interesting, inspired by the birds about tyranny and freedom from the perspectives of non-technically advanced beings. A deep topic and well presented. The Korobs fascinate me, they are all so family-oriented and yet they are also willing to engage in true and deep friendships with other species. They are impossible to offend and as smart as almost anything." taking a bite of the biscuit and chewing it. "I am impressed with the poem I didn't give it much thought at the time but it is an interesting viewpoint. Did you like it?"

Sihiryan nods, "the style was not my taste but it did bring me a sense of the feelings of the beings it was about." Looking at him for his response "Trecbeth?"

Smiling at her then with a gentle pulse on her hand with his he starts. "Well it is a interesting topic politically speaking. Is science's need to kill things in research worth the damage it does to the life forms it claims to be studying? To live we must kill, but for research alone on species that we don't interact with is it justified? Do we actually need to know what we can learn from it? I suspect every technologically advanced species has done at least some of this kind of research but at what level of sentient thinking do we stop doing it?" looking at them one then the other, "Our agricultural industries do all kinds of research on insects and bacteria in the soils and fluid to attempt improvements in our ability to produce foods. But we don't communicate with those life forms so who knows what they think about our experiments. Perhaps if we spent the same efforts to communicate with them they would help us produce better crops and healthier herds. It has never been attempted in our science".

Sihiryan smiles then chuckles, "I wonder if Provok has thought it through that deeply, or if he just thought of situation and wrote the poem. I will have things to talk to him about when I get back."

"Where are you going?" Shrehanker asks.

Sihiryan feels something prying in the way she asks and feels the emotion from her hand. It is cold, without connection, a business sensation, more than a question from the flow of the conversation. Looking into her eyes she sees the desire to get some information, 'Maybe it is just the drinks' she thinks. "I have three days of meetings with a delegate new to our systems nothing difficult but it needs my full attention. I should probably go now. It is getting late and I will need to look fresh in the morning." Sihiryan stands up and smiles at both of them then lets go of their hands. She looks at Trecbeth can you record Provok's show and tell him I want to watch it with him some time for me?"

Trecbeth shifts in his chair and gets up to embrace her, "Of course I will, it is always good to see you, thank you for coming out with us" as he gives her a gentle hug.

Shrehanker stands and hugs her too. "It was a joy to spend time with you. I will tell you about the waiter next time I see you, are you Ok getting home?"

Sihiryan smiles as she lets go, "thank you, yes it is close".

Surprise in the night

On the way out of the club Sihiryan sees a few friends but doesn't stop to greet any. She notices how intoxicated she is and laughs to herself about it. When she enters her room she goes directly to the shower undressing on the way then into bed. She had forgotten that Jay would be there until she gets into bed with him. She laughs to herself seeing that it is him sleeping in her bed but says nothing and gets comfortable to go to sleep. After a few minutes she starts thinking that it was good that Jay didn't wake up when she came in and that he must have needed the sleep to be sleeping so soundly. Then a few minutes later she rolls over and looks at his head on her other pillow and watches him sleep. She remembers when she first met him and he was astounded to be in her world. She thinks about the time she had to undress in front of him to get him to take his clothes off for the lab work. She thinks about his flirting with her afterwards. She thinks about how happy he seemed to see her earlier in the day. Then she started to remember him shopping and getting accustomed to Ramga under her guidance. She remembered the jokes the others made about him being sharp and a quick study but not knowing very much. Then she thinks about how young he is in her world and how old he is in his world. She realizes that she can't sleep and feels how intoxicated she is and decides to get her tablet and scan herself.

Slipping out of bed and getting her tablet form her pouch near her cloths by the door she sits down in a chair and starts scanning herself. After a few reading of various bio-signs and chemistry of her blood and her intestine's contents; she does an analysis and determines that she won't sleep for several hours unless she drastically changes her hormones and blood chemistry. She looks back over at her bed. She thinks to herself, 'if he was kyranin I would have sex with him and not think about it, he is a co worker but if he was kyranin that would not matter.' She looks around the room then scans herself to check her ovulation. It won't happen for twelve to fourteen days. She looks over at the bed and laughs. She goes to the kitchen and has a beverage from the cooler and fills the glass before walking back to her bed. Placing the beverage on the table near her bed, she climbs in and cuddles up to Jay. She pays attention to his responses as Jay reacts in a friendly manner to her without waking up. She has snuggled up to his side with her face beside his. Her lips on his cheek, with her left arm above his head and reaching to his opposite ear. Her body against his arm and chest and belly, her left leg beside his and her knee under his. Her right leg over and across his right leg and her foot on his left shin. Her right arm strokes across his belly and then up his chest. "Jay, Jay" she watches as he moves his face a little. "Jay" she sees one eye open. "Jay, I want to have sex with you now is that OK?"

Jay hears what she said to him and turns to look at who said it. "Sihiryan?"

Stroking down his chest slowly "I can't sleep so I want to have sex now with you so that I can sleep, is that OK?"

Jay starts to turn his head towards her and hears her say "you don't have to move, just relax and tell me that it is OK"

Jay is waking up enough to remember where he is and when he is and what he is dong there. "Yeah,, Sure, I guess, I will be Ok with that, of course we can". Jay heard him self say the words and starts to think about what he has said. 'What is going on here' he asks himself. He feels her hand sliding down his belly and toward his genitals. He feels her lips sliding up his cheek and hears her whispers into his ear for him to relax and stay still. So he does. Feeling her hand slowly brush over his cock he feels it beginning to swell. Feeling her hand slowly sliding down between his thighs, with her fingers brushing and stroking as they find there way down towards his knees Jay notices his cock lifting itself away from his scrotum, and as he feels her hand sliding back up to his balls he feels his cock lifting the blanket around it up off of him. He feels her hand working it's way around to get a good grasp on his scrotum and then it starts working the balls, moving them against each other inside his sack. He feels her breath accelerate as it warms his ear then she slides on top of him, keeping a good solid grip on his balls. The pleasure of her hand's grip on him, and the pull causing him to clench his torso a little.

She shifts her position above him and moves her left arm so that her hand is behind his neck and her forearm is on his shoulder. Her feet between his thighs and her knees straddling his belly she is stretched to keep her strong grip on his balls. With her hold of them she adjusts the angle on his erection to her opening moist hot cunt and slides herself back down consuming it into her. Feeling his cock inside her with the heightened sensitivity of the Korob drink and the grandillia sours she stops still for some seconds and says, "oh, wow, Jay, that feels so good." With her focus on her own feelings and the surprise of the richness of the sensations she tightens her grip on his balls without realizing it until Jay's clenching and groan alert her to his pain and she lets go of them.

'Uu, oohhwww" Jay released and started to relax back into the bed and can concentrate on the sensation of her on him again. The heat, the pulsing, and flavor that seems to be filling his penis, and the smoothness of her skin on his fill his thoughts.

He looks up at her face and sees her from that angle in the dim light and his heart softens as he realizes how beautiful she looks. "It does feel good, so good". Jay thinks as he hears himself say it 'what a dumb thing to say'. Realizing he is still half asleep he notices her starting to move.

Sihiryan feels the swelling of her energy in her pelvis and the change of her hormones building the fluids inside of her. Feeling his presence in her and the yearning to feel the pressure in all those hidden spaces within her depths. Tilting herself with her ass up and her belly against his then the other way, slowly lifting her belly like a cat hunching it's spine and pulling her pelvis up across his, then over to one side then around, slowly back down to the other side. Hearing Jay groan and his breath accelerate she worries that he will come first and she slaps him hard in the face. Then as he reacts with a shocked look she starts to lift and plunge onto him pounding his cock deep into her and as she grabs at his chest with both hands and moans a whinny whimpering groan laden melody with her eyes opening and closing. Sliding almost right off of him, then pounding down hard and grinding this way and that before the next near exiting lift.

Jay feeling more awake after the slap and distracted with the tearing on his chest of her surprisingly strong hands starts to enjoy the situation both in his mind and body. He realizes that she is using him to get what she wants and he is surprised at how much he likes to be a tool for her pleasure. His body still filled with the sensation of sleep is growing aware of the sweet sensations radiating out from his genitals, the smell of her juices exciting his nostrils out of that dream state and fully into the moment. Her toes on his thighs and the angles of pressure on his cock working to stir arousal deep within his pelvic region, Jay submits to his willingness to please. "Whatever you want, I will do it Sihiryan, anything you ask"

Sihiryan feels the surges of her arousal dwarfed by the body stone of the drinks and biscuits as her orgasm starts to build. "wwuim, uuoowwa, wwwwwaaa, Jay". The movement of energy in her groin makes her clench her vagina squeezing him, and her motions shorten and grind harder. "teeyuaa," holding her breath as she grabs his upper arms and changes her body angle to force it deeper as she thrusts. "wooooaaaa" slowing her movement to almost nothing. "JAY.. uOOOOOHHOOHHO. wooooaaaa" and a few fast grinds with pelvic tilts "thuia uuuua thuuia uuuuaaa" and she lets herself down onto him limpening herself with his still hard as steel inside of her. "oohhh, a second Jay just a second, then roll me over and fuck me hard."

Jay, feeling more awake smells her breath and recognizes the grandillia sour sent. He finds amusement in it but keeps his outward expression in check. Smiling to himself for a second before he rolls her over with him and positions himself on top of her, she is smiling up at him totally limp and sparkly eyed. Slowly sliding side to side and in and out as he watches her face Jay sees that she is focusing on the sensations in her genitals. He lets some of his body weight onto her pelvis and belly and watches her expression and sees the joy in her face. He lets himself down on her a little more so that his lips are only millimeters away from hers' and he feels her tongue slide across his lips. Jay starts kissing her and feels her body move under him as she kisses him back with more passion that he expected. Jay starts slow deep thrusting and grinding and squeezing her and kissing and looking into her eyes as best he can. He feels her vagina gripping him and senses the flavor of it soaking into him. He feels his own orgasm starting to build and his balls start to feel a glow. Then he feels her hands on his back sliding up and her pulling herself against him, her breasts squeezing against his chest and the heat of his fluids building a pressure that wants to escape into her. Clenching to hold his cum from going Jay slows his kissing and looks into her eyes more deeply as she squirms to bring his orgasm out with hers, she is gripping his back and gripping him with her mouth as her pulsing grows and he feels it ahead of his own. Her panting and squeezing starts to subside as his brain looses control and his buttocks take charge clenching it out one grunt after another squeeze of his semen out. His cock rings a soothing glow through his belly and back and then he only feels his heart beating. The look in her eyes staring into his of clarity and purity of spirit then he feels her lips nibbling at his and her feet sliding up the backs of his legs and onto his back.

"You said anything Jay" Sihiryan looks into his eyes, "I can't sleep yet, will you lick my genitals until I fall asleep, do you know how Jay?"

Jay looks at her sweet eyes and feels his limpness still fully inside of her. "Yes, if I get hard again do you want me back on top"

After kissing his mouth and gently scratching him on his back and shoulders "Yes Jay lick until I'm asleep and if you get hard give it to me however you like" and she spreads her legs wide to the sides and relaxes as Jay moves slowly down the bed kissing her breasts and belly before finding her pubic zone. As he slides his tongue into her folds Jay thinks about the grandilia sour. Licking her swollen ridges and slippery groves he asks himself if she will remember any of it the next day. The taste of her excites him, the way that she holds herself open slightly moving her pelvis as he touches her with his face pleases him. Realizing how much he is actually enjoying licking her cunt pulls his mind from the thought that she likely won't remember anything about it in the morning. After a few minutes Jay realizes that she has relaxed and also that he is hard. He climbs up the bed and sees that her eyes are still open so he lines it up and slides it in. She smiles and turns her head to the side and closes her eyes. Jay feels horny seeing that she is smiling so hard as she stays so still and totally relaxed. He slowly sides in and then back and forth and out again. Feeling that she is totally relaxed with his thrusting brings a calm into Jay that he is not familiar with while having sex. He tries to relax and thrust and probe and relax as he does it. In doing it he finds that he feels the contact between her skin and his and between her spirit and his more. Continuing the slow prying deep thrusts while hovering above her, holding his weight with his arms, Jay feels his orgasm starting to build, mostly in his cock. Looking down at her limp body and smiling face Jay starts to pay attention to how her boobs jiggle when his thrust's impact of reaching her interiors end causing repercussions through her flesh. Jay feels the tension in his arms and back and legs as he hovers above her so that his cock slides into her wide spread crotch without squashing her body at all.

Sihiryan feels her orgasm slowly building from her vagina and slowly spreading to her womb and all around her crotch. She relaxes the rest of her body as she focuses on the sensations of

Jay sliding into and out of her. Feeling the warmth of his hard cock gliding through her opening and deep inside, the shape of his head rubbing slowly on her interior builds the growing glowing sensations that are continuing to spread out from where her vagina is wanting to grip his hot cock. "Jay, I like it Jay, I want it like this, I like it Jay" then closing her eyes again and focusing on the sensations of him in her and what is being moved and what it is doing to the sensations of energy inside of her belly and bottom and around her opening. " uhmmmmmmnnn"

Jay feels the heat in his belly through to his back, from halfway to his knees to the tip of his cock, his balls seem to feel separate, surreal, and hot all at once and he hears her breath and make little noises. Clenching to hold it from explosion as it increases more with each slowing stroke. Feeling his heat throbbing and his arms burning to distract the greatness of the flavor of light in his belly, for one more thrust, for the way out, for one, more, thrust. Jay looks at her as he stops moving and it looks like she is asleep, he feels her hot vagina and it is throbbing and she is perfectly still beneath him. He isn't moving but the orgasm is starting to win. As he can still feel her throbs his escape his control and the sensation of a bursting dam change everything in his body the sensations of strain in his arms and legs are gone, only the bellowing of the strobes of liquid pulsing out into her is left. The sound of a feeling of it is all that he can hear, the receiving of it by her vagina is all that he can think and the sensation of his belly's fuzzy heat and that of his balls and his red numb cock glowing like a stream of lava from a volcano.

Jay gains his focus as the last pulses of his penis empties what his balls spent days making. He looks at her still smiling and not moving at all. "Are you awake Sihiryan, do you want more?" Jay looks at her and decides to pull out. As he does she does not move. As he lay beside her she does not move. He checks her breathing, it is good and she is still smiling, but has not moved. Jay shifts her legs together and arranges the covers so that she will not be exposed. Jay gets himself a drink of water and checks the time. It is not that late, not even midnight yet. He finishes his water takes a shower and goes back into the bed and goes to sleep again.

Jay awakes in the silent room, feels the silky sheets beneath and over him, he turns to see Sihiryan beside him, still asleep, still hasn't moved that he can notice. Jay thinks about where he is, back on Ramga, in a new lovers bed, going to go camping today, then to start a career on the Gyrekian moon. Taking a deep breath he decides that more sleep might be good and closes his eyes.

Jay wakes up again when he feels Sihiryan roll over into him. He looks in her direction and sees she is looking back at him with a surprised expression. "Hi, good morning Sihiryan, how did you sleep?"

Sihiryan looks at Jay for a few seconds and shifts to sit up on the bed facing Jay. "I slept well, and with you in my bed, how did you sleep Jay?" holding herself up with one arm and rubbing her eyes with the other. Then looking at him with stretched wide eyes. "I feel a little off, was I out late?"

Jay looks up at her "not that late I got back to sleep before midnight." smiling at her, "it seemed that you may have been intoxicated. I could smell the grandillia sour on your breath."

Sihiryan looks at Jay's face then at the tent forming further down. "I went for a drink with some friends, we danced and watched a show, but, I can't remember the details of getting home. Jay do you know what happened last night?"

Jay sits up, "so you don't remember coming in, and waking me up?"

She looks at him changing position to fold her knees under herself and straighten her body up. Looking into his eyes her hand goes to her crotch feeling it, "we had sex".

Jay with a worried expression "you asked me first, then ask for more, told me I could do what I wanted, then told me you wanted more too. When you fell asleep I covered you showered and went back to sleep. I was asleep when you came in."

Sihiryan looking at Jays face starts to smile, "Jay you look worried, if your performance was so sad that I fell asleep you don't have to worry, I won't tell anyone, only because I can't remember, though." Slowly turning her head from side to side

"Jay you are a Kiranin now. You have to have a reputation of being able to satisfy before a female will want to let herself fall into love with you."

Jay smiles, "so you actually don't remember?"

Sihiryan looks at Jay with a serious look for several seconds, "it is like trying to remember a dream, I feel there is something there to remember but I can't find the details. "Getting up and looking for her tablet, "I will see if I can find some clues to bring it back." She sits in the chair and works the tablet to see the last entries, the scans and analysis of her intoxication.

Jay puts on a robe from her closet and sits across from her "did you record us?"

'Hahahaha" Sihiryan looks up at him, "no Jay" smiling at him, "I scanned myself and I was high on a mixture of stimulants and psychotropic substances as well as wine. I used you for sex so that I could sleep. I am surprised that I can't remember any of it."

Jay looks back at her, "I liked it. I think it is common to not remember with the grandillia sours. Trentia warned me not to have more than one when I was under the sea with her."

Sihiryan looks at Jay for some seconds, "I actually can't remember Jay. In your species is it acceptable to have sex and still be just friends?" watching his face getting the look of deep thoughts, "Jay what I mean is are you going to be OK with it, that we had sex, and that we are not going to have a relationship that includes expectations around the topic of having sex."

Jay looks into her eyes, "that is a good way to ask, I understand the issue. Yes I am ok with it. I liked having sex with you but I have no expectations. I understand that although you like me as a being, that you have no desire to commit me to a relationship in your mind or in mine."

"But the sex, it was good in your opinion" she looks at him "and you would be happy to do it with me again?"

Jay looks at her sitting comfortably in the big armchair with her knees up and her feet crossed holding the tablet in one hand and the other totally relaxed on the chairs arm, naked in front of him. Jay searches his feelings about her and the idea of having sex with her as many seconds pass and he contemplates Heather, Trentia, working with her, leaving the planet in a few days for a long time, and says "At this time in our lives I would be happy, even excited, to have sex with you again. If you want me to I will, anyway you like, anywhere you want."

Smiling and looking him up and down a little, "Well Jay, if you are trying to get me excited the robe won't help, so maybe something to eat first. Then maybe later you can have your fantasy of having consensual sex with me will come to be a reality" putting one foot on the floor at a time she exposes her vagina to him and stand up in a very sensual motion arching her back to showcase her breasts as she takes the first steps toward the kitchen. "I have some pastries in the pantry and Mrruk in the taps." Seeing that he has started to follow she walks back, past him out of the kitchen brushing her fingers so slightly across his engorged but limp penis. "I will have a shower while you get our meal ready"

Jay smiles and starts looking for the pastries. Puts them on a plate and finds some cheese and fruit in the cooler to go with them. Taking two cups from the rack he tries the taps until he sees and smells the mrruk coming out of one and fills the cups. He thinks to himself that the mrruk tap is a small step forward from the counter top coffee makers on earth. Jay puts the pastries and mrruks on a tray and delivers them to her coffee table and sits across it from her sitting naked in the chair again.

"Jay do you remember me telling you that most Kyranins are naked most of the time at home." Sihiryan reaches for a pastry and puts a slice of red fruit on it, then picks up her cup of mrruk and slides back into the comfy chair. "If you are cold please tell the room to be warmer. Your wearing that robe is making me feel uncomfortable."

Jay looks at her for a second and takes the robe off, hanging it up back in the closet where he found it. "I do remember, I have not had a chance to adjust to the custom. In my mind presenting myself naked is suggesting that I would be interested in having sex."

Sihiryan takes a sip of the mrruk, and smirks. "Yes Jay, you have stated quite clearly that you have that interest." Then with a look of curiosity on her face "so the robe, to me, after hearing that statement suggested that you are conflicted, or dishonest about your words on the topic of having sex with me."

Jay looks at her, picks up his cup and has a sip. "I am sincere, it is the habit of being clothed from my world that causes my behavior." Sitting with his cup he leans forward to grab a pastry and his genitals are pressed against the cushion of the chair and his cock bumps over to dangle slightly down in front, with the scrotum still spread between his parted legs atop the cushion. Biting then chewing the pastry until his sip of mrruk washes it down he watches her watching his cock dangle and starts to feel it react to the attention.

"Did it hurt?"

"Excuse me?"

She nods toward his dick, "When they cut the end off" looking him directly in the eyes. "We studied the practice as part of understanding your physiology to make the adjustments to pass you as a kyranin here. The kyranin male genital is very similar but the skin never grows all the way up the tip. It is convenient that you were cut like that to pass as one of us, but it must have hurt." Looking at it again "did you have a choice?" Then taking a bite of the fruit covered pastry and squinting from the enjoyment of flavor.

Jay looks down at his now partly hard dick and snickers, "No, I was a child, about three or four years old, maybe younger. My parents said it had to be done and I was told it would be ok, that it wouldn't hurt much. I can remember the crying I did from the pain. And how stressed my mother was about it afterwards. She clearly didn't understand what would happen, it is cultural and parents make the decision. It is not a choice for most people. A few get it done as adults but that is rare. It was a huge trauma for me at that time. It was before I knew what sex was or that I would need my penis for sex. It took a few weeks to heal and it hurt until it did. It made me very conscious of my penis and fearful of letting anyone touch it or see it. It is a terrible thing to do to a child, to think that god made my penis too big so that it has to be adjusted made me question all of gods works." Looking up at her "It made me distrust my mother too because she told me it wouldn't hurt much."

Sihiryan looks at it again, "talking about it made it shrink again"

Jay looks down at his shriveled phallus, "yeah, the thought of having it cut and the memories of the pain are not that exciting, sexually speaking. Maybe that is why it is done."

Still looking at it "Kyranin genitals don't change size that much, I remember you were hairy too. Is that with all human men? Or are only some hairy like yours was?"

Jay thinks about it for a few seconds, "I am not an expert, I suspect they all have some hair, at least the adults do, but I am not an expert in that information. Next time I go back you can come and do a survey if you like?"

Sihiryan looks up at his face "haha, Jay, hahaha, that is funny haha hmmm" Smiling at him taking a sip she takes an obvious peek back at his cock. "Have you ever had this fruit before?"

Jay looks at it, "no" he reaches and puts a piece on his pastry and bites it, "umm"

"Yeah" Sihiryan says. "It grows wild in the mountains and is ripe about this time of year. If we are lucky we can pick some." stuffing the last bite of her pastry into her mouth she slouches back into the chair to chew.

"When will we leave for camping?" Jay asks.

Sihiryan continues chewing and lifts her cup to sip the mrruk then smirks, "first there is another fruit to be tried, story has it that it produces a special sauce if prepared just right." Taking another drink to finish her mrruk.

"What is it called," Jay asks then takes another bite.

Sihiryan gets up and slides the coffee table to the side and kneels down in front of Jay and looks at his groin, "Let me check something Jay" Pushing his knees gently apart with her hands, "Lean back so that I can have some light, Room - more light here."

As Jay looks down and leans back Sihiryan takes his penis and moves it side to side with a gentle grip then rolles it up to look at the bottom "I'm not sure Jay"

With concern in his voice Jay asks, "About what, what is it?"

She sniffs it and gently slips her other hand under the scrotum placing her fingers tips near his anal opening and rolling a nut between her thumb and her palm. "The word to describe it eludes me Jay, I'm not sure what to call it"

Jay leaning forward looking to see if there is some rash or something as her hands stop moving and hold their grips and she lifts her face toward his, "can you see it Jay?"

As Jay looks and asks "see what" he watches her looking very closely at it.

Sihiryan increases her grip on his scrotum and pressure on his perineum as she pulls his cock to one side and lifts it to point toward Jay's face and holds it still for a second, putting her right cheek on his leg and looking up at him so that he can see the end and right side of it "this" and she slips it into her mouth. As she slowly slides her snugly gripping lips down the shaft and drags her tongue over the head as forcefully as she can, she reaches her finger closer to his anus and pulls that ball with her thumb.

Jay's mind is boggled, He thought she was seeing something of concern and then the sweet sensation surprise with the shooting pain from his one nut and the growing question in his mind about how far she will move that finger as he presses his back into the chair and spreads his legs looking up at the ceiling then closing his eyes from the bright lights. Her suction as she pulls all the way up it with her mouth gripping his neck with her lips and working the top of its' head with her tongue before sliding back down and trying to swallow it this time. Then the other hand, it's fingers and thumb gripping the other ball with purpose and pulling it out to the side, stretching the epididymis to give a pulling sensation inside of him. Her changing the angle of her head and action from her tongue focus his attention back on his cock as she slowly slides back again to tantalize his neck and head with her lips and tongue twisting this time one way then the other before sliding back down for the suction and throat pressure on his now throbbing cock. Her fingers forging with the full force of her arm toward his anus, and as the tips enter he clenches. Feeling her teeth on his cock bring a shift in his body tension and her fingers find some depth to explore, His clench almost pushing them out again and a push of his nut with her thumb to under him causing another shift in his position and more exploration toward his interior. A slam of her mouth over him with his cock reaching the back of her throat as she pinches the other ball forcing him to relax his ass and let her get a grip inside his cavity. Her squashing his nut with her palm producing a warm rush from in it spreading around inside of him and the shooting stinging pain of his ball in her fingers causing his feeling of surrender and relaxing of his sphincter while she torques his cock with her mouth and now has her fingers spreading pressure inside his anus, pulling it forward and stretching its opening. Tears spontaneously forming in Jays eyes as he feel his orgasm flaring from his navel down. Heat in his sacrum and butt cheeks trickling down his legs. His weight on his heels and shoulders as he arches to submit to her hands' maneuvers while the warm nut and screeching ball hold back the process to ejaculate. He hears himself moaning and his heart pounding and the pain of his ball in her fingers extend the other sensations of pleasure as he starts to enjoy the sensation her fingers are creating in his rectum. With the increased speed of her mouth plunging and sucking on him and the fullness of sensations growing in his cock from it he starts to feel good from the shooting pain in his ball as her fingers pinch it one after the another against her thumb, still stretching the cord that carries it's products to his shaft that is swelling with heat. Feeling a gurgling sound within his own moans Jay notices that his semen is starting to flow, he feels it in his brain as a clear strand of thought connecting to his now numb balls and the twinges of pain from the one is balanced by the hot smoothness of the pressure on the other. His anus is throbbing faster than his heart is pounding and he feels Sihiryan slow down, and locking her lips on his nob, holding it by his neck as her tongue slowly and gently swirls the head making his sensation of the energy orgasm mix with the intensity of the sensitive seconds on the heads surface while ejaculating and shortly after. Her fingers relaxing and the pressure on his balls increase pushing the last of the orgasmic force form them into his shaft, extending the situation. His anus still throbbing, and with each pulse absorbing the full sensation of his genitals and bouncing them back into his solid shaft.

Sihiryan feels the bursting against her tongue and the pulsing in his shaft and tight around her fingers. Liking the way Jay is with it all she works his balls to get more form him and slowly sucks it all in as she carefully drags the tip of her tongue around on his engorged head, pinching his ball and squashing his nut so that he won't move from her grip, his intensity builds to a raw sensation and she feels his legs and torso starting to fade in their rigidity as he gasps and looks down at her working on his orgasming cock.

Jay fearing the way his ass and balls feel, the raw feeling on the head of his cock has him unsure if he is pissing or if she has rubbed a hot pepper into his cocks head, He wants more as the glow fills him from his knees to his ribs, his spine feels hot and his sacrum rings of Joy. As he feels the pressure release form his balls his orgasm feeling lingers from his navel to his thighs. She pulls out her fingers, releases his balls, and goes one long slow slurping plunge down and sucking him hard all the way off. He still feels the throbbing of the orgasm in his ass. The after glow everywhere else in his body is thick and sweet his heart beating slow, big bursting thuds and he relaxes his legs and back more. The feeling inside behind his genitals is still intense, warm, tingly, full, and new to him. He takes a few breaths and watches her stand up smiling down at him and walks to the shower and washes herself. As she is finishing he walks to the shower and washes himself.

He thinks of something to say. "Did you figure out what to call it?"

Sihiryan looks at him with a surprised expression, laughs and replies, "only the sauce, MMMM"

Jay still feels the sensations inside of his anus after his shower. He notices that his balls are sore and his cock is aching. He feels alert and ready but tired and shaky. "Can we have some nutrients before we go to the forest"

From the kitchen she answers, "I'll make us something to get our energy back." opening the cupboard with medicines and herbs in it she picks through and builds two smoothies for them. She makes them up and pours each of them into two glasses and brings the darker one into the bed area. "Jay, come here and drink this. It is good if we have a nap after drinking this. I will turn on the rejuvenator and that will speed the effect of the mixture" she goes to a panel by her closet and slides her fingers around on the screen.

Jay takes his drink from the bed stand and drinks it. "The flavor is not that interesting"

She walks back toward him finishing hers. "It is not for the flavor, it is for you health and strength." Nods toward the bed, we will nap for an hour so that it can work then we can have the one for flavor and go to the forest." Flipping over the covers and climbing in she gets comfortable. "We can cuddle or lay apart, what do you like?"

Jay finishes the drink, puts the cup down and sits on the edge of the bed. He searches his feeling. After that experience he feels a little shocked and disturbed, he reflects, and feels that he liked it. He looks at her, "lets cuddle" and climbs into the bed with her and snuggles up to her back.

She wiggles a little then rolls over snuggling face to face with him. "I actually like you Jay". Then slowly kisses him on his lips. Smiles and closes her eyes.

Jay ponders her words for a few seconds. He starts thinking that she must mean more than just as a friend, then with reflection on all their interaction, or maybe not. Jay decides that how he feels is what he should think about and feels his eyes closing and sleep taking him.

Bleep, Bleep.

Jay looks around, sits up "Sihiryan, what was that noise"

She looks up at him, "the rejuvenator has a timer, let's get moving Jay. The glasses in the kitchen can you bring me one? The other is for you". Sitting up on the side of the bed she looks at the closet. Then walks to it and pulls our several garments and throws them on the bed. She looks at them as Jay returns with her drink and she reaches for it without looking at Him. Feeling it in her hand she takes it, and then a drink from it. "What do you think Jay, which one do you want to see me in for three days."

Jay looks at them then at her then at them again. He points at the middle one, I like that color it goes with your eyes best", then takes a drink from his glass. "What will I wear?"

Sihiryan looks at him, Jay that is easy, you only have one outfit so far, you will wear it." picking up the others and putting them back in the closet she says, "get dressed as soon as our glasses are empty we can leave."

Jay takes a sip and go to get dressed. With his close on he finishes the drink, puts the glass in the sink and goes to the door. Slips on his shoes and looks at Sihiryan putting on a different outfit. "That looks great", he says to her from across the apartment.

She turns and smiles then takes some foot ware from her closet, puts it on, downs her drink, leaves the glass on the coffee table and walks past Jay to the door. Stopping as the door opens and looking at Jay, "ready, got your tablet?" then stepping out into the hall and toward the elevator.

Jay follows, "are we in a hurry?"

Stopping at the elevator she turns to Jay, Looks at him for a moment. "No Jay" Then looks at his puzzled face. "How is it going to be with us for the three days Jay?"

Jay looks at her. "I'm sorry, I don't understand the subtleties of your culture, What ever it is I want to make it up to you" he

looks at her as the elevator opens and she breaks their gaze
to step in.

She hits the buttons and they start going down. About half
way down she elbows him in the ribs softly. "You should flirt
a little at least"

Jay looks at her, leans and sniffs her hair "mmm," but can't
think of what to say.

She steps back to face him straight on, "Jay, is that a flirt where
you come from?" slowly turning her head side to side as the
door opens, "I'll teach you, you will learn." As she gestures for
him to go out first with one hand she softly touches his ass
with the other.

As Jay steps out he turns his head with wide eyes looking at
her.

"Hahahaha, You didn't know," she says, "It will be good Jay,
you are a fast learner." Walking beside him through the
corridor and foyer to the street she says "Jay, Kyranins don't
let pleasantries or kind deed go un reciprocated, there is an
silent etiquette to return helpful actions, or gifts or kindnesses
as soon as the opportunity appears." Then after looking over
at him a few times. "Sex too."

Jay looks across at her as they start down the stars to the street. "Oh..." he realizes that he is expected to do something "My bad" looking around at the street "It won't happen again."

Sihiryan waves at a taxi and it starts to slow down and turns towards them.

Jay asks, "Can the taxis hover over the water?"

As the door opens she looks at Jay, "yes" and she gets in.

Jay asks the taxi as he gets in "Taxi could you set the security for viewing and listening to our interactions only my highest security level and higher for the duration of our time in you?"

The Taxi responds, "security set"

"To the lake by the park please" then looking at Sihiryan with hungry eyes, "Taxi hover over the lake to give us a good view of the waters edge on all sides" as the taxi starts to move Jay climbs across the taxi and first kisses her on her mouth, then stokes her breast with his hand then reaches inside her jacket and un buttons her pants.

"Jay" She says.

"Take them off " Jay says as he slides her to a position that allows him to be comfortable. He hears a giggle come from her as she slides down her pants then pulls one leg out of them. Jay gives her a serious look and slides his nose down into her folds, using his arms he separates her legs to give him self better access and starts to rub his face into her crotch. "Can you see the lake yet" then grips her labia with his lips to spread them. He strokes her ridge between them with his tongue slowly, firmly and comfortably. As he hears her sighs and breaths of approval to his actions he feels her juices starting to flow. The flavor indicates to Jay that it is time to allow his thumb to slide over her vagina's opening and soak up some sweetness. He feels her body tense and legs widen as it enters. His mouth still gently working around where her clitoris should be, a few strokes inside with his thumb and the fluids are dripping. Sliding his thumb out and into her anus Jay hears her soft squeak with his fingers spread on her sacrun and his thumb pressing and exploring the other side of it from her rectum wall. Jay slips the long fingers of his other hand into her sweet tangy vagina as his lips and tongue continue exploring the ripples and bumps between her folds. Stretching and rolling his fingers where a human woman's g-spot would be Jay is hoping to find her some joy. His tongue tastes a new flavor as she starts to quake and he hears a little moan and feels hands on his head pressing it harder into her. Starting to expand the motion of his thumb and the fingers of his other hand as he presses harder and slightly more vigorously with

his tongue. Feeling the grip and pull on his hair Jay
changes the position of his tongue and notices the spot she had
him looking for. Feeling a new texture on her inside with his
middle finger he spreads the others two and slowly grinds the
one into the spot. The clenching feeling on his thumb and
twisting stretching that starts in her pelvis widens the area that
his tongue is loving to lick. With a force from her hands
grinding his nose into her, he hears her grunting several times
as his face and hand become soaked. Keeping his tight grip on
her sacrum he removes himself from her genitals for a few
seconds and watches her face, Keeping the grip on her sacrum
he watches and as she starts to relax more and as she opens
her eyes Jay goes back in. First to the vagina, with the fingers
reaching another way this time, bumping and stroking the
cervix, as the vaginal cavity starts to widen his lips go back to
the clitoris with solid slow strokes and he turns his hand back
to the G-spot to slowly grind it again, feeling the hands on his
head.

"uuaannnm, wwwwoo uuuannmm wwwooooUnnnummmn"

Jay can feel a new level of saturation in his mouth, on his face
and in his hand as she quakes several times and stops with a
fuller relaxed breath pattern. Jay retreats again to wait for her
to recover and as she starts to open her eyes again Jay starts
sucking and licking her cunt hard and fast then working his
thumb further in and pulsing her sacrum while his fingers
start to alternate from her G-spot to her cervix and back. His
face grinding rhythmically over her clitoris and the rest of the
as her hands grip his hair and grind him into her self harder
and deeper, her legs shifting, gripping his back and her toes
grabbing for something. He feels that she is crunching without
taking a breath.

"ehuuhuua, ehuuhuua, ehuuhuua, ehuuhuua, uwwwaaa huoooha wwaoooo hhhhhhhhooouuu hhhh. Ohh, Jay"

As his wet face feels her relax and wiggle back onto the seat. He thinks for a second and starts licking and sucking at her crotch and thigh tops,

"No Jay stop" She says as she lay totally relaxed with her arms at her sides.

As Jay lifts his wet face to look at her he says, "I didn't want your pants to get soaked when you put them back on." looking out the window at the park around the lake "Taxi can you let us out near those four birds on the grass field over there between the tall trees and the edge of the lake." Then looks at Sihiryan, "I will wash my face in the lake before talking with the birds."

Sihiryan looks at Jay, "Birds?"

The taxi lands and the door opens. Jay steps out and looks around as Sihiryan steps out beside him. Jay holds her hand "They said they would take me to a good place for camping, if I was going to go."

"Who said" Sihiryan looks at Jay then at the birds.

Jay looks at her as they start walking across the beach toward the birds "do you remember when I was on the social media for taking a tour on the birds. Well, the next time I saw them I mentioned that I might be going camping in the forest and they said they could show me the good spots"

Sihiryan looks at the birds and stops walking and grips Jays' hand to stop him too. "Jay, lets go for a quick swim first, I don't want to smell like sex when we start talking to the birds."

Holding her hand and stepping back towards her "Ok, in the lake?"

She smiles at him and start walking towards the water. "Strangest thing Jay, I feel like I can taste sour on my skin"

Jay looks at her as they walk to the edge of the water. He watches her as she lets go of him and starts to undress. Looking up and down the beach Jay sees that no one is taking notice of her encroaching nudity and he starts undressing too; then follows her into the water. Remembering about the large shelled creatures in the lake Jay asks, "Is it actually a danger that the shell fish can be near to the shore?"

Sihiryan, up to her neck and scrubbing herself, looks at him with wide eyes, "only if we swim out a distance. They only come to shore in the cold seasons." looking at Jay slowly walking in deeper as the water reaches his navel. "Are you worried Jay, do you think I am so delicious that they will risk being eaten by a bird to just get a little taste of me?"

Jay smiles at her and makes his way to stand just next to her and whispers in her ear, "You do taste good"

"hahhaahh, Jay, you are such a sweetie." as she grabs his head and pulls him over and shoves him sideways to that he has to swim a few strokes to get his balance back. She watches him and when he is on his feet she goes back to scrubbing herself. "I was worried about you; that you would drown again, like you did in the sea, hahaha" and smiles looking into his eyes.

Smiling back and nodding, Jay gives himself a scrub in the water too and swishes out his mouth. "mmm, there is a · smooth flavor to the lake water, what is it?"

Sihiryan looks at the view of the tall buildings in the city across the lake. "It is the lake's flavor Jay, they are all a little different." and starts walking back towards their clothes. The city is so majestic from in the water here. It is so beautiful isn't it Jay."

Jay looks at it as he walks out of the water and stops with his thighs still submerged. Seeing the various colors on the buildings in the sunshine as it shimmers across the lake. He looks at the kyranins down the beach, and at the trees and back at the buildings again. "Yeah, the colors, I never actually appreciated them before, they are painted in such a way. Each one different, each one with a style of it's own. Humm, the hues of color are, they are, I have never seen some of those colors before."

Sihiryan looks at him then at the buildings "The amburst don't see the colors they say. They say they watch the sunrise like it is a viewing screen, and they say they talk about it like something is happening that is better than a sports event, but when I watch it, there is just the sun flashing a little as it comes over the horizon." Looking at Jay as he is still looking at the tall buildings across the lake. "Maybe our eyes are different, maybe they see things differently?"

Jay still looking at the buildings and remembering how they looked as an amburst. "I guess so" turning to look at her and thinking 'I wish I could tell her about my time as an amburst'. Looking at her naked on the beach doing some stretches in the sunshine Jay smiles and remembers his feelings for Trentia, from a few days earlier in his life and four years ago for her. Feeling the breeze evaporating the lake from his skin he decides to do a few stretches too as he dries before getting back into his clothes. After some various movements he starts doing a Tai chi form as he continues to watch Sihiryan doing what looks like yoga movements.

Sihiryan stops her stretching and starts putting her cloths back on. "Are you dry yet Jay? I bet it took a long time to dry when you had all that fur!"

"hahaha, ha ha, yeah" as he stops his movement and walks to his clothes. Shirt first then as he stands up with his pants he notices Sihiryan looking at his crotch. "Something of interest there?"

Sihiryan changes her gaze to his eyes, "I think part of it washed off Jay, it seemed like so much more earlier. I hope I didn't swallow any of it, are you OK?"

"hahaha, no, Yeah I'm Ok it shrinks from the cold, it will be big soon enough hahaha"

Sihiryan looks at Jay with a hesitant seriousness in her face, "is that true, it is not like that for us, I thought our adjustments covered all things."

Jay looks down at his stuff before doing up his pants, "well, that is still mine, it is still part of what I am, I guess that part won't change, I hope it won't anyway" and takes a closer look.

Sihiryan smiles and chuckles as she steps toward Jay and brushes her hand over his hinting that hers is available to be held again, "lets go see the birds" then as Jay takes her hand and they start walking, "I don't know if they will remember you Jay, it was a long time ago and things have progressed socially with the birds and us since then, they even come to our big sports events and talk about them in the bars with us once in a while.

Jay smiles at her and nods, he thinks how attractive she is with her hair wet from the lake. "Yeah, but they will still know the forest well and can get us there comfortably." Looking about forty feet ahead he sees that two of the birds each have an eye on him as they approach.

Sihiryan mentions, "we should ask to be near a place to bathe, with ample food, fruit, roots and berries, and water that we can drink nearby Jay"

Jay thinks about it and smiles at her, "have you talked to many birds?"

Sihiryan looks at him with a puzzled expression, "no".

The two birds turn to face them as they get about 10 feet away then the other two look them over pretty good too. They all give each other a glance and look back at Jay with one eye each and the other eye at Sihiryan. The lighter brown, one second from the right speaks first. "Hi, Good morning"

Jay stops walking and smiles looking into the birds' eye. "Yes it is, Good morning to you too. My name is Jay and this is my good friend Sihiryan. How are all of you doing this morning?"

The one on the right shifts her stance and looks them over a little better and the one on the left responds. "I am well thank you for asking, my name is Brackshess" and with a wing tapping and pointing at the others starting from the closest to her, "Chrenns, Jartsel, and Kretiksal"

Jartsel looks at Sihiryan "it is an honor to meet you Sihiryan"

Chrenns bends low to bring her head the same level as Sihiryans' "Sihiryan, that is a strong kyranin name, it is a pleasure to meet you. I don't think I've seen you here by the lake before."

Sihiryan feeling a little odd, "n-no, I seldom come here to the lake"

Kretiksal settles into the sand and adjusts her neck to be at the same level as their faces too. "That makes sense, I have seen you going in and out of one of the towers a few times, Jays' tower but never here at the beach."

Jay looks at the birds as the other three also settle into the sand "how do you know which building is mine?"

Brackshess replies, "Well Jay, after your tour everything changed for us, we all know where you live. And don't worry we won't drop you off on the roof and get you in trouble again."

The other three birds laugh as Sihiryan's jaw starts to drop a little and she turns to look at Jay. "You all know who he is?"

Jartsel looks at Jay and responds with one eye focused on Sihiryan's eyes. "If Jay says you are his good friend we will all soon know you as well."

Kretikal says "Don't take it the wrong way, he isn't a hero or anything. We just don't have much to talk about, your sports and stuff, you see, well they don't really interest most of us you see, so odd kyranins, like Jay, and the strange things they do, and their friends end up coming into our conversations."

Brackshess breaks the silence after a few seconds, "actually Jay, we were worried that none of us saw you for a very long time. And after the drowning at the beach and other stuff the speculations of your demise got your stories told a lot"

Jartsel asks, "Where have you been Jay"

Jay looks at Sihiryan then answers "I was off world for a long time, I was on a planet that is not affiliated with the alliance. It is good to be back. But I am only here for a few days."

Chernns looks at Sihiryan "so he came back to take you with him to some far away place, careful, he will load you down with eggs then take off all the time, males are all the same."

Kretiksal laughs, "I don't think she is so naive to let Jay catch her like that. No offence Jay but we saw you come out of that lake and your, uhum, masculinity, well it won't capture her heart either"

Sihiryan starts to laugh, "hahaho ho ho, now girls, lets not hurt his ego"

Brackshess looks at Jay, "so you are a male, that is what they said but after that swim I thought they were mistaken!"

The other birds laugh hard and Kretiksal steps over to rubs Jays' back with a wing, "don't worry Jay we can keep a secret. Just put out the lights before you undress and your future will be OK".

Jay starts to laugh too and smiles at Sihiryan then asks the birds, "well, the reason I came over wasn't to be insulted, but now that I am here I am enjoying it. Is it possible to give us a ride into the forest? We want to do a little camping. I heard that you would know the best spots. We are hoping for a place with ripe wild fruit and berries and leaves that we can eat and good drinking water and a place to swim that is safe for us." Jay looks at them looking back at him. "By the way have you seen my old friend Quarraktutu?" then looking to Sihiryan, "it was just the cold water that made it shrink, really". Then at the birds, "your angle of view made it look smaller than it was".

The birds start laughing again and stand up nodding at each other. Chrenns says, "Ok you two climb on me and we will find you a good spot."

Jartsel says, "I will go tell Quarraktutu you are here for a few days" takes several steps away and takes off.

Sihiryan asks, "Both of us on your back, is that comfortable for you?"

Chrenns nods, "Yeah I'm training for the race so it will be good for me"

"What race" Jay asks.

Brackshess looks at the others then one eye at Jay and one at Sihiryan. "We don't like others to know about our culture so please don't mention it to the social media story collectors. When we come of age one of the rights of passage we can choose is to race with our peers around the planet twice. It is a big event for us all. But it is a cultural secret and we should not have mentioned it to you."

Chrenns looks at them then at Brackshess, "sorry mom." Then she squats back down, Get on you two I will show you two spots over the mountain in the valley that are both just what you ask for."

Jay gestures for Sihiryan to climb up first and sees that she is not sure how to do it. Bending down "step up on my knee and grab her neck feathers and pull yourself up".

Sihiryan sees Chrenns nod and squat a little lower for her. She does as suggested and swings her leg over and balances on her back and neck then feels Jay pull himself up behind her and slide up to her back. She feels a little surprised as Chrenns stands and jumps and starts flapping all in one motion. Seeing Kretiksal on one side flapping and Brackshess on the other looking back at her.

Kretiksal winks at Jay "I think I know the spots she is thinking of, they are secluded and seldom visited at all. You should have a good peaceful time there."

Sihiryan turns her head a little to one side, "Jay this is amazing. I can't believe how fast we are climbing."

Jay holding her with one arm and some neck feathers with his other hand, "it is, and the views are fabulous."

As they start to cross the forest beside the city Chrenns starts to turn a little to the south, then higher. After many hard flaps Kretiksal and Brakshess are falling behind as they continue to climb. Jay looks back and sees the city behind them and the sea shimmering behind it. He looks out to his left and looks at the patches of cultivated lands inter laced with forests, mountains and lakes. Looking to the left he sees a large lake and wonders if it is the lake that he spent some time over with the kyranin couple. He looks ahead and sees an area of sharp mountains and steep hills. Bringing his mouth to Sihiryan's ear, "I think we are going in there"

Chrenns answers ,"yes the two best spots for you to see the forest and have some quiet from the city are in there"

Sihiryan turns her head to smile at Jay then looks forward again. "I was going to get the taxi to take us into the hills near the city Jay. Asking for this gift of seeing the real forest is much more than I would have considered, Thank you Jay" Then talking louder, "Thank you Chrenns for taking us into the deep forest it is an honor to be shown such places."

Jay thinks about what she said and asks, "don't kyranins often go into the deep forest?"

Shaking her head. "No Jay, the farm workers seldom go far from their farms into the wild and only some of the city dwellers ever go into the forest parks near the cities." turning to look into his eye. With a smile she says, "Jay this is an adventure for me, not a usual camping trip."

Jay thinks about it. "Yeah, where I am from only a few of us actually go into the wild places. It will be interesting." then thinking for a moment. "Will there be any dangerous creatures?"

Chrenns turns her head to look at Jay with one eye for a second as she starts to go into a slow dive. "No. You are Kyranin, nothing on this planets surface will harm you." Then shifts her wings to turn and steepen the dive slightly. "Do you see the tiny lake between the trees, with the meadow to the left and the waterfalls further up the valley, the tall grass, between the Bruktdu trees, that is where I will show you first, then if you want we can look at the second spot past that crystal peak" as she nods her head to the tallest peak on the right side of the valley. Changing the angle of decent again as they gain speed into the area. Leveling off her decent at about 200 meters above the ground and gliding over the valley's gentle slope from the tall peaks, "see the variation in the trees, the darker ones are nearest the streams, the smaller stream is better for drinking and the other has pools for swimming and bathing in. Look over here," as she turns toward the edge of the valley, closer to the peaks. "See that fog under those Bladcol trees?, there is a hot pond there, fed by a spring up the slope a short way. The source pond is hot enough to cook the fish in. But the lower ponds, the ones near the valley meadows are good for bathing in the winter." Then turning further up the valley souring about 10 meters above the trees' tops. "This area has tree fruits but they are high in the trees," turning back down the valley with a few flaps of her wings, "the other side has several berry and fruit trees and they are easy to get to. The animals that live here only eat about half of the fruit so they won't mind how much you eat. The berries get ripe in the lower valley first and as the season changes they can be picked up to the peaks. Now is about the right season for the meadow areas over here" nodding to the place she earlier indicated. "Do you want to go down, is this good?"

Sihiryan says "I like it here"

Jay adds, "This looks perfect" then watching as they slow down and start a fast decent. Jay tightening his grip on Sihiryan and Chrenn's feathers sees how close her wings come to the branches as she flap slowing their decent to a hover before she extends her feet to the ground.

Chrenns takes several steps turning and looking around before she crouches to let them off.

Jay swings his left leg over her back and slides down to land with both feet and looks up as Sihiryan makes a similar dismount. "Thank you Chrenns" looking around in the forest. "In a few days when we want to go back to the city how can we contact you or another for a ride?"

Chrenns looks at Jay then up, "oh, my mother and Kretiksal are here" as she nods to them and they dive down at them.

Sihiryan steps tightly to Jay as she watches them coming almost directly for them. Feeling Jay's arms around her as she sees them swoop past, turn and land about ten feet on either side of them.

Chrenns says to her mother, "Mom, they are asking about a ride back, how can they find a bird to take them back when they are tired of the forest?"

Brackshess looks at Jay and Sihiryan, then at Kretiksal, then at Chrenns. Then taking a step forward and looking all around at the forest looks at Kretiksal again "well"

Kretiksal looks at Brackshess and at Jay then at Brackshess again, "well what do you look at me for?"

Chrenns looks at her, "You are the oldest and wisest of us three, you should have an answer"

Kretiksal stares at Chrenns for some seconds then looks around at the forest. "Well, she looks at Jay, and takes another step as she looks at the forest again. Then she looks at Sihiryan and swallows looking back at Chrenns. "I don't have a tablet so they can't call me."

Brackshess laughs, "it isn't a problem. They can just walk back."

Jay starts laughing. "We thank you so much for the ride. If you are in the area in two or three days would you please check on us?" feeling some tension in Sihiryan's shoulders, "and if it is convenient for you or any of your friends could you come and take us back to the city in two or three days?"

The three birds smile at Jay. Kretiksal nods "So you are starting to know our humor Jay"

Sihiryan states, "Better than me, I was getting worried"

The three birds start laughing and nodding at each other. Brackshess looks her in the eye. "We live over the mountains in the next valley. You will see some of our friends flying over regularly and if you yell loudly we could hear you. When you wave for a ride you will be taken wherever you want to go Sihiryan. I will come and check that you are warm enough at night and if not I will show you some caves up the hill that have hot pools inside."

Sihiryan looks at her "thank you Kretiksal"

Chrenns says, "There are green snakes that are friendly, they don't bite but you can't eat them they will make you sick for days if you do. "If you have any questions before we leave? It was joy giving you both a ride, it is the first time I have given a ride to anyone."

Jay smiles, "thank you, it was fabulous"

Sihiryan says, "I never would have know, it seemed like you were very comfortable with it"

Chrenns chuckles, "Well, it was you who took the risk, I have wings so I am safe at any height".

The other birds laugh and Jay starts laughing too. Sihiryan looks at them and smiles. The birds nod as they choose a direction to take off between the trees. Then all at once they jump and start flapping, with a flurry of swirling winds raising leaves and blowing Sihiryan's hair the three of them disappear between the treetops. Jay and Sihiryan turn to each other and open their squinting eyes and smile.

Camping

Sihiryan takes a step toward Jay still smiling she says, "That was more than I thought it would be."

Nodding, Jay smiles and looks around at the forest then at her as she steps closer to him, "now what do we do?"

Sihiryan takes another step putting her self about 40 cm in front of Jay. "Well, usually when we are camping we go naked. The first thing I want to do is find those caves with the hot springs in them. What do you want to do Jay?"

Jay looks at her starting to undo her clothes and asks, "What about insects? Are there small insects that will bite us here in this forest?"

Sihiryan looks at Jay with a confused expression as she takes off her top.

Jay starts undoing his shirt "where I am from the insects bite in the forest and it makes our skin itchy."

"Oh" Sihiryan smiles as she takes off the rest of her clothes. "I thought you were making an excuse, no there are no such insects here. Some bite but it is not noticeable. Here it is the snakes that can be trouble. They like the heat but their skin can cause a rash, only the yellow ones" bending over to put her foot-ware back on. Then turning to look into Jay's eyes. "If you see or smell a yellow snake don't let it touch you".

Jay takes off his pants and rolls them up. "Smell them?"

Sihiryan, "Yes smell, it is a foul aroma like the material of new shoes!"

Jay is bent over putting his shoes back on, "oh," as he stands back up, do they bite?"

Sihiryan smiles, "no they are friendly". Looking Jay up and down as she pulls out a strap from a corner of her tablet and hooks the end on another corner of it and slips it over herself to hang across her side, "Maybe they see you as I do, they just want to use you to keep warm at night"

Jay laughs and smiles at her. "So should we start up the slope to find the caves?" As he looks at her tablet and finds that his also has a tab with a thin line that extends when the tab is pulled. He makes a strap by attaching it as she did then puts it over his head to let it dangle on his side like her.

"No Jay, I want to do that, but lets find drinking water first, and then some food sources."

Jay looks surprised by her statement. "Good idea" and he looks around at the forest then back at her, "I think the stream is that way", pointing down the slope of the valley. "It was hard to keep track when She was showing us the area."

Sihiryan looks around and nods, "I agree. We can leave our clothes here, ,,, or lets put them on the branch of that tree", as she points to a tall one with light green leaves. There are only a few like that in each valley so it will be easy to find later." Starting toward the tree, "we will keep out tablets with us."

Jay asks "for safety?"

"No for work Jay, I have to bring you up to date on the past four years remember?" smiling at him and slowly turning her head back and forth, "is it true Jay. That joke about your species, when the blood goes down to the little head there is not enough to supply the big head's brain?"

Jay looks at her as he realizes that he is at half-mast. He smiles, "Good joke" takes another step toward the tree. "I had forgotten about that, I was excited about camping and still a little surprised about last night and this morning." Then seeing her turn to look at his junk, "well maybe some truth in it".

Smiling at him as she stops by the tree, "Actually Jay I have always thought of you as attractive but never would have considered anything because we work together. Last night surprised me too, and I don't remember. But this morning changes things for me between us. I like how we were together and am open to more, after we find water and food though. Kyranins always take priorities seriously."

Jay looks at her expression and realizes that she is actually slipping an important cultural lesson into their relating. "Priorities first aye, good with me" takes the clothes from her hand and with his he stretches up on his tiptoes to slide them onto a fork in the branch of the tree. "Is that good?"

Looking up she smiles "should be". She looks all around at what she can see of the valley from there. Then works the screen of her tablet for several seconds. "OK Jay, you were right the stream is that way. You want to lead?"

He looks at her screen as she turns it for him then points at where they are and then to the creek. He looks at her and smiles, "sure. Follow me." Starting through the tall grass and between the bushes across the meadow toward the thicker forest ahead. Jay feels the tall grass stroking his legs as he walks through it. Feeling it without the buffer of his leg hair seems odd to him. The taller blades and stalks are at his chest level so he notices the tickle of it brushing under him as well. The leaves and branches of the bushes and shrubs feel gentle on his skin and cool. He sees an odd-looking fury creature with six legs about 8 meters to his left and stops walking. It looks to be bigger than a big dog. "What is that?" he asks as he points to it. Sihiryan walks up beside him stepping almost through him, grabbing his arm and putting her other one around his back and her hand grasping his ribs in the front.

She looks at it in silence for a few seconds then whispers to him "it is a jywodip, they eat small animals and snakes and berries. They live high up in the big trees. They taste good but can't be farmed and there is only a short season to hunt them. They don't see well Jay. If it smells us it will run. If we try to catch one, it will tear us up with it's claws and try to bite our necks off. A loud nose will send it up the closest tree so it is best to not be near a tree when we make the loud noise."

"Are we going to make a loud noise?" Jay asks

Sihiryan, looking around "over here Jay," as she guides him between two large trees then seven long steps past them. "It will go up one of the trees and here we can see them all." turning him so that they get a view of all the large trees near the jywodip. "Ready, yell on the 4. 1,, 2,, 3,, FOUR HWHWH"

"HAY RAAHH" Jay yells as he sees the thing jump and turn and dart one way then the other then up a tree like if it was pulled up by a giant elastic band. "fua, that is fast!"

"hahahaha, ya Jay haha, they are fast haha, I hope we see it again tomorrow"

Jay looks at her "is it that funny?" then looking up the tree as she is still laughing, "where did it go?"

Sihiryan looks up at the trees, "we won't see it again today, they travel from tree to tree in the canopy. It won't stop running for a few minutes." They are non-communicative beings verbally and our biologists have studied them in depth. Their threshold for hearing is high, so if they hear something it is a shock to them, they react with fear and escape, it is fun to watch but it is safe for them. They don't mind. If you get a young one you can make friends with them like a pet but because they can't hear they don't make a good pet."

Jay smiles at her still holding him and in the silence hears the gurgling of the stream not far away, "can you hear the stream over there?"

Nodding she start to walk toward it "lets go" taking the
lead she glides with long swift strides between the shrubs and
bushes, gracefully bouncing over large rocks and logs. Jay
follows surprised at how agile she is. He can see the creek and
she stops at its' edge. Takes off her shoes and walks in, gets
down on all four and brings her face close to the water to smell
it. Then straightens up with her knees still in the creek and
looks at Jay, "Smell it Jay"

Jay looks at her naked kneeling in the creek and takes his
shoes off. Not wanting to seem judgmental he follows and gets
down on all four in the water beside her. Then brings his nose
to the surface to take a whiff of the water. To his amazement
he smells a sweet earthy cool tone of aroma and notices how it
soothes him. Looking into the water from inches away he
exhales and takes another whiff, slower this time. "My god, it
has an effect on all of me"

Sihiryan has again brought her face to the water with her
hands on the bottom of the creek and puts her face into it for a
few seconds. Pulling out and turning to Jay "take a drink Jay.
Taste it"

Jay feeling the coolness of the water on his hands, wrists and
legs sticks his mouth into it and sucks some up into his mouth
and swallows it. Then sits back onto his heals in the creek.
"Yeah, the flavor, I can't explain it. It is something almost
surreal to me." leaning forward again and sinking his face into
it to suck some more up he leans fare enough so that his eyes
are submerged. Jay looks into the water with his eyes open

and sees the glistening of the stones and pebbles on the bottom. Lifting his head to look at Sihiryan "the colors under there are different too."

"Yeah" Sihiryan agrees, "The mountain water has an energy in it that effects the spectrum of light that we see and changes how we perceive it." Sitting back on her heals and looking at him. "Our science has studied the effect to understand it. There is no useful purpose that is derived from the effect but it has taught us that the energy that is in mountain water is real, that the effect of the energy on the water is real and that we all have the ability to enjoy it. From the work done to understand the energy and its' effect we expanded our science of energy, specifically subtle energies, that we previously ignored. Our science experimented for hundreds of years with subtle energies and now we use it for space travel and communications and healing therapy. It has helped us to develop inter species communications and exploration of our own planet and others. All of this because some of our ancestors opened their eyes under the mountain stream water like you just did."

Jay looking at her sitting in the water, "the water is cool but I don't feel like I am getting cold."

Giving Jay an odd look then bending down for another drink. This time putting her head right in it and splashing the water up on herself soaking her back and belly then standing up and flipping her hair out of her face. "Common Jay lets go get some food."

Jay takes a drink, then lays down in the water and waves it over his chest and belly before getting up to follow. She put her shoes on wet so Jay does the same. He picks up his tablet and follows as he slides its' strap over his head again. "How do you know where to find food?"

About 3 meters ahead of him walking toward the sunbeams between the trees, "In the meadow Jay. That is where the best berries are."

Jay watches her moving and how her muscles flex as she makes her way swiftly up the slope over logs and rocks and around the shrubs and trees. He thinks of Reggie on earth, such a different culture for Reggie to be in. What an adventure he must be having. What hardship he must be enduring. Then focusing on getting over a steep section and past a bush with thorny leaves. Jay thinks he sees some light in the forest to his left, stops and turns his head. He looks between the trees and up them too. Then at the shadows and the shrubs, then starts walking again and in the corner of his eye he sees a twinge of blue moving light again. Looking sideways a few times as he continues to follow Sihiryan he can't seem to see what the light was. He can see Sihiryan about 12 meters ahead stopping in the sunshine at a bush and looks to the side again between the trees and sees the dim blue light beside a tree, then it is gone. It looked to be about 2 meters high and narrow beside the tree. Stopping to take a good look he sees nothing except the forest and all the life in it. The large flying insects, some little fury things up in the trees and some other types of fury things under a few of the bushes, a brown snake, and a long lizard like thing on the side of a tree, about 40cm long.

"Jay" Sihiryan waves, "this way, they are ready."

Jay walks to her and starts picking and eating the berries with her. "They are good"

Sihiryan looks at Jay, "these are similar to the ones that they make snnnt sauce from. That bush has longer flowers and is only on the tallest mountains. You like the snnnt sauce; the berry is slightly different too but the bush is almost the same other than that."

"I don't see any flowers here", Jay says and pops more berries into his mouth.

Sihiryan smiles. "In the winter the flowers come out. These ones are only out for a few weeks and are good to eat. The snnnt ones are out for a long time. They are good to eat but taste bitter and are four times as long as these ones. The ones on these bushes have no flavor and make the digestion fail for a few days."

Jay picks and pops a few more berries into his mouth and smiles. "What do these berries do, are they nutritious or do they have an effect I should know about?"

Smiling back at him, "they are called sivent berries, they are good in cooked pastries and are nutritious. They do make the heart beat a little harder and constrict the veins ever so slightly." nodding her head for him to follow, "these other ones are good too. They are bigger and with a stronger flavor."

Jay traces her steps to not step on the small bush patches on the ground as he looks to the almost blue shrubs a few meters away. "What are they?" Jay looks at the tubular protrusions from the stem of the bush. There is a frilly leaf where they start and they protrude about 9 cm off the trunk, and off of the thicker stems of the bush. He watches her face as she slowly smiles and chews the protrusion that she had picked with her eyes close. Jay decides to try one even though he didn't get an answer yet. Pulling one off a branch he takes a bite of it and feels the juices of it spreading over his lips and tongue, then his gums and throat. His eyes close and his mind goes to the sensation of sparkling warm gummy slightly sour and sweet sensation as it sooths it's way into the flesh of his mouth and face. "Is this safe Sihiryan?"

As she takes another piece and stuffs it into her mouth, "sort of Jay"

Jay takes the rest of his first one and looks at her slowly chewing her second "sort of, what do you mean sort of?"

"mmmm," she turns to him and forces her eyes open, "it is such a delight to the palette that it is hard to stop eating them."

Jay looks at her as her hand picks another without her eyes breaking contact with his. "What does it do to our bodies?"

Putting her third one in her mouth and closing her eyes again to chew it before answering. "Well" slowly chewing some more, "you may notice that there are only about 20 of these on this bush" Then stopping to enjoy the sensation again. "If I eat them all I will get a mild euphoria and not be able to sleep for a full day." Then swallowing it and all the juice from her mouth, "a few won't do much"

Jay picks another and pops it in his mouth, he feels it spreading and filling his face with joy, the soft sensations and warmth and the urge to keep his eyes closed cause him to savor the situation and the texture and the aroma until he has chewed it to juice and pulp and swallowed it all down. "But is it nutritious?"

Sihiryan smiles at Jay, "slightly, it has vitamins to help your night vision". Looking at the trees then back at Jay, see the tree with the many fingered leaves, the fruit from those is very nutritious." turning toward the tree, "lets get some of those"

Jay picks another and takes a tiny bite of it as he starts walking behind her. He looks at the trees and sees what she means by multi fingered leaved, like a maple leaf, or cannabis leaf. It is the only one like it he can see. As they approach he sees that it is filled with brown flowers and green fruit. When they get closer he sees that it has two fury creatures that like the one they scared with the sound earlier. He sees her walking toward the part of the tree that the furry thing is in. "Sihiryan, stop."

Stopping in her tracks she stays perfectly still and slowly reaches for her tablet.

Jay continues, "There is a jywodip up in that tree, actually two of them."

Sihiryan with her tablet in her hand looks up into the tree and sees them, she nods and checks her tablet and steps back four steps then yells as loudly as possible and records the two jywodips bolting back and forth before climbing up out of sight in the tall tree.

Jay walks up beside her and looks at the tablet. She plays it for him and then again in slow motion.

"Jay, can you see how fast they move and how they grip the branches with their claws and palms?" Then changing the screen to show a close up moving image of one of it's hands grabbing and branch and letting go after it's body shifted. "They are so fast and so graceful."

"Yeah" Jay nods, "and you say they are delicious too."

"huhaha, Jay you like to make things funny" giving him a sincere look, "You know that these creatures live in tribes in the canopy and each tribe has it's own language. There is a basic greeting that all tribes share but most of them know the languages of all the other tribes within three days travel for them. They have cultural events where they meet in very large groups three times a year according to the alignment of the moon and sun. They play musical instruments, both string and wind, and they have been doing the same ritual dances for as long as they have been recorded. There has never been an incidence of war between two tribes and they mourn their dead. Six legs doesn't make them a lesser species than us."

Jay looks at her contemplating her words. He starts to blush and looks at the screen then up at the canopy. "On my world we don't give much respect to any other species. The whales are known to have several languages, one for each pod and most know up to seven of them. But we still hunt them with technology that they have no chance to escape from." Then looking into her eyes, "the whales have bigger brains than we do and may be smarter too."

"Do they taste so good that it is worth killing them?" she asks.

Jay looks at her, "I don't know, only a few people eat them, mostly they are used for their oil. I don't know what it is used for."

Sihiryan smiles at Jay, "the jywodip do taste delicious. The only time they can be hunted is if they are too many for the food in their area and then the hunting must be done with primitive weapons. It is over seen by ships in orbit to prevent suffering from a bad kill. If their is a serious wound that will cause a slow death the officers in the ship will deliver a beam to end the jywodip's life without pain. The beam leaves the tissue unaffected so the jywodip is still good to eat." looking at him, "we too are a predator species and will eat other sentient beings, not too different from yours Jay, but our respect for life is more developed."

Jay smiles and takes a deep breath. "I hope my species isn't found by anything that thinks we taste good." he looks around in the forest and across the meadow beside them. How well will my skin do in the rays of the sun all day?"

Sihiryan looks at him, "I can't imagine any problems, why?"

Jay looks up at the clear sky "On my world too much exposure to the sun will cause a burn to the exposed surface of the skin."

Sihiryan takes his hand and starts walking to the meadow, "not here Jay, lets take a nap in the sun, it is good for your blood, it causes a detox of the organisms that grow in damp dark places."

Jay follows. After a short distance she lets go of his hand walks in a circle looking at the ground and lays down in the grass, face up, eyes closed. Jay looks at her laying down in the grass and weeds and does the same a few feet beside her. The grass and weeds beneath him feel odd at first then as he settles into a comfortable position the warmth of the sum fills his attention. Taking slow deep breaths he feels his body relax and starts to enjoy the mix of aromas filling his nose. The dirt offers his olfactory and totally new scent. Like ground granite and charcoal with a mild accent of the mix of sulfur and compost. The sent of the grass, freshly broken beneath them sweetening the air and the wafts from the flowers and trees as the breeze graciously swirls through the valley. As he is feeling his muscles releasing and his body settling against the ground Jay exhales, "this is nice".

Sihiryan starts "So Jay, a lot has changed since you left. There was a long time, two years, when the Amburst restricted access to the sea for off world speices. Our own security forces triple checked all travel and visitors form other alliance worlds and special permission was needed to arrive on Ramga from non-alliance planets. Every living being on Ramga was scanned by the Ryberian special security agency and all records of communications were also searched for hidden data streams. It resulted in a totally new level of scrutiny from all security workers. There is new satellites monitoring the arrivals and departures of vessels form all alliance planets. There are scans done from satellites of all comings and goings between cities as well as scans done of any suspicious activities or behave patterns concerning technology. What this means Jay is that you have to know what to stay away from to avoid getting scanned too many times. Jay if you get scanned six times for being in suspicious situations the protocol is to have a constant scan on you for the next months until it is determined why you were flagged as being suspicious. Those who have chosen this investigating work are a little excited to do it, they enjoy looking at details and trying to find something that may lead to something that could be something that needs to be investigated further. They are actually perfect for the job but it will make it terrible if you are investigated."

Jay listens to the quiet of the forest as he thinks about what she said. He takes a breath, "so, I need to avoid being suspicious?"

Sihiryan reaches over and holds his hand, "yes".

Jay, feeling her gentle grasp responds with a shift of his hand to hold hers. Being so relaxed he feels the tone of her hand in a new way, he feels her from an emotional perspective. He feels her worry for his safety and her kindness motivating her to want to keep him safe, her courage to be with him and her joy to be close with him. Then he feels it arouse a warmth sensation growing in his heart. He focuses on her hand and it's grip on his again. He notices that he likes the physical contact with her. Realizing his distraction from their conversation he goes back to it, "what should I do".

"It is easy Jay" she turns her head toward him, looking through the grass and weeds to see his face, "always be aware of technology installations and don't go near them. Don't travel without communicating allot about where and why you are going, and act like you belong to Ramga, act like a Kyranin." gently tugging his hand "if you were a kyranin right now, what would you do?"

Jay is laying flat on the ground and looking at her as he thinks about it for a few seconds. His limited knowledge of Kyranins behaviour only takes a few seconds to review. Rolling onto his side, towards her he smiles and shifts his body across the ground closer to hers. He reaches with his free hand and strokes his fingers down her side, across her thigh and across to the far knee. Looking down at her smile he shifts again and kisses her face. Seeing her smile growing and her body relaxing he kisses her again, softly on her cheekbone. Then again on her eye brow, this time ending it with a slight grip from his lips tugging softly on her eyebrow.

"That feels interesting" she says as she brings her hand up to stroke his chest. Gliding her fingers up to his throat then down toward his heart before sliding under his arm to his scapula. Looking up into his eyes as she smiles and tugs him toward her, "the jywodip do it clinging to each other while hanging in the trees Jay" and she pulls herself up against him. She feels Jay arcing his back slightly and tensing his arms to take her weight. Gripping his shoulder on the other side with her other arm she lifts her torso off the ground pulling her face toward his. "You are strong Jay"

Jay smiles and feels her lips reach his. Enjoying her kiss he starts to feel her slowly sliding her left leg up his thigh, her knee reaching his lower ribs, her calf sliding over his hip, and then her heel roaming on his sacrum. The pressure on his sacrum brings a strange feeling through to the front of him and his genitals accept the excitement. Filling them with his attention Jay notices a feeling of swelling.

Sihiryan shifts her lips to Jay's neck, sliding her tongue to his earlobe and whispering something in kyranin that the translator fails to respond to. Jay feels her teeth gripping his ear and tugging slightly as her other leg slips up his; her heel finds the small of his back. He stretches his neck to get his lips onto her trapezius and feels her belly and breasts gently pressing up against him. With one heel on his sacrum and the other exploring the small of his back while she continues to whisper and lick and nibble at his ear; Jay starts shifting his arms and body to take her weight. He feels her grip on his shoulders and back increase and her genitals touching the bottom of his. He feels her body shifting against his as her teeth on his ear pull his attention to what she is whispering.

"swereera sheeeaarooon chhoooww" She glides her moistening genitals against the end of his hardening cock, "awuoooooo shshshiyasises" gripping him to slide her opening onto his head, sliding it up and down to get it ready.

"mmm, I don't think My translator is working, but I like what you are saying" he says as he shifts his body and arches his back slightly to carry her weight better. Feeling the sensation of her hanging from him and pressing up against him is getting his heart pounding. Enjoying her whispers and nibbling while he adjusts his pelvis to find some comfort in the area where her heels are digging into his bottom back. The warmth on his cock as she slides herself against it brings a yearning within his guts.

Sihiryan lowers her top, gently sliding her nipples across his chest as she shifts to bring her head to his other ear. "It is an old dialect that is not shared with other species Jay". Pressing her wet cunt onto his almost stiff penis. With a second push and shift of her pelvis then a third and it slips in, a gyro and thrust and it is all in. "I've got you Jay!" as she lowers her upper body and shifts her head to look him in the eyes. Slowly shifting her pelvis as she smiles at him.

Jay smiles back, he starts to move his pelvis and he feels her finger nails digging into his back. He looks into her eyes as she continues to smile and gives him a wink.

"Stay still Jay, be in a comfortable position and hold it, I want to have it my way. Enjoy the forest and the view and relax as much as you can."

Jay feels his heart pounding as he is on all four with her clinging to him. He starts taking full deep breaths and tries to relax as he notices her slow constant shifting and slight sliding on his cock. Feeling that he is only mostly hard he tries to relax more of the muscles that he doesn't need to keep his position. Her breasts' hard nipples gently stroking his smooth chest as she slowly contorts her body beneath him. Feeling the grip of her heels and hands shifting as she works herself against him Jay strains his focus to do as she asked. Continuing to stay relaxed he looks up at the forest and feels her mouth contacting his neck. Listening to the sounds of the leaves in the breeze he hears her breath from her nostrils as it warms his neck. Looking at the tall grass around them Jay's mind splits; filled with the panoramic beauty of the meadow, and noticing how the moisture on his cock with warm slow twists and squeezes feels. His efforts to not react to the tantalizing stimulation on his neck slowly fail as his mind fills with lust and desire. As he starts to bring his focus to complimenting her movements with his she digs in her nails.

"No Jay," kissing his lips so tenderly, "enjoy the forest and let me have my way".

Jay stops moving as he looks into her eyes. Seeing the softness of pleasure in them he swallows his passion and settles into a comfortable arch, shifting his arms to relieve the beginnings of fatigue. Thinking to himself 'I like this' as he takes a slow deep breath through his nose and looks across the meadow through the grass. She slowly working his neck with her lips and tongue and grinding to fill herself with his large loaf. Jay again is distracted from his views of the valley as the sensations in his half hard cock slowly increase. Looking at the mountains to his left Jay starts thinking about his interactions with Sihiryan for the past several months at his training and work on Ramga. Remembering her calm excitement to see him understand a new thing and eagerness to have him start a new training, or to practice what he had learned. Feeling her clinging to him as she pleasures them he feels the emotions starting to swell up in his heart for her, as a friend and teacher and work mate. He feels his attraction to how he trusts her and respects her. He feels his guts lusting for her, and he feels the warm glow of compassion and community for her filling his chest. He feels the strain in his arms. Shifting them again as she starts sucking harder on his neck and grinding over his full almost flaccid phallic. The feeling of warmth in his pelvic partly disguised from his muscular tension to keep his back arched. Jay notices that his body is having an urge to start crunching his pelvic to thrust into her. He feels the shifting in his testicles that happens when his semen starts to flow. Taking a deep breath Jay forces his mind to relax as much of his body as he can. Focusing on relaxing and adjusting his arms as the swelling of heat starts to spread in his pelvis.

Sihiryan wrapping her neck on the right side of his and pulling harder with her heels "Jay, do you want me Jay. Do you lust me Jay, will you give yourself over to me if I asked?"

Jay asks himself 'what does she mean?' and says, "I do, I will".

"Relax more Jay, "oooh", biting his clavicle and grinding harder.

Jay feels his arousal spreading the feelings migrate from his pelvis through his torso and up his spine to his head. Trying to focus more on relaxing, his mind going to his cock and feeling it still only half hard but tingling with a vibrant warmth; he forces a calm into it. Focusing on his breathing, slower and deeper, then his feet and ankles and calves. Relaxing them as best he can, working to ignore the ripping rolls of heat floating around in his thighs. Feeling her squashing her breasts into him as she grinds even harder starts a pressure in his heart that he feels flowing down his arteries to all of him. The sensation of heat from her stroking onto his cock spreads into his pelvic bone and balls. He hears her soft grunts and she sucks and slobbers on his throat all as he steadies his breaths and body and feels how he does feel about her.

Sihiryan almost orgasming tasting Jays sweat and gripping his straining muscles and bones. She smells his perspiration and the ground and flowers of the meadow. She feels him inside of her, soft and full going where she wants and filling her the way she likes. Feeling the rumbling in her vagina and the heat from her kidneys flowing through it as the glow of her clitoris enjoys the pressure of her grinding his belly and pubic bone. The warm tingle of her breasts squashing as she likes on his chest and the pounding of her heart form the exertion of pulling her body up against his. The adrenalin giving her increased awareness of the sensations and expanded alertness of her surroundings as her waves of delight start to build. Digging her fingers into his scapula and "eeuuoh, uuuoohaa,"as she starts panting as the swelling heat tingles out from her groin and belly engulfing her with a blurring sensation of burning bliss that sweeps slowly through her torso and head then seeps into the straining muscles of her arms and legs until she feels it in her fingers and heels. Then opening her eyes and looking at Jay looking back at her, She let her limbs relax and lowers herself to the ground beneath him. "Jay"

Jay looking down at her and feeling the sensations where her hands and feet were, "yes?"

Smiling at him she says nothing. Slowly letting her legs straighten and her arms find comfort stretching out to the sides. She looks at his face and eyes and the sweat dripping from him; still firm. She smells the secretions form her on them and the sweet sap of the trees in the breeze. Still experiencing the sparkling soft throbs of her climax she takes a deep slow breath, "Jay" and looks at him again as she thinks about what she did and how she feels.

Looking down at her and wondering if he should get up or lower himself on top of her "yes Sihiryan, how are you doing?"

Looking at him for a second as her smile grows. She feels the ground beneath her and embraces the view of the sky behind him, "Jay" she says again as her orgasm is finishing and the arousal is still filling her mind and body, and she sees the expression of not knowing what to do now in his eyes. "Jay," as she raises her knees and spreads her legs, and softly says "fuck me now Jay".

Feeling his orgasm almost ready to flow, Jay looks at her so ready and smiling up at him. He looks down at her spreading legs and his half hard dick pointing at her soaked vagina. Lowering his pelvis to place his cock correctly he slides it in. The zing of ecstasy on his cocks skin surprises him and he hold still for a second as he looks into her eyes. Almost drooling he lowers himself to kiss her lips. Seeing only her lips move to greet his he knows what to do.

Sihiryan liking the pressure of Jay now on top of her as she spread limply under him is responding only with her kissing. Feeling her orgasm energy starting to build again as Jay squeezes her shoulders with his for arms, framing her face with his hands and allows his full weight to rest on her torso as he grinds and thrusts. His cock still not rigid Jay works to fill her with each tilt of his pelvis. Feeling his desire and yearning and caring for her in his heart as he looks at her and enjoys her kissing him back. He feels his orgasm starting to bubble up in his legs and buttocks, He feels the sweet heat tingle in his cock and he feels his heart thudding so hard. His mind filled with joy of how close he feels to her, the kyranin that has been so helpful and kind and fun to be around. His body so filed with lust and desire. Distracting himself with the ground beside her head and the smell of the grass Jay stays off his ejaculating as his surging billows of pleasure fill his guts and groin.

Sihiryan feels her own orgasm resuming it's tingling flows of syrupy warmth through her relaxed body. As she feels Jay's heat radiating from his cock into her, she kisses him. With her flaccid body being pressed by his crunching tense form and his grinding thrusts bump hard and push her she focuses on relaxing and feeling it all. The growing intensity of her orgasmic energy swelling up spilling slowly through one part of her and then another, the elevated glow not quite peaking as she explores his kiss and thinks about how Jay is, how they have been at work and how much fun she had working with him. Feeling the growing glow and now noticing that Jays' cock is changing, it is now harder, poking not filling and prying not pushing. "Jay"

Jay hears her say his name and looks into her eyes as he feels the blood leaving his brain. He feels the bursting of his groin into her and the waves of glory in his guts and he sees her eyes and the smile in them and she is kissing him again as he empties his first shot of hot semen into her. He feels her grabbing him with her arms and legs and squeezing him and pulling at his shoulders as he squirts again. His heart releases tension and a tear comes from his eye as he feels the emotion of his love for her, and he squirts again. He feels his erection with a slippery sensation around it as she works to help his slowing thrusts and he squirts again. The sensation on the head of his penis takes lead in his mind. It's zing thickens, and rips through his nervous system; causing his muscles to stop responding. Then her squashed form awakens and she grinds him with her insides as the zing grows to press through to his brain. Continuing her action on his throbbing phallus Jay feels his emptying, and the emotions he has for her replacing what he is releasing in the physical. The glow of her orgasm is still perking as she finishes him with a few more twitches of her pelvis. Their mouths still touching continue to kiss as she cuddles him from below. He again holds their weight liking how she is clinging to him as the pounding glow subsides and his attention notices the meadow around them.

Looking at her smiling back up at him Jay doesn't know what to say.

Savoring the moment Sihiryan takes a slow deep breath and continues to cling to Jay. Her tense body squeezes him out as she listens to the sounds of the forest and Jays' labored breathing. "Jay" she says with a soft tone, "would you like a bath in the creek now?" Lowering her self from him onto the ground and watching his face "it is a tradition in some mountain kyranin tribes to do a ritual after sex between friends. Would you like to try it?"

Jay looks at her starting to reflect on what she just said. 'This is an interesting culture. I truly have no idea what she means' he thinks to himself. "Ok, can you explain what you mean"

"Oh, Jay" taking another deep breath, "we are friends, we just had great sex, at least from my side. We won't have a romantic relationship but I want to bond with you because the sex was great." smiling at him and looking into his eyes to see that he is following her thought. "We can go rest in the creek water and I will give you some physical therapy that will help you body and make me feel closer to you in a caring friendship way".

Jay walks his hands back and shifts his body to be erect from his knees, "sounds good".

Sitting up and moving her arms to take the weight of her shoulders, "If you feel the sex was great and you don't want to crave me after we part ways you can return the therapy, I will tell you what is expected and normal."

Taking a deep breath Jay looks in the direction of the creek. "Do we go to the creek now then?" as he stands up and offers her his hand to help her up.

Taking his hand and standing with him, smiling at his face and waiting for eye contact before saying "yes, you lead"

Jay turns his head and feasts his eyes on her naked body. He still feels the tingle of the orgasm and the intensity it had fills his attention as he looks at her. Thinking only of her and the past few hours with her Jay takes the first step toward the river. Noticing an aroma sweet and pungent subtly wafting around him. "That scent, what is it?"

Sihiryan looks at him with the sun glistening off of his skin and the sweat drops rolling down his sides from his under arm. "That is us Jay" as she turns her view toward her genitals. She sees the sheen of the fluid running down her legs and takes a slow inhale form her noise. I haven't ovulated but it almost smells like I did. Then smelling her shoulder, "I smell sour"

Still holding her hand and walking toward the creek, "you were drinking grandillia sours last night?" as he stops and turns to her. Bringing his face to her neck and sniffing, "you do smell sour" then licking her shoulder with a long wide sloppy stroke of his tongue.

"Jay, I'm not a sample of food"

Jay is looking at her with a serious expression. "You do taste sour."

Her eyes open wider and her expression starts to look serious and questioning.

"At Trentia's families home I was told that the only way to wash the sour off was with the fluid of the sea."

A surprised look transforms her face and she starts to smile, then a step towards the creek and a tug on Jay's hand "come on, the ritual will be good for us."

As they are getting settled into the creek Jay sees the blue lights in the peripheral of his eyes again. Jays thinks about the blue light as he does what she tells him. Sihiryan gets him to lie down so that he is almost submerged in the water with his face out so that his ears are in the air. His arms and legs placed so she can easily move around them to massage him. Her instructions for him to relax and not mind the cooling of his body while she does the ritual gets an agreement form Jay. Starting at his right hand she massages him with pulsing squeezes up the arm and down his side, then down the outside of the leg to his right foot.

"Jay as I work on your foot think the thought again and again that you will move forward in your life without regrets or attachments to the past. Say to yourself, in your mind, the words I step forward as life continues."

As Jay is thinking the mantra she meticulously works all of his toes of his right foot, twisting and pulling and squeezing them. Then moves to the rest of the foot doing the same. She starts massaging up his leg and says, "relax again, and when I get to you genitals Jay. Then think about everything we did sexually until I stop and start down the other leg".

"Ok" he responds. Thinking about the effect the mantra will have on his unconscious mind Jay finds it easy to relax until her hands are squeezing the top on his thigh. He feels the reflex of his genitals to the attention on his thigh and prematurely starts thinking about all the sexual things that they did. He remembers being taken by her in the night and what happened in the morning and in the taxi. Then her grip on his right testicle fills his thoughts. The pressure is firm but just short of giving pain, he feels the fear shooting through him and decides to focus on the ritual. Feeling her squeeze his nuts with one hand and carefully wash his penis with the other he works to remember all what they did. Her strokes on his epididymis and the gentle scrubbing on his neck and head fade to the background of his thoughts as he recalls the various activities on his bed, in the chair, the taxi and the meadow. When she shifts to her hands to stretch his sack and manipulate his perineum. He keeps focusing on the details of the sex. When her finger slips into his anus he takes a deep breath and forces his mind back to the sex they had, and tells him self that he can focus. Then her massage toward his interior increases to a prostate manipulation, and more fingers. Straining to focus and relax Jay finds pleasure recalling the details of what they did sexually. Jay's mind starts to hold both the anal pressure and manipulation with the memories of sex at the same time. Her stretching of his scrotum and the pulling and pushing and slow rubbing on the inside of his rectum with the pinching and pressing on his prostate have Jay's mind mixing the thoughts, like they are being aged. Jay tries to focus on the sex memories as the cool water and her fingers find their way around in his ass. Barely noticing the limited stretch on his scrotum he works to pull his mind back to the memories. Her hands shift again and the other one starts up his ass while the first moves to his cock and pubic area.

Jay starts to find pleasure in having Sihiryan's fingers working the inside of his anus, She works silently moving her hands again and working his testis on the left until she tells him to relax as she moves down his other leg. At his foot she gets him to do the mantra again then up the other side to his other hand. Jay thinking it is over, as he feels totally relaxed in the creek, closes his eyes.

Sihiryan straddles his chest with her feet and placing her hands in the creek lateral to his hips slowly lowers her cunt to Jay's mouth. "Jay, lick me as I suck on your cold limp cock. Don't stop relaxing, and think the mantra as you remember all the things we have done sexually".

Jay's eyes open and he sees her anus between his eyes. Then feels her starting to press her slippery opening to his mouth. He feels her mouth grabbing at his soft shriveled cock and decides to do as she said. Slipping out his tongue and gliding it up over her folds and into her willing opening, then down to her clit he feels the suction of her slurping on him. Remembering the taxi his enthusiasm to please her is sparked. Remembering to relax as he works to aliven her sensations he feels his own starting to emerge. His body cool to the core and as relaxed as a limp noodle he feels sensations from her mouth through his hose to his lower back; a dull sensation of moving fuzzy joy. Soft. Cool. Gentle like a breeze on your face that fails to move your hair. Continuing with his tongue tasting her and feeling the contours as he remembers the chair and what he did not expect. He feels his slowing heart beating harder and a swelling in his cock. Jay feels that he is only full not firm but the sensation he can feel being so relaxed is surprisingly pleasing to him. His mind a little soft, slow, distracted, from the cooling body temperature Jay finds his focus drawn to the fluids he tastes as her salty pussy is quashing his lips. Remembering to focus on relaxing and the memories as he slides and slaps his tongue over and into her. The sensation of possible climax is building slowly as Jay remembers watching her shower in the morning and then the activities the night before that she couldn't remember. Feeling the pre orgasm glow expanding in his cool relaxed body stable but sweet. Jay takes his mind to the pleasure of the sensation he finds sweeping his tongue. Noticing that her folds are becoming fuller and almost rigid, and a slight tangy flavor slides into his mouth. Feeling the heat of her on his full limp cock and dripping into his mouth a wave of sleep starts to slide past his focus and his dreams start to appear through his conscious thoughts. The vision in Jay's head of wildly fucking on a bed starts to seem as real as the flow of the creek over his limbs. Her pelvis now moving too much for his tongue to keep constant contact his dreams of her start to merge with dreaming or other females, and other activities. Jay feels like he is watching a movie of himself having sex in the water on a beach on earth. The pull on his cock awakens his awareness as he feels her pressing her pussy a little more onto his mouth and he extends his tongue again to find her clitoris. Her clit finds his tongue and her mouth sucks harder. Jay hears some sounds from her and works his tongue as his dreams starts to come back past his thoughts, dreaming of having a rock hard and plunging her with it as her opening starts to slide over his nose. The discomfort awakens him again as he realizes that he has little control over his body movement. He lay there relaxed as she brings him closer to the sensation of orgasm. An orgasm he can't believe will ever happen with his body in this state.

Jay notices that the scent and flavor of her vagina is changing, sweeter, tangier, and it is hot on his face. Then it stops and the action on his cock gets more focuses. He feels sleep taking him and then only feels the sensation on his cock. The smooth suction and slow sliding lips squeezing it, up, and down the head rounding the roof of the mouth then the pushing sliding tongue moving it as it swells and throbs, still hardly firm. The ache in his balls and back feeling familiar and calming and remembering the joy of waking up with her in the morning, and the swimming and washing in the lake, and a heat in his shaft. In his soft shaft, slowly sparking around inside of it as the sensation of her on his head intensify, like hot peppers in the mouth the sensation grows to fill his shaft from end to end then the flooding pulses, slow and empty but pulses of pleasure as his mind's images fade to blackness

Sihiryan feels the cock get softer and tastes the fluid that it produced. She gets up and looks down at Jay. Seeing him with his mouth open laying on his back all stretched out in the shallow water. She smiles and looks at the juice on his mouth and laughs out loud. "Jay" she says, "JAY". Then looking at him for a few seconds before looking for the best way to move him. She takes his arms and pulls him slowly out of the water and onto the grass at the edge of the stream. Looking around she estimates how long the sun will be directly on him before the shade of the trees will come into play. She takes a deep breath and looks him over before taking his pulse and smiling. Then turns back to the meadow and goes to collect their stuff and makes a camp place, with a small place for a fire and an area to comfortably sleep beneath the stars. She goes and gathers some berries, fruit, flowers, and roots for their dinner. When it is all set up she makes the fire and goes back to Jay; sits down beside him and jiggles him a little. "Jay, dinner is ready" and jiggles him again. Looking up at the sun and

seeing that there is still maybe an hour before the shade
will come to cover him she shakes him again "Jay".

Jay is in a dream of him and Heather on the moon with a
group of aliens picking cheese and sipping wine. He hears the
loud echoing call of his name from the sky as it opens up in his
left eye. Seeing the light of the sun and the trees above he
forgets the dream and looks at Sihiryan. He sees her smile,
then her eyes and her breast. Realizing that she is female, and
naked he opens his other eye. Jay looks up at her still not
awake and can't think of where he could be. He looks at her
then around at the trees and sky. He hears the creek and
recognizes her voice, then her face. "Oh,,, what happened?"

"Hi Jay, I prepared our camp would you like to rest a little
longer?" she asks.

Jay starts to sit up and starts to remember what put him to
sleep at the same time. He sits for a second without
responding. "Well, I think I can get up. How are you doing
Sihiryan my friend? Did the ritual work for you?

"Hahahaha, I believe it did Jay" standing up and offering a
hand for Jay to hold as he gets up too. "You did well in the
water Jay".

"Did I" he looks at her with a smile and a hesitation, "I felt Like I was getting hypothermia and lost consciousness several times. I couldn't actually move at the end. I was shocked that I could orgasm in that state.

"How do you feel now Jay?"

Jay looks around and takes a few deep breaths still holding her hand. "Dizzy and exhausted. How was it for you?" looking her in the eye and smiling; now not completely sure if it is a dream or if he is actually on Ramga.

"Jay it was exceptional for me. It is rare for a city girl to get a chance to try the ritual. It has always been a fantasy for me," smiling at him, "It was everything that I had hoped". Turning toward the meadow and tugging his hand, "lets go eat".

Jay steps to follow feeling the hollow ache in his back, and shakiness in his legs.

Jay sits by the fire and looks at the food then at the area that is fixed with lots of leaves, then at her. "Is that our bed?"

Sitting between him and the food, "Yes Jay, are you wanting more action already?"

With a worried look on his face, "no, no, I'm good"

"hahaha, Jay eat" as she hands him some fruit. These will get your digestion started. The order we eat this food is said to be important to bring your energy back"

They eat the fruit then she asks if he will be willing to do his side of the ritual the next day. After some questions and assurances that he won't have to worry that she could die he agrees. They eat the flowers and roots then start talking about him going to the moon.

"So," Jay asks, "what will my work be on the moon?"

"Well, from what I understand Herfermks has created some position in the bureaucracy of their records department of one city on the moon where you will correlate various records of events in the development and growth of the city." She gives him a long hard look, " I can't understand why but he insists that it is very important."

Jay looks at her and thinks about all the secrets he is keeping for Herfermks.

Sihiryan looks back at Jay "I don't see from your personal history that you are well disposed for this work or that the moon needs it done." Looking to the side quickly for a second then back at Jay "do you have a interest in political history or social development?

Jay thinks, then as he looks in the direction that she looked, says "well, I do find both topics interesting but am not sure that I am well suited to this work." looking back at her, "did you see something over there?"

She looks at Jay, "a blue glow, in the corner of my sight. It is an energy life form that is folklore from our mountain kyranins. Most of us think it is only a myth."

Jay looks at her for a second, "have you seen them before?"

"No Jay it is just an anomaly of light during sunset and dawn".

Jay looks at her with curiosity "I saw it earlier today as well".

Sihiryan turns to look into Jay's eyes, "You saw it earlier, when?"

"When we first started walking in the trees and then a little while before the ritual. It was like you, just a flash of it in the corner of my vision." noticing the seriousness of her expression he asks, "should we take some scans with the tablets to see if we can find out what is actually causing it?"

"Good idea Jay" she says as she gets her tablet from its' pouch. Working the screen for a few moments as Jay finds a spot to sit in the middle of a berry bush and starts eating some of them. "What do you see?"

"Well, there are some energy signals indicating mass and movement but the volume trajectory and speeds don't make sense. It is like they are and then they are not, and then they are at a different place."

"What do you mean by volume?" as he gets up and walks toward her.

Looking at Jay then at the forest to her left then back at Jay "see that big tree, about half way up to the first branch there is one according to the device."

Jay looks then looks away so that the spot is at the edge of his vision and he focuses at the center of his field of sight. Turning his head slightly back and forth, "yeah, look forward and let the edge of your vision pass the spot. I can see I slight flash sometimes as my peripheral vision crosses it."

Sihiryan looks straight at it then works the screen of the tablet and tries Jay's method of looking not at it. "Yeah, interesting, just a slight glow sometimes in the corner of my eye," looking at her tablet again, "It seems like it is out of faze or something."

"Oh, that is interesting" Jay says. And takes his tablet from the pouch. He turns it on and he walks toward her. I'm going to send a message to Herfermks, can you send him your data from the scans?"

"Yes, why?", as she starts to work the screen to send the data to Herfermks.

"He told me something that makes me think he will want to know about this" Jay steps right beside her so they can both see each others screens. His screen gets a reply from Herfermks first then as they are reading it her screen gets a picture image of Herfermks looking at her.

"Hello Sihiryan, the face shifts, Jay you can't see it but it has light that is visible on the edge of your vision and Sihiryan you think it could be out of faze?" he asks.

They both nod, he hesitates to answer for a second, "Well, I will get myself there soon, maybe in the morning?"

"Yes" Shihiryan says as Jay shrugs and nods. Then Herfermks face disappears from the tablet.

"It has been a long day Jay, do you feel up to looking for the cave with the hot pool before dark?"

Jay looks at her, feels his body's fatigue, looks around the meadow and asks, "if we must but can't we just stay here and go up there in the morning?"

She looks at him and smiles, "we could, but that hot pool will make you feel better by morning."

"How so?" Jay asks as he starts to wonder what she means.

"It's the salts and minerals in the hot springs Jay. They relax and strengthen the body. Can you make it? It won't take long." She starts working the screen on her tablet.

Jay looks around at the hills behind the forest. He can only see them in a few places between the trees. He looks at Sihiryan and then at the tablet as it shows a map of the valley. He sees the shapes of the terrain and the stream and the red dot up one side of the valley. "Is that it, the red dot?" He asks.

"Yes" it is about a 10 minute walk, not steep and the bushes don't look too thick." Looking at his face and smiling, "well?"

"Ok lets go, what about our clothes, will we need them?"

"No", She looks at him with curiosity, "you can grab them if you like but we won't need them, the cave will be warm and the bushes aren't thick or prickly." seeing a calm face of agreement on Jay she smiles and says "come on, this way," then turns and starts walking.

Jay thinks 'if I don't need them' as he looks for the tree with his clothes. He thinks he can see it across the meadow. He turns and follows Sihiryan. He watches her gracefully make her way between the bushes and trees and into the forest. Picking up his pace Jay follows about six steps behind her. Watching the

ground to choose where he steps while keeping her in
view he makes his way up the shallowly sloping hillside.

She stops. Jay sees her working her tablet and looking around.
He stops beside her and looks at the tablet, then at her. "Are
we lost?"

"It says it is right here" she looks at him then back at the tablet,
"we are standing in the pool according to this."

Jay looks at the tablet and then looks around. "It must be
under us" he says and looks back down the slope in both
directions. "Huh, well, maybe in those thick trees" as he points
about 30 feet across and down the slop a little, " if the entrance
was there we wouldn't be able to see it unless we went into
those trees."

Sihiryan looks where he pointed and nods, and starts walking
down toward the trees. "I hope you are right Jay".

There are some thick bushes before the trees and she turns to
go around them as the slope steepens. Jay hurries to catch up
as she gets to the trees. The branches of the trees interlace so
she pushes them to make a way through.

"There it is" and she crouches to go into an opening in the ground on the steep slope behind the trees.

Jay pushes through the branches and sees her foot disappearing into the darkness in the opening. "Sihiryan? Can you see in there?"

"It is dark Jay". Then she asks the tablet to shine brightly.

Jay sees the brightness coming out of the opening and crouches to get in through it. "Wow it is bigger in here than I would have expected," Jay says as he takes several steps down into the cavern.

The light from the tablet glistens off of some of the cave walls while others remain dark. The dirt floor is worn smooth like a pathway. The sound of water trickling is the only sound as they stand still and look around.

Sihiryan starts walking again, "this way Jay" taking the light with her.

Jay starts following as he takes his own tablet out to use it as a flashlight "can you see it?"

She stops and stands still as Jay comes up beside her. She looks over at Jay as he looks at her working the front of the tablet as the back shines at the floor and the water just in front of them. "It is warm and safe." She says as she reaches and holds Jay's hand. "It is not too deep" looking up at his face, then squatting to put her tablet down so it shines at the ceiling of the cave.

Jay watches her and takes off his tablet and puts it beside hers. "Should we jump in?"

"The tablet said the rock on the bottom are sharp away from the edge. It is about 3 times as deep as your height, it won't taste good but it is safe to swallow a little bit. I think climb or walk in is better. There are a lot of minerals so you will float very well in this pool" Sihiryan moves her hand a little, "lets do it Jay" and slips off her shoes then steps into the water.

Jay Takes his shoes off and steps in as she does. He feels the warmth. He also feels a sensation of something happening with his skin on his foot in the water and stops. "What is it doing to my foot?"

Sihiryan takes another step in and another as she gets thigh deep and is now facing Jay. "That's from the minerals being absorbed by your skin Jay. It is good for you. Come on in and float with me."

Jay starts taking more steps as she does until he is chest deep and she is floating beside him. He feels his feet light against the bottom and takes another step forward. To his surprise his feet don't stay on the bottom and he topples over to float. His legs coming up in front of him as he maneuvers to keep his face on the top. "hahahah, this is great."

"Isn't it!" still holding his hand as she is spread out like a starfish on top of the water beside him.

Jay lays back straightening his body then relaxing until he is comfortable. Looking at the ceiling Jay notices that there are some occasional movements taking place above them. "Sihiryan, what is up there on the ceiling, I saw something moving"

Sihiryan looks up for a few seconds. "Nothing to worry about Jay, things live in caves, but there is nothing dangerous in here. Accept me Jay, I could turn off the light and let go of your hand and you would be alone in the dark"

"hahahah, well I guess I better not let that happen." Jay turns his head and sees her looking back at him with a smile on her face, half in the water. "Thank you Sihiryan" with a gentle change of grip on her hand and the look on his face, "I am so grateful for your friendship and teachings." Then not finding more words Jay just looks into her eyes for some seconds. The silence of the cave is only broken by the distant sound of water trickling. "Is it safe to sleep like this?"

Sihiryan hesitates then says, "It is common for us to sleep in floating hot ponds Jay." Tell you tablet to set an alert call if we break physical contact and to shine brighter than mine until we answer the alert". Paddling with one hand to start them both turning in the water, "Then we can sleep without getting lost from each other. Oh also tell it to alarm if we drift 30 feet away from it or if anything large comes into the cave."

After Jay gives the commands to his tablet, closes his eyes and takes a few deep breaths as he focuses on his hand and it's gentle grip on hers. Feeling how few muscles are actually needed to keep a slight grip on her hand he focuses on relaxing the other muscles in his hand and arm. Then imagines that his grip will stay steady until she wakes up. He intends it consciously and accepts that it is easy for his body to do it while he sleeps. Jay takes more deep relaxed breaths as he feels his skin pressing against the water and he is looking up into the darkness of the cave. Jay starts to daydream about his situation, being on another world, camping, naked and sleep takes him.

Some short time later, in his dream, Jay finds himself floating between several blue light bulbs with tropical trees and berries amongst them. The lights are looking at him and talking to each other. In his dream Jay starts listening to the sounds the light bulbs are making and he hears it like music that sounds like a trickling stream. As he focuses to hear it he starts to wake up. As his eyes open he remembers where he is. He feels her hand in his and sees the slight reflection of light from her tablet on the ceiling of the cave. The only sound he can hear other than their soft slow breathing it the sound of the trickling water in the distance. Jay takes a few relaxed breaths and thinks about his situation. Four months from earth, about, he saw his spouse two days ago for the first time in four months, and is floating in a subterranean pond on a planet filled with aliens. Good aliens and great food. He feels a tension building in his chest as he starts to wonder if it is all actually real. Turning his head to look at Sihiryan he sees her sleeping, with her mouth open a little, floating, only partly out of the water. Jay starts taking more slow deep breaths and concentrating on relaxing again, he drifts back to sleep and into his new dreams.

Jay hears a sound and the room lightens up revealing the roots on the ceiling as his eyes open. He feels Sihiryan grab his hand gently as he hears her voice.

"Jay" she says, "Oh, I was dreaming of the blue light beings and I woke up. I forgot where I was and let go." Gripping her hand to his snugly, "It is odd to be in here. It's so quiet."

Jay looks at her and asks, "tablet how long have we slept?"

Jay's tablet responds "six hours and forty three minutes."

Sihiryan asks, "Jay how long is that?"

"Not long enough" it won't be light for a while yet.

"Would you like to see the night sky?" Letting go of Jay's hand, still on her back, and paddling with her arms she moves toward the tablets on the shore. "Come on Jay it is really interesting to see them in the night."

Jay thinks about how they looked from the city then thinks about how they are more visible on earth from the countryside. "Ok" as he rolls over and tries to swim toward her. He notices how thick the water is about two feet deep beneath him as his hands push through it. With a few strokes he makes it to the shallows and stands up to walk the last few steps out onto the cave floor. "Strange water"

"Ya" Sihiryan replies as she picks up the tablets and hands Jay's to him. Pointing hers around she finds the opening and starts towards it.

Jay, still half asleep puts his tablet into his pouch, and puts it on and puts on his shoes before following her. As she crouches to go through the opening, Jay watches the light coming around her showing the edges of the opening. He climbs out after her into the thick trees and hopes they can find their way back in. He looks up into the forest above them. "Well, I guess we will be going to the meadow to see the stars"

Sihiryan looks up in various directions, "unm, good idea Jay," She turns off the light from her tablet. After a few seconds she starts walking down the slope.

There is moonlight enough for Jay to see the forest and the ground. He starts to follow. "Will we come back here to sleep more?" He asks.

"If you want to Jay, or we can sleep in the meadow."

Jay keeps following her, as he thinks about the temperature and how he feels, wet, naked, but not cold. When they reach the meadow there is a slight breeze, but Jay still doesn't feel cold. As they walk out into the tall grass Jay can see the stares above them. So many so colorful, many of them flashing and moving in various directions. "Wow"

Sihiryan stands beside him looking up, "yeah, it is worth the walk to see them without the city lights isn't it Jay?"

Jay silently watches then, "the fast moving ones, are those ships?"

"Yeah". Sihiryan says then points. "That orange one there, that one is a sun about the same as by your planet". It has no life planets though. Then pointing to a blue one near to it. That is the one near the moon you will be living on. It looks blue from here because of the debris sphere at the extreme of that solar system. It is closer to white when you look at it from the Gyrekian moon. Then pointing far to the other direction "that is Vwortex's sun".

"Can we see my sun from Ramga? Jay asks and starts looking for another orange one.

"No Jay, your sun is so far away that it can only bee seen from space. "Actually Jay, until the ryberians told our science teams about your world and it's sun we didn't know it was there. We had never look at anything that far away. It was impossible for us to go there so we didn't care. The amburst agreed with us but the birds said we should learn what ever the ryberians are willing to tell us about. So we started a small science brance to study planets like yours.

"are there other planets like mine?" Jay looks at her with curiosity.

"like yours in that we don't have the technology to get there yet." she smiles at him and holds his hand. "Jay, without Herfermks secret efforts to start this branch and fund it from the ryberian's alliance shush

funding accounts, our research of your species would have never taken place. It is basically about three hundred years of his efforts to get your planet know to our science and about fifty years to get us to a situation that we can bring a few of your kind here."

Jay looks at her for a second, "there are others?"

"Were" she says. "Some didn't make it through the training, we had to send them back after cleaning their memories. One got caught on his third day. He tried to go out in public and got into a fight with some vworktex soldiers. We fixed him up and sent him home. Two women worked out, they are on assignments. One other man is working with us back on earth already."

"Reggie told me that he had trouble interacting with humans often." Jay looks at her, "does he report back often?"

"Reggie came back two years ago" Sihiryan says, "he can't tell us anything about his time there as it could effect our choices here that can effect him making it back to here." looks into Jay's eyes, "It is complicated with time travel and decision making. That is why the ryberian that sent you back has been stripped of his time privileges for six hundred years. Apparently it is one of the few crimes that ever happens on ryberia. That one of their own will do unauthorized time travel."

Jay thinks back to the incident. It was only a few days ago for him. Thinking about what he had said to him and Trentia before sending him back to earth. "I am surprised that he would take such a risk for me."

"Well apparently you are well liked, It was an open trial and he had support for his choice to do it, but it was not authorized, and so he was still partly punished." She looks at Jay, " I wish you could tell me why you are popular with them, It must be an interesting story!"

Jay looks at her as he remembers what they said to him at Crenshaws. "What would have happened to me if he hadn't sent me back when he did?"

Sihiryan raises her eyebrows, "It could have been tricky Jay." A lot of off world beings were researched and a lot of minor things that no one actually wanted to find out were discovered. It was a difficult time for any being without full legitimacy of their situation." Then a little laugh, "Jay you would have been put into stasis and studied for a long time before we would have been able to retrieve you." Squeezing his hand and looking into his eyes, "I was upset at first thinking that we could have saved you with some simple cover up, but after the events with security and the constant reestablishing of new protocols and new agencies doubling up on scrutiny and then off world military research to double check details. I realized that if he hadn't done it you would have been in stasis for at least a month, maybe still in some secret facility somewhere."

Jay feels his heart quicken, "I, I didn't take it that seriously! I guess I owe him a debt of gratitude."

Smiling at him "Jay from what I understand he is well liked for what he did among the ryberians, even by those who sentenced him for it. And for a ryberian that length of punishment is not so bad. His punishment is only that: none of the time travel technology can be worked by him, but his friends can take him to anytime they or he want to go to. I am not suppose to know these things but I have been made privy to a few secrets from ryberia"

Jay looks back up at the stars. 'So many, what is happening on all those worlds to all those species?' he thinks. Then thinking about the feeling in his body, "where will we go back to sleep now?"

Sihiryan lets go of his hand and looks around on the ground. She starts pulling up some of the tall grass and putting it into a pile, "help me Jay, take the tall soft grass and we can make a bed." Clearing an area about five meters by five meters they make a decent pile of the grass and she gets onto it. "Come here Jay"

When Jay gets down and lays on the grass beside her she snuggles up to him then says "roll this way and cuddle my back Jay, I want you to keep me warm."

As they snuggle and shift to get comfortable Jay is still thinking about his narrow escape of stasis. Once they are comfortable together on the grass Jay turns his head just enough to see the stars. Sihiryan feels the movement and does the same and takes a deep breath as she relaxed to fall asleep. A few breaths and Jays eyes close too.

The sun comes up behind them and is warming Jays back before it hits the corner of his eye. His eye opens, then the other. Finding himself naked with a woman in the forest he thinks for a second about where he is. Remembering the previous day he relaxes and thinks about his time since getting back to Ramga. He feels her move and starts to lift his arm off of her until he feels her grasping his forearm to hold it over her.

"Good morning Jay" She says to him, "can you smell the forest?"

Laying still, and relaxing again Jay takes a long slow sniff "mmm, yes and something different too"

Sihiryan sniffs the air with out moving. Then sniffs it again and sits up and looks around. "JAY" as she look behind him.

Jay turns and looks. He sees a large animal with long teeth showing and long arms with long claws. He turns and gets up as it does the same. He holds Sihiryan's arm and says, "What is it"

Sihiryan stands as he does and starts slowly stepping backwards away from it. "A Wearoda" holding Jay firmly as they are backing away from it "they don't usually show themselves to us. They only eat meat Jay and it is looking at you"

Jay watches the thing as it steps toward them keeping the distance constant as they back away. Jay watches as it looks at him then at her. "Will the loud noise work with this thing?"

"I don't think so" she looks at it looking at them with a puzzled expression in its' eyes. Then she sees it look into her eyes.

It makes a sound "krerannian," then it looks at Jay and sniffs the air then back at her, then at Jay and it moves closer.

"Should we call the birds?" Jay asks.

'The birds?" Sihiryan pulls out her tablet and starts working the screen, "we don't know how to communicate with these wearodas"

"QUARRATUTU" Jay yells, then again "QUARRATUTU" Jay notices the wearoda giving him a puzzled look and stepping closer again. "It is pretty big"

"Jay it seems to be drooling as it looks at you". She says as she starts clinging to him with both arms.

They hear the hard flapping of wings in the distance. The three of them look up. Jay looks back at it first and motions Sihiryan to start backing up again with him. But it moves forward with them slightly closing the distance without looking toward them until it can see the bird coming. Then it moves much closer in an instant, putting its' face within a meter of Jays face. Squinting and sniffing and drooling at Jay, then looking at Sihiryans arms around him and looking past Jay at her. It looks puzzled when it looks at her and looks back at Jay and licks its' lips with it's long snake like tongue.

The birds swoop over their heads and one starts flapping hard to climb and starts making loud bird sounds as the other lands making a tight triangle with them and the wearoda.

It looks at the bird like it isn't important at all, then back at Jay as a drip of saliva falls from it's mouth.

"Shit, I make it hungry" Jay thinks aloud, "what does it see, it looks at you differently than me".

"I agree, I don't know, you skin is a match to kiranin according to our scans" Sihiryan says.

"Maybe the water last night washed something off?" Jay suggests.

Working the screen still, "uuuum, nothing shows here, I'll call Herfermks."

There is more hard flapping and two more birds swoop past then three come from the other direction diving into the meadow. The three of them look as the three birds land so close to them that the wind tests Jays' balance.

"Jay" The middle bird says as it turns to focus an eye on him.

"Quarratutu?" Jay says, " how are you doing, it is good to see you"

Quarratutu looks at Sihiryan and then at the Wearoda then at Jay again, "Well Jay I am doing better than you, your are not doing to well I think, to me it looks like this wearoda wants to eat you"

"Yeah, I am a little worried about that actually" Jay looks at him then at the other birds and then at the wearoda. "What should I do?"

Quaratutu steps a little closer to get almost between the wearoda and Jay "Well Jay where you bragging about how tender and juicy you are?, you know if you were it is only fair that he should at least get a taste".

"Nope, didn't say a word to,,, it" Jay says then continues, "I don't know if this is a good situation for humor my friend"

"I will talk to him for you Jay. We have a treaty with them concerning the amburst and kyranins and the guest species that are part of the alliance."

Herfermks appears a few meters from Sihiryan and then reappears in the same place facing slightly differently. Turning to Jay, Sihiryan and then to Quaratutu. "Hello, Quaratutu, Jay, Sihiryan," Then turning to the Wearode and taking a low bow and growling out some sounds, then turning to wave and nod at the other birds. Herfermks Holds up his tablet then works it with his fingers for some seconds.
"Jay, Sihiryan, ask your tablets to load the wearode language data from my tablet to you ear communication equipment".

The wearode looks at Herfermks and starts growling out some sounds as Jay and Shiryan talk to their tablets and the birds watch Herfermks nod and growl back at the wearode. Jay starts to hear words in place of the growls.

The wearode replies to Herfermks "yes you are a ryberian and I acknowledge your right to visit our planet and respect your freedom hear through our agreement with the birds. But our agreement is with them not you ryberians. No insult intended but we have no formal or informal relationship with your species." It looks at Jay this one is not a kyranin. It is not any alliance species that I am aware of. So as soon as the kyranin female lets go of it I will eat it and we will all be happy"

Herfermks looks at Jay and Sihiryan and then at the Wearode, then at Quaratutu.

Quaratutu looks at Jay then at Herfermks and then at Sihiryan as she has both her arms around Jay. Quaratutu looks at the wearode and introduces himself. "I am Quaratutu, I have seen you and your tribe in all the mountains of this region. Is there not enough food for you in the forest now?"

The wearode replies, "yes, Quaratutu, you are a noble known to my tribe from the first days of the treaties. I and we all have never broken our agreements with your flocks. I honor our peace. This thing is not part of any agreement so I want to sample its' flesh for my morning meal. I won't harm the female kyranin that is keeping it still but when she releases it I will have my meal."

The birds all look at Jay with one side then the other. Quaratutu gives Jay a close look then a sniff of his head. He looks at Sihiryan holding him and then looking at the wearode. "Do you have a name sir?"

The wearode looks at Quaraktutu for a second, "we don't need names, we know who we are".

Quaraktutu looks at the other birds as they shrug their wings and look at Jay again. Then he looks at Herfermks. Then at Jay, Then back at the wearode. "What makes you think Jay is not a kyranin?"

The wearode looks at Quaraktutu for a second and nods his head at Jay, "the glow, the glow is not like any other species I have ever seen." Then stepping sideways to have a more direct look at Jay without the bird being in the way. "And the thoughts he has, they are more random and shorter. When you listen to the thoughts of this one, it becomes clear it is different."

Quaraktutu looks at the wearode and says "so you see something in the energy around him?"

Herfermks starts working his tablet again and periodically looking at Jay.

Quaraktutu looks at Jay then says to the wearode, "we can't see what you see in his glow. But I know this one. I have known him for some years and he is OK. We like this one. We don't mind that he may look a little different. We like him."

The Wearode looks at Quaratutu as Herfermks is working his tablet. He takes another step to improve his position to pounce on Jay. He sniffs the air, and licks his lips.

"Hi, I am Jay, I am interested to find out what my glow is like. How do I look different than other kyranins?" As he give a friendly look to the beast.

It looks at him, "well Jay are you delicious or just tasty, oh, no need to say! I will find out any minute".

Sihiryan looks at it. "This one is my good friend. I won't let go of him."

Herfermks says "would you like to come to another place and do some hunting with me?"

It says "come on, don't make me wait. I will find this one alone some time and he will be my food."

Quaraktutu looks at the wearode then steps between Jay and the wearode. "Ok, I like this one, I don't care what he is, I like him and he is under my protection. You eat him and you will have me after you."

"Come on Quaraktutu. You were a legend once, but now you are just an old bird. Sure you are as big as me and once you were as fast but now, now you don't really want to match claws with me. I will eat him, this Jay, and that is all."

The other birds step up. "My name is Grembits and I am one with Quaratutu. He is not alone to retaliate for damage to Jay"

"My name is Rertha and I will protect Jay too"

The wearode stands and walks between them. "You are so many and so helpless to stop me. What will I do after, when I see him alone, in the city, by the sea, or here in my lands. Why do you all care, what is this thing that hides to look like a kyranin?"

One of the birds from the back walks forward, "should we fight for him then, if you kill all of us now you and eat him, but if we win we can eat you?

The wearode looks at all of the birds and asks, if not him what will I eat?"

Hefermks interrupts "You like to eat living things correct?"
He watches the wearode nod. "Well so do I, If you like I will
take you to a place with lots of wild things that are tasty and
nutritious, even some that can give you a challenge to catch.

"Take me? How? I don't see your ship. How can you take
me?"

"Ryberians have tools that the others don't know about. I can
take you anywhere and have you back with you belly filled so
fast that you may think it was just a trick, except for the flavor
still in your mouth and the full feeling in your belly. This one,
Jay, he is special to us, it is complicated but I can't let you have
him. If it is a new flavor you like, come with me. You will be
glad that you did."

The wearode looks at Jay again then at the birds, then at
Herfermks, then at Jay. "You are the one they call Jay. I can see
that you are not one of them but they can't." Then looking at
Quaraktutu, "it is an honor to meet you Quaratutu." Then he
looks at Sihiryan and says to her "this one is not or your kind,
He can't fool me." Then at Herfermks, "ok take me to that
place, lets see what this ship is about"

Herfermks walks over to it and holds out his arm to it. "Touch
my arm and we will travel." As he touches Herfermks arm
they fade to nothing.

The birds look at each other and then at Jay and Sihiryan. They see the worried look on Sihiryan's face. Quaraktutu looks at the other birds and then at Sihiryan. I don't know where Jay is from but he is welcome here, and if you treat him like a kyranin so will we. We watch the strange things that go on with your work mates and we understand how complicated your off Ramga situation can be. We won't start rumors. He looks at the other birds "Is that how we all feel." Quaraktutu watches as all the other birds look at him and nod. Quaraktutu looks at Jay and Sihiryan. "I guess I won't see you on the public media again soon Jay."

Jay smiles at him, "I don't know what to say".

Sihiryan looks at the birds and at the details of their feathers and beaks and eyes. "Hello Quaraktutu, I have known Jay since his first arrival on Ramga and I do accept him as one of us. I am saddened by the fact that he won't be among us for long though"

"Well" Quaraktutu takes a close look at Jay "I hope you have time for a beer before you leave Ramga, it will be good to see you in the bar again Jay."

Jay looks at Sihiryan to see her smile and nod.

"Tonight we will go back to the city and tomorrow he will have the afternoon to do as he pleases." She says.

The other birds start taking off and Quaraktutu says "do you remember how to find the place we first met Jay? We will be there tomorrow shortly after mid day."

"I will be there" Jay says.

Quaraktutu jumps and flaps hard pounding them with wind as he burst up toward the trees' tops then circling once before following the other birds.

"That was interesting" Jay says as he turns to look at Sihiryan. "I didn't know that Quaraktutu was a famous bird. He was the first one I ever met." The others that came with him seemed much younger and didn't say much. Usually they all have a lot of things to say."

Sihiryan looks at Jay for a moment. " I don't understand what the wearode meant by our glow. I don't see it."

Jay looks at her for a second. Trentia told me that each species has some kind of light anomaly that she can see around them. She seemed to indicate that all amburst do see it. It is like the blue light beings for me, I can only see it a little bit once in a while." Jay looks at her and tries to refocus his eyes and look beside her in an attempt to see her aura. "On earth we call it the aura. Some humans can see it all of the time but most have to learn how to see it. Most never learn how to." Jay smiles and shrugs, "I guess if we don't see it then it doesn't exist for us. There is technology on earth that can read it and extrapolate what is happening with the body's health and emotions and thoughts from the energy in the aura. Or so they say. Our official medical industry has nothing to say about it?"

Sihiryan looks at Jay, "you have technology to see the glow and understand what it indicates but your medical industry doesn't use it?"

"Uumm, Yeah, there are several technologies and healing systems that our official medical industry won't use or accept. Some of them have been in use for thousands of years." Jay looks around the meadow. "Lets get some berries".

"Are you hungry Jay?" she smirks, "what about some live food?"

Jay laughs, "hahaha, well, as long as it is not me!"

Sihiryan laughs a little then harder until she has to stop herself to catch her breath. " ha ha ha, That was good Jay. No there is some worms that grow under the roots of those shrubs" as she point to a patch of scrubby looking, low to the ground, bushy, thorny, kind of blue broad leafed plants with thick stems and branches growing in soil that looks like it has been turned recently.

Jay looks at her hesitating to respond, then finally after some long seconds of silence "worms you say, worms ahy?" then looking at her with a questioning expression. "Mmmm, no, no I'm happy with just berries."

Sihiryan looks at Jay "You should try one Jay, they are delicious."

Jay looks at her to decide if she is serious or not. Thinking that she is, "maybe you should test them first. If you can convince me they do taste good when you are actually eating them I will try one."

She looks at him for a second them smiles, "haha, Jay, do you not have tasty worms on your world?"

Jay looks at her, then thinks, 'am I closed minded about foods?' Still looking at her smiling at him, "actually in the part of the world that I am from, children make cruel jokes about making others that they hate, eat worms." Starting to smile back at her "It is not something that they would do under any circumstance. I have never eaten one."

Taking a good look in all directions she says "well Jay, there are no human children here to make jokes at you. Now is your chance to see what they are all missing out on."

Jay starts to laugh, he laughs harder and his knees bend, as he laughs harder tears start to come to his eyes and he tries to say something, then still laughing he sits down. "haha hahaha, oh ha ha ha Sihiryan, ha ha that is so funny."

"What" she looks at him laughing so hard sitting naked with tears on his face and looking back at her. "Ok Jay I don't understand the issue of worms but it can't be that funny. hehehe" She laughs a little too.

Jay takes a breath, "I can't explain hahahaha but it is that funny to me." He looks at her and takes another deep breath to help him consolidate his emotions. "Maybe partly I am reacting to the situation of almost having been eaten myself just a few moments ago. But the thought that the most disgusting thing I have ever imagined having to do as a child, is something that I actually will want to do often after trying it now, that is mind shatteringly funny to me. Partially because you could be right, I just might actually like it. Hahahaha"

"Well then Jay, lets get some and you can try."

"hahaha, no, no not just now hahaha." Jay looks up at her and asks, "can we eat anything else first please, I will have to think about it a little before I can try the worms."

Sihiryan offers her hand to help him up "sure Jay, come on, lets go get some roots from near the creek, and some cane cores."

After eating and washing in the creek, a nap in the sun, and savoring the peddles of a few flowers they agree to climb to the ridge of the tallest side of the valley to see the view.

As they approach the top Jay starts thinking about the worms. He remembers that finding a worm in an apple he was eating as a child and being scared that part of it might have gotten into his stomach. He remembered the fear that the worm was searching around in his stomach and doing what worms do. He thought how silly it was to be so worried. Looking forward he sees the sky between the trees just ahead. "Is this the top?" he asks.

Sihiryan turns her head toward him then back and takes a few fast steps further then stops. "Ya, I think it is, she looks through the trees on both sides and says, It seems to be the highest point on the ridge then looks down in front of herself. It seems to be steep on the other side Jay, careful when you get up here."

Jay takes the last few steps to stand beside her and looks down the slope on the other side. Taking another step forward then holding onto a tree's branch and leaning forward to look down the slope better. Yeah it seems to get very steep." turning he steps back up to stand beside her. They are both bobbing their heads to see the view between the trees and their branches. Jay can see between the hills in one direction to the flat lands past them but can't see any cities. "I can only see wilderness".

Sihiryan holds his hand and looks around a little more, "yeah."

Jay takes a step back toward the valley, "Should we go back down?" feeling her follow, and still holding his hand he says "I have been thinking about eating the worms. I guess I could try it"

She looks at him and keeps walking.

They walk a few hundred meters before she says anything. She explains that the worms are best in the morning, that they come out to bask in the moonlight and the moist air but by mid day they are hard to find and not as juicy if you can find one. Jay listens to her talk about them like they are a rare treat that should be savored. Like the worms are a special thing to get to eat and that he did miss a great chance to try them. 'I guess she actually wanted to share the experience of the worms with me' he thinks to himself. Jay, not knowing whether to feel relieved that the worm eating opportunity was missed or to suggest that they hunt for worms the next morning, says nothing as they walk back to the meadow.

As they enter the meadow Jay sees Herfermks sitting with the wearode in the grass. He takes a few fast steps to get beside Sihiryan and softly says, "They are back".

Real friendships

She stops and looks around the meadow as Jay points in the direction of the wearode and Herfermks. She nods, takes his hand, makes a gesture for them to go toward then and starts walking. Jay follows. As they get close they can hear Herfermks and the wearode conversing about their hunt.

"Hello sir" Sihiryan says as she leads Jay toward them.

Herfermks stands, "Hello Sihiryan, Jay. Our friend has given me the honor of his name. He is willing to accept you Jay as a guest of the alliance and as such regard you as a non food species even though he is correct to assume that you are actually not included in any treaty or contract or agreement to give you such protection. He has also agreed to have the others of his kind to give you the same courtesy. Jay I hope you don't mind but I told him that you would let him lick your skin to know what you would have tasted like."

Jay still holding Sihiryan's hand looks into Herfermks eyes to see that he is serious, then at the wearode, then at Siheriyan. He lets go of her hand and as he starts walking toward the wearode he says to Herfermks "if you have given your word to him I will do it."

The wearode looks shocked as Jay walks directly up to him. It sniffs Jay's belly and face with his large snout. Looks into Jays' eyes and then over at Herfermks. "I see; he is so brave, and trusting of you my friend." He looks at Jay. Looks at his legs then belly, then his face. "Turn around Jay I will lick your back."

Jay smiles at him and turns looking at Herfermks as he feels the wide wet tongue of the wearode slide across his back. Smelling its' breath and feeling the tingle of its saliva drizzling down in a few spots. He turns back to face it. "Well, don't take it the wrong way but I hope I taste terrible."

Herfermks starts to laugh. Sihiryan lets out a little hit of a chuckle too.

The wearode looks at Jay with wide-open eyes for a few seconds and makes a grinding growling sound and starts to smile and nods his head. After a few seconds it stops and silently smiles at Jay. "Well Jay, you taste OK". My name is Gruembft. If my kind approach you, mention my name and that we are friends. That will be enough for them to treat you, as I will, as a friend. Jay I am glad we met. Although it could have gone badly for you it has been a great advancement for me, and my kind. In the time I have spent with your friend I have learned many things. It is an honor to meet you Jay. I will take my leave now so the three of you can visit without me." Looking over to Sihiryan, "I thank you and your species for all that it does for us. I truly had no idea. Thank you. If you ever need us we will come to your aid, just ask as the bird do." and he stands turns and nods at Herfermks, smiles and starts trotting toward the trees.

Jay watches him go and turns to Herfermks "what a change in attitude".

Herfermks says "he was so much easier to find agreements from after he had several good meals." then looking at Sihiryan "what about the blue light beings?"

She takes out her tablet and scans the area, "they are not showing up now." Holding her tablet out toward Herfermks, "see if you can locate them.

He takes her tablet and works the screen for a few moments, then takes his out and holds it on top of hers and works on it's screen. "Huum, I see they were here but they keep a good distance from the wearodes. That is interesting. The wearodes can see things that my scanners hardy pick up and some things that were unknown to our technologies." he looks at Jay and holds out his hand toward him. "Your tablet please Jay" As Jay hands it to him Herfermks starts to fade and changes position a bit.

"Can you find them now?" Jay asks as Herfermks hand reaches Jay's tablet. Herfermks stacks Jays tablet under Sihiryan and his. He mutters something half under his breath and works the screen on his again then taps it's screen several times. "Well they are interesting, we will have to wait until the wearode is further away then they will be more likely to come forward so we can interact with them.

Jay asks, "Come forward?"

Hefermks notices that Sihiryan has an inquisitive look on her face. "Well, they seem to almost be out of time. It is as if they are in a wider spectrum of physical reality than us, and out of synchronicity with our time matrix. I have never seen anything quite like it."

"So they are not fully in out physical reality?" Jay asks.

Herfermks looks at Jay then at Sihiryan then works his tablet some more. "Not quite" Herfermks says, "it is more like we are almost able to peek into their reality from this more limited one. But from what I can detect of them we can only access their reality even to perceive it while they are in our presence here in ours".

Jay looks at Sihiryan "well, I guess it is all up to them then. They have to want us to know about them or they can simply avoid us and we will never learn about them."

Herfermks look up from his tablet at Jay and Sihiryan. Hesitates and says, "yeah, that is about it. From what I can tell from my scans they will know that I scanned for them, they will know that we talked about what I learned from those scans. So they will either not meld into our reality while we are in an area of it. That is what they seem to do about the wearodes. Or they will make it clear of their desire to contact us, or continue to ignore us."

Jay looks at Herfermks. "Well, is there a way we can leave them a message that they could understand? I can understand why they may not want to interact with the wearodes, maybe they are concerned about what flavour the wearodes would consider them." Jay makes a face with tight lips and raised eyebrows, "If they know we are friendly with the wearods and now posses technology to find them and track them they may not be so friendly to us. Leaving them a friendly message or invitation to be friends could be in our best interest." Jay sees the looks on Sihiryan and Herfermks faces. "If they have a vaster reality than ours they may have ways to affect our reality that we will not have control over."

Herfermks looks at his tablet and works it with his fingers. Sihiryan gets close enough to Herfermks to see what he is doing on his screen. Then she taps her tablet to the bottom of his and starts working her screen too. And they both nod as they continue to work their tablets independently.

Herfermks stops and looks at Jay, "what would you say?"

Jay looks around the forest and then at the ground as he thinks for a moment. "Thank them for their tolerance and interest in our reality and ask them if they would like to have communications with us," nodding his head he adds, " I think making the point that we are varied species that cooperate with each other may make us more interesting to communicate with."

Sihiryan looks at Jay, her tablet then at Herfermks, "It makes sense to me. If we found out that four collaborating predator species just found a way to scan and track us we would make preparations for war. If we don't make a friendly introduction we could have a big problem soon."

Herfermks still working his tablet starts slowly nodding. "Yes, I can produce a message that they should be able to receive, but I can't be sure they will, or that they will pay attention to it."

Jay asks, "If they notice the message will they understand what it means right away?"

"Humm", Herfermks looks up from his tablet "good question Jay, they may not expect us to communicate with them. I will place the message in enough situations that they can't ignore it. I will have the reception of it monitored so that we can know when it is noticed and when it is reacted to. I will search folklore to see if there were ever communications with these being in the history of the alliance and if there was; I will research those interactions to see what we can expect." Putting down his tablet he sits on the ground and pulls a canister out of the pouch on his side. He opens it and looks inside then looks around the meadow, "this is really a great place to spend time on Ramga" and has a sip from his canister. Licking his lips before continuing "I hope the messages work. We may not know for a long time."

Jay asks "don't you think they will respond right away?"

Having another sniff of his canister, looking at Jay for a second before having another sip, then looking at Sihiryan. "We don't know what they know Jay. Without knowing what they know it is uncertain how they will see our invitation to communicate. For instance, they may have had science teams studying all of our species for thousands of years. Or they may be more like the wearodes than we are but can't actually digest things from our reality. We will wait and see. Maybe they will finally find us interesting enough to invade now that they know we are intelligent enough to attempt communication with them."

"So you like the meadow?" Sihiryan asks as she walks toward him. "I like it too the birds chose a great spot for us", and she sits in front of him but to his left.

Jay sees the hint and sits with them making the triangle about equal with them. "I like it here too". He looks at the worried look on Herfermks face. "I don't know if I want to stay here the full 9 years but I do like it here."

Hefermks looks across at Jay and smiles "yes, I like the way you think Jay. How are you doing with being back here Jay?"

It is good, I was only gone one day so it is, well actually it is a little odd that things changed so much, but somehow it seems the same to me. I wasn't really that familiar with how it was so the changes don't seem that different. I am starting to look forward to being on the moon for a few years." turning to Sihiryan. No offence Sihiryan, I love your company and Ramga but the pace of new and exciting events is starting to make me a little jittery."

Sihiryan smiles at Jay and says nothing.

Herfermks smiles and nods at her. "Jay you have handled stress excessively well. I have been asked about your ability to deal with the events by many researchers. It is good that you realize that it is effecting you."

"It's ok, I don't mind the stress, mostly I see it as excitement. But I have to admit there have been a few things that I worried about." Nodding his head he says "the wearode, that was difficult for me. Thank you so much for turning him to see things differently."

Sihiryan say,s "we wouldn't have let him eat you Jay, he has no idea how fierce we are."

Jay bursts into laughter, "yes we are a fierce lot aren't we, but I feel that with his long claws and teeth, and with his vastness, that he may have had a claw full and a bite of me if it came to violence."

Herfermks laughs, "yes Jay you are likely correct. He is surprisingly fast for a creature of his size. Hunting with him was a joy. He can move as well as anything I have ever seen. I think he was right when he told Quaraktutu that he was no match for him. And cunning, he taught me a few new tricks for hunting. I too am glad he was wise enough to understand his need to let you and other guests of ours to live." He smiles at them. "What will you two do today here in the forest?

Sihiryan picks a flower and puts it in her mouth and starts chewing it.

Jay says "I think she may have some more things to tell me about how I need to behave so that I don't get investigated and we will find some wild food, and rest and play." He looks at Herfemks "Oh, there is a hot pool in the cave up the hill, it is good for your health to float in it."

"Jay I am heavier than I look, I may not float in it!"
Herfermks says. Taking out his scanner and fiddling with it,
"humm, I might. I will like to try this, will you be going back
there today?"

Sihiryan says "we could" and she gets up, "come on lets go
now" and starts walking.

Jay looks at Herfermks and sees him watching Sihiryan as she
walks away from them. Jay starts getting up to follow her.
Herfermks stands as Jay starts to walk and walks beside Jay.
"That was quick" Jay says.

"Yes" Herfermks agrees. "I can't get accustomed to the look of
the back of a female without the tail. You think I would, but to
me it looks odd." After a few more steps, "I don't mind you
and her relating the way you do, I know that Kyranins are like
this openly all of the time. If you want to be with her while I
am here I can look the other way Jay."

Jay thinks about what he just heard as he walks with his friend
for a moment before thinking what to say. "Well thank you sir,
I don't think She will want to do anything while you are here
with us."

Herfermks turns his head to Jay, "should I leave?"

Jay looks back silently for a split second then starts to laugh. "hahaha, No, no, that is not what I meant. We are happy to spend some time with you. We won't feel like having sex while we are visiting with the three of us. At least I won't. The activity of conversing with good friends is a priority for my species. I think it is for the kyranins too."

"You know Jay, the situation of my work takes me to many cultures with species of various social development. I wanted to be sure that nothing would be awkward," Herfermks says. "Jay I could tell you some stories that would shock you about what is normal in some places. I know things that happen on earth that are repulsive are kept hidden. This is part of what gives me hope for your species. Not that it hides it but that it has to be hidden from those who would object."

"What do you mean?" Jay looks at him.

"Well Jay" Herfermks says "you know about the various forms of physical abuse, forced work without reward, and segregation and oppression that takes place on your planet, the terrible things that happen to some children, the senseless killing for entertainment, the executions to free up property for financial gain. Those things Jay, in the countries that could stop these things, most of the humans have no idea of the details of how and where or how much it is happening. The events are hidden form them. They urge their governments to prevent these atrocities and believe that they are not happening in their parts of the world."

Jay thinks for some seconds as they walk. "I hadn't thought too much about it Herfermks" after several steps, "I see what you mean. I agree. If all humans actually knew how much these things were happening they might do more to prevent it." Jay gets a serious scowl on his face and looks at the ground for a few steps. I don't know how to help to change things there. The systems are so complicated that wield control over human media and publicly shared information. I don't know what could be done."

Herfermks puts his hand on Jay's back. "Let me look for some things that could be done while you are on the moon Jay." Herfermks looks ahead "where did she go?"

Jay points "behind those trees is the entrance to the cave with the pool." as they approach the trees in front of the cave opening Jay asks "would you like to go in first?"

Herfermks bends down and looks between the branches, "No Jay. You go ahead I will see how you do it then I'll come in."

Jay pushes through the trees and crouches to go through the hole. As he does he looks back behind him and can't see

Herfermks. He goes a little further until he can stand up straight then a few more steps and turns on his tablet light. "How did you get in here?"

"Well Jay, I watched you clamoring in that hole like a vermin in a burrow and I thought it was too small for me. So here is where I entered the cave; will that dirt from the entrance walls stain your new skin Jay?"

Jay smiles and laughs, "stain my skin, hahaha"

Sihiryan tells her tablet to brighten and calls to them "boys, the water is fine come on in."

Herfermks look around the cave, I think some food and snacks would be appropriate and fades out of view, then back in with a table and a tall cabinet. He folds out two side of the cabinet to expose some plumbing controls and pulls out a shower-head near the top. Walking around to the back he opens a door and exposes some towels stacked inside. He strokes a few buttons on the side and a light glows from the top and spot-lights shine in various places on the cave walls. He turns to the table and points, "some kreptigs for you Jay, and these on this side, under the glass, that is for me." turning to Sihiryan, "Wine?" waving his hand over the table, "I have many of the snacks that you like here and a few things that you can't get on ramga to try."

Jay looks at the variety of snacks on the table and the selection of wine in the box under it and smiles. He takes off his pouch and takes a kreptig in his hand putting the end of it into his mouth as he walk toward the pool. "mm, it is good, would you like a bite Sihiryan?"

Sihiryan floating all stretched out, "maybe latter Jay. I could enjoy some music though"

Jay turns and sees Herfermks working the screen of his tablet and hears the sound of a band softly playing some music. It is odd but soothing to Jay's ear. He smiles to himself as he enters the pool and hears Herfemks stepping into the water behind him. "Sir the rock may be sharp in the deeper water."

"Thanks Jay" Herfermks says and dives into the pond from knee deep making a slash and disappearing into the water where it is deeper.

Jay takes a few more steps, and finds him-self starting to float a little as his chest is entering the water. He turns and leans back and his feet and knees float out. He relaxes and his head sinks so that his ears are part out of the water, just enough so he can hear. Working his tongue to get the rest of the flavor of the kreptig he starts to think about how effective the technology is that they used to change his form. "Sihiryan, is the technology that you used on me to make me into a kyranin used for medical repairs also?"

Sihiryan paddles with her arms so she can see his face before she answers. "No, actually it is still secret from the kyranins."

Herfermks surfaces and tries to float like them.

Jay asks, "wouldn't this technology provide great enough health benefits that it could be considered as something that should be shared for the benefit of the alliance?"

She replies. "We have talked about that with the various health authorities on ryberia and research has been done. Not to try to get it used that way but to be sure that we are within correct use of technology if we have to explain things that it is being used for. As it turns out it would only provide a slight statistical improvement in the overall wellbeing and longevity of Kyranins or Ambursts. Our own medical systems are effective and well implemented."

Herfermks asks, "Are you talking about the form changing technology we used on Jay? It is not as effective on all species Jay. If we use it on ourselves there is a slight risk of side effects each time, so that if we use it more than 10 times the accumulative risks almost ensure some minor deformity that

takes decades to recover from. Actually a few ryberians
have died from using it too much. For the amburst it only has
a temporary effect most of the time, lasting maybe a hundred
years. With them the side effects start to show after four or five
uses. The kyranins don't change back as easily so once
changed they are stuck with the effects. If they use it ten times
they have perception shifts that seem to affect their ability to
learn new physical skills. We do use on many species, for some
medical emergencies. It can be the difference of life and death
in many situations and we use it without explaining what our
medical technology is in those cases. But it is too dangerous to
share this type of technology with most species. The
experiments that they would do to try to understand it better
could have wide spread repercussions through entire planets,
and the resulting aftermath could destroy the alliance and
many of the species that thrive in it now."

Jay thinks about it, thinking how earth scientists experimented
with bombs and lobotomies, and electro shock therapy and
torcher, and GMO foods, he starts to nod his head. "I suppose
it is best to keep the more dangerous tools away from the
babies."

Sihiryan looks at Jay "what?"

Jay looks at her, "On earth we have to put everything that can
harm a baby out of it's reach before it learns to stand up or it
will inevitably find the dangerous objects and do something
with to hurt itself. Maybe do something very dangerous to
others as well. It is a concept that only parents have to think

about. As a result the children are in danger whenever the parents take them to any other environment. It is like with his technology, it is safe if he uses it but if it gets in the hands of the less benevolent, or the less meticulously careful it will make unforeseen problems for the users in a short time."

She looks at him, "A metaphor. It suggests that many members of the alliance are babies?"

Jay looks at her. "It reflects a similarity of relationships between those who control the environment for infants and those who have an opportunity to control some aspect of the environment for ambitious externally motivated beings."

Sihiryan looks at him for a second, "do you mean us Jay?" as she starts to smile at him.

"Not specifically us, but yes I do mean us!" Jay continues. "I know that my kind would do some stupidly thoughtless experiments to start with; then try many other things in their attempts to correct the damage, if they had something like this technology. Hahaha, it wouldn't be long after getting some technology like this that my species would find a way to have a catastrophe with it. Hahaha, I am sorry to find it so funny but it is so serious that I can only laugh. When I think about the hysteria of those involved with it, and some of them trying to find a way to make some windfall profit from a side use of it. They would risk anything to get a result that could have a market. Hahaha you have no idea the things that could happen if this technology was learned by the powers in control on earth now." he looks at Herfermks. "For the first time I actually understand what is meant by the old proverb – with great power comes a greater responsibility."

Herfemrks strokes one arm so that his body spins part way around and his face is in view of Jay. "It is such a relief to hear you say that Jay. Your world is a safer place because of your clear thinking."

Jay looks at the cave ceiling and listens to the music. He listens to Sihiryan and Herfermks joke about what various species would try to do if they had the technology and about what the results of the use of it would bring about. He feels the pressure of the thick water against his skin and the sensation that the salts and minerals cause in his skin. Looking over at Herfermks he realizes that he actually is not floating that well. He sees that Herfermks' face is only out of the water enough so he can breath and talk. There are bits of him that do show above the water but not much. Lifting his head to look at himself he sees that he is only about half submerged. Jay thinks about how dense Herfermks body must be compared to his. He looks at Sihiryan, she is floating like him, about halfway out of the water. "Herfemks? How can your body be so much more dense than ours?"

Herfermks looks at Jay "It is my chemistry Jay. My cell membranes have a lot more minerals than yours. My bone's matrix has more metallic minerals than the calcium based crystal of human bones. My DNA has more than two strands, the space between the electron clouds that hold my molecules together is slightly less as a result, and the nucleuses of my atoms are on average much bigger. More mass, more of me for the gravity to pull on, that's all. Its is not complicated Jay." Turning his head to look at Jay, "why do you ask?"

Sihirian looks at Jay too, curious to hear his answer.

"Well" Jay starts, "it is interesting to me, all of it, the cultures, the various species, the history, the politics, and the science. But it is more interesting when it is to do with those that I know and care about. I am a spiritual being but I don't believe in mystery. I know that there is some reason for everything to be the way that it is... I guess I am just constantly curious."

Herfermks turns his head back to look at the ceiling again "that is what makes you interesting and useful Jay."

Sihiryan shifts her view to Herfermks for a second before looking back at the ceiling to relax fully again.

"That is interesting, I never thought about it before. But that is what drew me to get to know you better when we first met Jay, your curiosity. Not all being are curious you know. The vwortex don't seem to be. The birds are only a little. The amburst, some are and some arn't. Kyranins are only curious about things that they find pleasure in. Well most of them, the ones that go in for science are curious or is it the process of researching that they enjoy. Herfermks do you see kyranins as curious?"

"A little" Herfermks pauses, "I have only seen a few creatures as curious as Jay though. According to the information that Reggie collected a lot of humans are curious like Jay. But not all of them are benevolent with what they learn." He rolls on his side then treads water slightly for balance with his neck and head out of the water. Since the treaty with the pixies Jay, it has been possible for us to study your species and planet more closely. Since they are actually the technologically dominant species from your world we are able to classify your species as a species of interest and they have granted our science departments full access to do as we choose, hahaha, they have no idea what they gave us. Lucky for you it is only ryberia that has a treaty with them, they haven't actually joined the alliance yet, we are still within the scope of the in term arrangement that you helped me get." he makes eye contact with Jay before continuing. "Jay it seems that most of the species on your planet are highly susceptible to learned or imprinted behavior patterns as infants and youth. This is why things don't seem to change for the better."

Jay is looking into his eyes and thinking about what and how he told him. He thinks it must be more important than it sounds or he wouldn't have told him in this manner. "Ok,. That is good to know, what can I do with this information?"

Herfermks swims to the shore and takes a shower using the tall box he brought and starts to towel himself off. "Jay think about it a lot, that is always a good start to a great outcome." He steps over to the table with the towel draped over his shoulders. He licks his lips as he looks into the glass tank with his food in it. Then reaches to a bowl and takes a kreptig and crunches it. "There isn't a lot you can do yet Jay. Time will give us opportunities and when you are ready you can do your best."

Sihiryan turns over and floats face down for a moment then swims to shore and walks to the table. "Thank you Herfermks this is a great choice of foods. Will you have trouble justifying the expenses to the department?"

"No I paid for this and the delivery myself, from Ryberian accounts, from ryberia.

It is a little thank you gift for all your friendship and kindness to me and to the others on the teams these many years."

Sihiryan picks up and eats a few snacks and then looks at the shower, "Is there enough water for us too?"

"hohoho, yes Sihiryan, have a shower there is towels enough too." He smiles.

Jay comes out of the water and walks to the table. He looks at the various things to choose from. He recognizes a few and takes something he knows he likes, a pastry with fish in it that was cooked in a slightly spicy sauce. While savoring it's flavor he watches the creature in the glass that Herfermks is likely going to eat soon. It has very short fur, a head that moves like a turtle's and four legs that move like a spider's, no tail. "What is it?"

"Well," Herfermks laughs, "the curiosity can't be stopped. They eat grass and bugs, they don't communicate with their own species. If you eat a leg first they look with curiosity as you chew and sometimes try to reach to bite the edge of the wound. They can make sounds and some do seemingly randomly. Most don't. They are tasty, a little sticky in the throat but only for a minute. If they are cooked they are poisonous to us both. The things that live inside of them would give you a slow painful death if you ate one raw, but those things are easily digested and very nutritious to me. They don't move fast so they are a good snack to keep around. They bread very often and give birth every few weeks."

"Rabbits and rodents are fast breading on earth like that, they are food for many species. But both are very social creatures." Jay says.

Herfermks takes the glass lid off and picks up the creature with his other hand, replaces the lid and steps well back from Jay and the table. "You won't want its fluids on your food Jay" as he moves back a few more steps. "The planets that these grow on are good for hunting, nothing there is intelligent. Some creatures are dangerous though. There are three planets with them. Some hundreds of thousands of years ago a species that controlled and farmed on all three planets got into a serious civil war and used weapons with radioactive and toxic after effects. The results are three planets with genetically similarities. Each planet has some of it's own species and many that are common to them all. The slight variance in details of the species from planet to planet suggests that there was some travel for a long time after the war. But none of that species survived. Now none of the creatures on any of those three worlds has much intellectual capacity. The one with the most ruins is too radioactive and toxic to eat from still."

Jay looks at him for a minute thinking about it as he watches Herfermk petting and playing with his food. "Wow. That is unthinkable, that they wiped themselves out. Are you sure they didn't get attacked from some other place?"

Herfermks says "We checked, we went back and watched." he makes a face and shrugs and looks at his food then takes a bit, like you would bite a sandwich. As he chews he looks at Jay watching him and the still living creature. The creature doesn't seem to be bothered by the wound from Herfermks bite. He swallows. "It was shocking to see the escalation of the atrocities and the stupidity of the leaders through it all. It was like they believed that they would gain some great value from defeating their own species; and they would do, they did do the most unthinkable things to each other." He takes another bite.

Jay looks at the creature, still moving in Herfermks hand, it is not trying to get away or seeming to be in pain at all. It is dripping and looking around. It looks at a part of itself dangling between Hefermks fingers and tries to get its mouth there but can't reach. Jay hears a phrase in his head 'the meek shall inherit the earth' and he feels a shiver go through him as Herfermks takes another bite.

Sihiryan steps beside him toweling her self off and he thinks and says "my turn" and goes to the shower.

"Tasty?" she asks as he is putting the last of it into his mouth.

Nodding as he chews he point to the table and swallows. "Anything you like?"

"I would like most of it but I can't eat that much?" turning back to face him she smiles, "I am so honored to have you do this for me Herfermks. It is so rare that we get to do anything other than short meetings and training tutorials. I am melting inside with your tone of friendship.

Herfermks looks at her for a second. "Don't expect it all the time. You know I put work first too often."

"You do" she says and takes a pastry from the table and pops it into her mouth, smiling at him as she chews.

"I do enjoy your friendship too, and your work is always so complete. I haven't ever praised you for it have I?" he steps toward the table and picks up a napkin. "I have thought about it many times while off on projects that were going well because your part of the job was done so competently. Thank You Sihiryan for all of your many efforts. I hope to continue to enjoy your work companionship for many years, and I will happily be your friend there after."

Sihiryan finishes chewing and turns a little to be more directly facing him "I agree sir, I will be your friend for the rest of my days, anything I can do for you just ask and it will be done."

Jay walks over as he towels himself off "this seems a little formal to me, is it culturally correct to be formal when talking about friendship?"

Herfermks looks at Jay as Sihirian starts talking. "Jay there is nothing more permanent than friendship, it is like family except from a choice rather than from breading. Lovers come and go, we all have families and they will help us if they can. A friend will do what ever you need done even at a risk to them selves. A friend wouldn't ask you to put yourself in danger for them. A friend will always be happy to see you even at a bad time. It is a feeling of love that has nothing to do with sex that actual friendship makes, or is. To admit these feeling is a formal event for Rybreians."

Jay finishes drying himself as he listens and thinks about what she said. He puts the towel over one shoulder and steps to the table and takes a bottle of juice and pours some into a glass. He lifts it to his mouth and has a sip. And walks to the far side of them from the table and looks at them both. "On earth, in the culture where I am from, friends are sometimes what you said but not always. Some humans are fickle with there friendship it only lasts a short time, while it is convenient. I hope one day that you will feel the bonds of friendship with me as I do with you both."

Herfermks reaches to the table and picks up a flask, takes off the lid as he looks inside and his smile grows, then looks at Sihiryan to see her nod at him. Turning to Jay and smiling as Sihiryan gets herself a beverage from the table, "Jay we feel your friendship and we feel it for you too" he lifts his glass and looks to Sihiryan.

Sihiryan smiles at Herfermks and then looks directly into Jays eyes,, lifts her glass and says "Jay I am your friend, for as long as you live."

Herfermks says "Jay we are friends and I will keep you alive a long time." Making a gesture with his beverage "should we drink to friendship."

"Here hear," Sihiriyan says as she makes a gesture with her glass.

Jay smiles and straightens his posture lifting his glass to eye level "to friendship."

After they drink Jay asks "where did you get the 'here here' from Sihiryan?"

"It was in a report from Reggie. We had him working in several places on earth, England uses that for your drinking ritual in formal situations he said."

Jay thinks of Reggie, on the fishing boat, and starts to laugh. "When I came back to this time I left Reggie on a fishing boat waiting for me to come out of the bathroom. Hahaha he had to use the toilet and that was three days ago for me now. In my time line he will be waiting many years."

Herfermks looks at Jay, "we will get you back to the same moment you left he won't have to wait long."

"I know that he will find me getting out of that room almost right after going in but I am still new to the time thing and the idea of me being here camping and then having a career and stuff while he is waiting for me to come out of the bathroom seems pretty funny." Jay smiles.

Sihiryan looks at Jay for a second, "Yeah, I get it I can see how it has humor."

Herfermks looks at the floor for a second then at Jay, then at Sihiryan so he is waiting for you to come out of the bathroom after ten years so he can go in and relieve himself, hahaha, yes haha, I see it I get the humor now, that is funny when you think of it like that, hahaha, and Jay you are likely not certain that you will make it back right? He may be waiting a long time."

Sihiryan turns her head a little sideways and looks at Jay, "That would be funny, how long do you think he would wait before going in if you don't come back?"

Jay laughs, Not too long I hope, one of the others would probably come down to use the toilet too then he would have to explain why he is waiting to use a washroom when it is empty."

Herfermks looks at Jay "what others?"

Jay replies "I had to talk to him and wanted to help him learn more about human behaviors and interactions so I took him out on a boat fishing with a friend and his brother-in-law. We caught some fish then the captain took us to a cove beside a beach to have lunch. That is when he got the answer to send me back."

"a captain? Did you leave him with the military?" Sihiryan asks.

"No it was a charter boar, it is a title for anyone who controls the operations of a boat, a water going vessel. It is a private boat. The captain makes his income from taking humans out on the water to catch fish. We caught four, one each. Reggie seemed to like it and was getting better at making conversation. When we first met he was not very good at it. He told me it was difficult for him to know when to say things."

"When you get back you can help him for a few days while we are organizing your work there then."

Herfermks says and then slowly finishes his drink as he watches Sihiryan looking at Jay with a curious expression. "What are you thinking Sihiryan?"

"About the thoughts in Jay's mind; how Reggie is stopped in time while Jay is here for so many years, and poor Reggie's bladder is wanting relief."

"hahaha, when you put it like that I can see why Jay laughed so hard" Herfermks says and smiles at Jay.

Sihiryan turns to Herfermks and looks very serious. "It can cause a lot of difficulties when one time travels and changes things."

Jay says "it can be confusing for those who travel too, and dangerous too I suspect."

Herfermks nods, "a lot can be affected if we are not careful. When I travel there is a team that watches what is affected from back on ryberia. If there is anything that causes a discrepancy in the normal activities of living things the causative events are found and I have to go back and correct them. It does get confusing sometimes for me. So I only travel in time when it is very important." and he gives Jay a look of seriousness.

Jay responds, "Really, so is my time travel form earth to here, now also watched?"

Herfermks nods and says "there are safeties in place for all time travel that is why when some unauthorized time travel occurs the traveler can loose their right to time travel." After a short silence "one time I arrived on a world and was attacked by three locals. They tried to rob me! The entire incident was observed by several hidden local beings so I had to go back seven times to clean up the mess. They were going to start a religion about me, they raised a small army to defend against me, one of the attackers died and his children weren't born and thus did not become the great benevolent rulers that started a dynasty of peaceful governments in that area for the next thousand years, One of the onlookers was killed for being insane when he first mentioned the incident, then after the others confirmed the story those that did the execution were killed, and as a result the village became polarized and never prospered into the city that is now a great capital of the most socially advance part of that world." He smiles and looks at Sihiryan "That was a long time ago and now I am much more carful."

Jay takes some more treats from the table and pops one in his mouth. He gives a nod of surprised satisfaction to Herfermks as he chews. Sihiryan looks at the table and takes a snack from Jay's hand and pops it in her mouth. Herfermks smiles and picks up a lidded bowl from the table and holds it out between the three of them. He looks at them both finishing their chewing and opens the lid "would you like some local worms, I caught them this morning."

Sihiryan looks at them, "they look still fresh" as she puts her fingers in to lift out several. Dangling them in front of her face to look at them for a second, then her mouth opens and she puts them in. I few movements of her jaw moving and "mmmm."

Jay feels his heart pounding. He knows he wants to but the fear of the unknown is trying to freeze him. His hand reaches and his fingers go into the bowl as he watches, the feeling of the moist comes between his fingers, then as he grips them, they wind onto him. He feels the fear from them as he brings his hand toward his face, up above his eye level. With a deep breath Jay looks at them, tilts his head back, opens his mouth, and in they go. Closing his lips to pull them from their grip on his fingers Jay feels them moving in his mouth. On his tongue, against his cheeks and he feels the vibration of their terror as he starts to bit down into them. Then the juice from them comes into his mouth, as his second bite happens he starts to experience their flavor. His eyes open wide and "uummmmmm" some more chewing, and a swallow. "Oh my god! Those are delicious. I would have never guessed a smooth succulent slightly sour flavor, that almost tingles."

Herfermks looks at him and hastily dumps the remains of the worms in his own mouth, and chews as he starts to smile.

Sihiryan looks at Jay with wide eyes, "we'll catch some tomorrow morning Jay."

Herfermks adds "You looked so excited with the flavor of live food I thought I better have some before you hand grabbed the rest Jay. Was that your first time eating live food?"

Jay thinks for a second, "that I am aware of. I have eaten yogurt but I don't think bacteria counts as live food does it?"

The three of them talk about various foods and beverages as they slowly finish the food on the table. Then they talk about getting Jay to the Gyrekian moon and Herfermks packs up his shower and table and leaves with them. Sihiryan and Jay make their ways to the creek for a refreshing bath then to the meadow to lay down in the sun before it slides down behind the mountain. They watch the stars coming into view as Jay talks about earth and Sihiryan makes comparisons with situations on alliance planets. When the moon is high and Jay starts to feel his eyes closing they go back to the grass bed. Jay gets comfortable and Sihiryan snuggles up beside him. In the morning Jay wakes to hear the sound of some small creature eating the grass of the bed near his head. When it sees him move and open his eyes it bolts. Jay closes his eyes and goes back to sleep. When he next awakes he feels cool where Sihiryan was against him. He sits up and looks around at the grass and shrubs. Then he listens and hears soft foot-steps from the between trees to his left. He watches as Sihiryan appears from behind some bushes and trees.

"You are awake", she says as she continues toward him. "Let's go get those worms Jay."

Jay looks at her walking towards him, naked, looking great to his still blurry eyes. He thinks about where he is for a second and as she walks closer smiling at him he considers what she just said. 'Worms' he thinks 'are we going fishing?' then he remembers, 'worms to eat' "Oh." Then remembering the day before in the cave, "oh yeah, the worms" and he starts to get up. Looking around for his clothes he remembers that he has been naked for two days, in the forest. 'I could use a coffee' he thinks to himself. Standing and looking around as she reaches him, steps up close, and gives him a hug and a kiss on the cheek. He smiles at her and says "good morning, too bad we can't have a murrk right now"

"A little sleepy Jay?" giving him a little soft slap on his butt, "wake up my friend, it's time for worms!" grabbing his left hand with her right she starts walking towards the shady side of the valley with Jay in tow.

Jay stumbles his first step and catches his balance to make a few fast steps to get beside her.

"Breath Jay, it will help wake you up faster. We got about an hour until the worms are going to hide from the sun. They are not all good to eat so you will have to pay attention to what the good ones look like. The ones with a green sheen are ok but not as tasty, the ones with a slightly blue sheen will leave a sticky feel in your mouth unless you eat them with the grimbin flowers, the small pink ones in the patches of round leaves close to the ground. The ones with a clear sheen are the good ones. The ones with a yellow sheen will make you feel like vomiting for the whole day. So look carefully before you put one in your mouth."

Jay takes another deep breath and says, "clear sheen is good, colour sheen is bad. I'm going to eat worms. Haha hahaha."

"And you are going to like it Jay" Sihiryan laughs, "I'm like a childhood friend but in reverse Jay. I'm older and want you to eat worms because you will be so glad you did." She turns and smiles at him, "and if you mention having eaten worms to any kyranins they will envy you and want to come with you next time so you can show them how to get the good ones."

Jay laughs. "I want to eat them. If I was more awake I might talk myself out of it so lets find one quickly".

Sihiryan laughs and looks at Jay with his effort to open his eyes more than a squint. She sees some large flat rocks between some shrubs and asks "Jay look down here" as she lets go of his hand and gets on her hands and knees. "See under these branches" as she pulls them up "see them on the rock?"

"Yeah" Jay says

Picking one up and holding it out of the shade in front of him, "what color do you see on the sheen?"

Jay looks at it as the sun reflects off or it. "It is... hard to tell I don't see any color."

"yeah, its a good one" and she pops it in her mouth. Pointing at another one.

Jay picks it up and looks at it, "I think it has blue."

She picks up another one, "Yeah, that's not a good one this is though and she pops it in her mouth."

Jay put the worm down and grabs another one. He sees her take another directly to her mouth. He looks at his closely and thinks it is clear. He starts moving it toward his mouth.

"Do you trust that worm Jay?" Sihiryan asks

He holds it up between them to look at it as she leans toward him; he repplies "Yes" as she grabs it just before he pops it into his mouth "hey! That is my worm."

"Mmm" and she bites it in half, "you don't want this one Jay! Look at it all sticky and squirmy. What will it do in your mouth Jay?

Jay looks at her and grabs it pulling what is left of it out from her loose grip "that's my worm, I want to eat it" and he pops it into his mouth and laughs with his smile then starts to chew. His eyes close and he sits on the ground as he savors the flavor. Then looks at her for a second before he turns and starts looking under the next bush over. He finds some and then more until they both have eaten their fill of the little things.

Sihiryan suggests they go to the creek to wash and Jay takes the lead through the trees. As they are sitting in the creek to wash off the worm slime Jay offers to do the ritual for friendship for her. Sihiryan looks at Jay and with a smile and a sincere explanation she declines. Jay is surprised but with the explanation that it would be a ritual for him, that she already had done it for her, and that she was feeling pretty good about how well it worked.

"Thank you for offering though Jay. If you feel you need to do it to be ok with us not being lovers again now we can do it", she adds.

"No" Jay said "I am comfortable with our friendship" he smiles at her, "I will always feel closer to you because of our physical intimacy but I understand that will be just friends now."

She looks at him for a moment. "Maybe sometimes we can be lovers but not for a while Jay, I don't want anything serious that could influence my ability to do my work. We will be working together and I want to be able to focus on what we are doing with work, not be thinking when we will be able to do what with you in me."

Jay smiles at her and nods his head. "Good point. I would be thinking similar thoughts." He stands up and walks out of the creek, "what should we do now?"

Sihiryan stands in the creek and looks around. She walks out of the creek towards the meadow and looks around then turns to Jay, "I am satisfied with our camping experience. If you can't think of anything you want to do I am ready to go back."

Jay looks at her with the sun at her back and searches his mind for desires, "mmm, no, can't think of anything should we go get our clothes first before we call the birds?"

Sihiryan replies "sure" as she turns and starts walking to the big tree.

Jay starts to follow thinking to himself as he walks. 'I still am not fully relaxed with seeing a naked woman. It is so programed in me that a naked woman means I should want sex. It can't be natural. In nature we would all be naked. It must be learned. As babies we think nothing of nudity, it is only after we learn to talk that we are taught to cover up our genitals, it must start from that young. I remember at about four I was curious, I was curious because women sat down to pee and had no penis to pee from, I was curious about that. Then I saw TV movies, the innuendo of sexual attraction. It seemed so special and important in the movies. There was a lot of mystery and that made it interesting. But I still didn't know about sex, so, it was as a pre teen time, maybe I was 9, no younger maybe 6, mm no 5! The other kids.. Yeah, Billy down the street saw his parents doing it that's right, we talked about it often that summer. By the end of the summer I was craving to do anything with a girl. We got some playboy or penthouse magazines, yeah. I remember, I didn't get what all the fuss was at first. I thought it was just some moms in a magazine until they told me that these were not moms!, The were play-boy-bunnies, center folds, Miss August, Miss June , Miss July.' Jay smiles to himself walking across the meadow several steps behind Sihiryan. 'I do remember', he thinks to himself. 'I wanted to see every girl I met for the next several years naked. And I had them so high on a pedestal because they could become a center fold model and be so special, or a mom and it would be wrong to think what I was thinking of them. That's why I was so shy with girls all the way through school until I was about 16. All those years of desire, those impressionable years, my entire youth I was fixating on what a naked woman was. All my friends seemed to be doing the same thing.' He looks ahead at Sihiryan as she approaches the tree. He sees her naked as a friend without any sexual content in his thoughts. He watches as she walks and turns to reach for the cloths exposing a full view of her genitals to him and his eyes are pulled to her hand trying to reach the clothes. With a quick few steps towards her and the tree he says, "here let me get them I'm taller." Noticing his urge to help his good friend and realizing that he has no feeling at all about her being naked in front of him. As she steps back to allow him room to stand under the branch he goes up on his toes and with a little hop he grabs them. He hears her laugh and looks to see her looking up from his genitals to his face.

"I always like the way they bounce when males jump." she says.

Jay smiles, "yeah, they are funny things dangling down there aren't they?" and he looks at her handing her clothes to her. He sees that her nipples are hard. Looking up into her eyes he smiles and watches her as she takes the clothes from his hand and smiles back at him.

She gets dressed and looks up. She sees a bird crossing the sky at a great height and says to Jay "there's one".

Jay starts to wave his hands in the air "I don't see it" He looks at Sihiryan as she point to above the mountain across the valley and Jay turns, still waving his hands.

Sihiryan asks, "Where did it go?"

Jay stops waiving and puts his cloths on as fast as he can. As he is doing up his pants there is a swishing sound and moving air and then the sound of flapping wings. The bird lands almost between them.

It looks at Jay doing up his shirt buttons, and then Sihiryan putting on her clothes. "Did I land too fast?"

Jay stops what he was doing and looks at the bird, "I'm not sure, it was fast but how did it feel to you?"

The bird looks at Jay then turns it's head onto one side and continues to look at him. "Felt good to me what about the two of you?"

Jay look at Sihiryan and then back at the bird, "well she is usually ok with being seen naked, but if it bothers you then maybe you did land too fast. From my side it seems like you landed just about perfect." Then turning to Sihiryan as she is putting on her top, "What do you think, did it seem like he,.." then Jay stops talking and looks at the bottom of the bird, then at the beak and back to Sihiryan

"Did it seem like he landed too fast?"

Sihiryan looks at Jay then sees him wink at her. "Well,, I could have been dressed when you arrived, but you are here now and I am happy about that,, so, uummmm, No, you landed great." She looks at the bird.

The bird steps back. And looks at both of them. "Hey, that's not fair, I'm the one who is suppose to give you a hard time."

Jay chuckles. " I'm sorry. My name is Jay and this in my friend Sihiryan, What is your name sir?"

"Shyruk" looks at Jay for a second then "well, what were you waiving for?"

Jay turns to face Shyruk, "Shyruk, we would like to go back to the city, Shiyhra. Is it possible for you to take us? We would be very grateful if you could."

The bird scratches the ground a few times, then steps toward Jay, "well, first you joke at me, then you want a long ride for two. What if I don't feel like it just now?"

Sihiryan looks at the bird and then at Jay, "If you are not going that way please forgive us for the discourtesy of what ever we did. We will ask the next bird that comes by."

"Oh, you two are good" Turning his head side to side. "If I don't give you two a ride I will be know as the bird that didn't give Jay a ride for the rest of my life, they won't even say my name any more."

Jay says to him, "oh come on, you just gotta work on your game a little, you can get a joke on us before we land, look at us, a couple of Kyranins, no feathers, no wings, how hard can it be to come up with something. You can do it. You just got off to a slow start that's all."

"Yeah,,, ok, sure hop on" as he sits on the ground so they can climb on easily.

Jay climbs on first and Sihiryan climbs up and pulls herself tight against him. Shyruk stands and stumbles a little, "Oh Jay, you are heavier than I thought, how much did you eat up here? I think you are the fattest kyranin I have ever given a ride too".

Jay says, "hum, good insult but there is no humor in it." Pats his feathers, you gotta work on the humor aspect of what you say, insulting me only works if you leave enough latitude in what you say that it can be made into something funny."

Shyruk stretches his wings and bends up and down working his knees, "it will be funny to the other birds if I can't get off the ground with you on my back."

Jay starts to laugh, "Ok good one, you got me lets go."

Shyruk jumps and flaps hard, he starts to go up then before he gets to the tree tops he starts to level off then drop a few feet, "um, I, never had this happen before Sihiryan, I can't get up."

She starts laughing so hard that she can't reply. Shyruk gives a few good flaps and they rise above the trees and up towards the mountain peaks at the edge of the valley. Then turning he takes a bit of a dive to pass over the meadow and circles around before starting up again. Then turning in the direction of Shiyhra. Climbing as they leave the wilderness area. Climbing more and more until Jay starts to feel cold from the altitude. They are above some puffy clouds, looking down between them at the agricultural lands and the small towns. Jay notices that there is patches of forest that are connect with each other by wide strips of trees and shrubs.

Jay asks "can we go a little lower please I am getting cold." then turning to Sihiryan, what's with the trees connecting the patches of forest?"

She looks at him then back down at the view as they start to loose altitude to the level of the puffy clouds. See the water inside the patches Jay? There are streams that connect the small patches of wilderness all over the planet. To have a health stream there must be trees and forest plants and forest life so the soil will be alive, or the stream can't stay healthy. By keeping the streams healthy we also give the animals migrations paths that are comfortable so that they can be healthy too."

Jay looks closer trying to see between the trees. "It is a thick forest over the streams, I can only see the water a little bit here and there."

Sihiryan says "in some places the water is several meters underground. But to be health the forest must live above it. The subterranean world is part of the world too Jay, it cohabits this world with us. There are life forms there that are never seen on the surface. The steams are our only connection to them. If the streams get damaged from our developments we have seen that the subterranean life is effected for a very long distance up and down the stream, and sometimes in adjacent subterranean areas."

Looking at the strips of forest he sees the web like grid that they make in all directions across the planet in view beneath them. He thinks to himself 'wow, how humane, to consider the details to keep the planet health for all life forms. I wish my world would do this'. "That is commendable, what was the cost?"

Sihiryan hesitates, "what do you mean Jay. Costs?"

"What was the difficulty, the extra efforts, the lost productivity, from making these areas?" Jay asks.

Sihiryan hesitates, Then says, "Jay it cost nothing to leave these tiny areas alone. If we destroyed them it would have cost us our environment, our food chain, out clean water, our relationship with the other species, the permanent use of the natural water for drinking. It was only a gain to leave these tiny areas alone." She gives him a jiggle, "Is this concept new to you Jay?

Shyruk asks, "can you see Shiyhra on the horizon?

Jay and Sihiryan look forward and look at he towers of the city poking up between the peaks of the hills and the towers of white stone protruding from the land. "Wow", Jay says "that is incredible" as he watches the city get close the angle changes and he start to see the sea behind the city, the mist on the sea and the glow of the fluid. "Sihiryan, have you ever watched the sun rise from the beach when the mist is still thick on the sea?"

"Jay!" she says, "that is what the amburst always talk about for their first year out of the fluid. It is nothing, I have watched it many time, no big deal. I guess if you have never been out of the fluid it might look like something special. I wouldn't recommend getting up early to go down there for it."

Jay remembers his time under the sea. "Have you ever been to Akwerts?"

Sihiryan hesitates to answer, "no"

"It is really something to see. They have suits so you can swim like they do, well not as good but you can get around with them." Jay turns his head to look at her with one eye. "You gotta make time for it Sihiryan. You will love it, it is so different it is hard to describe."

"I have never been invited", Sihiryan hesitates, "well, since I was young, a amburst friend from education wanted me to visit him at his family home... I haven't seen him for years, decades"

They start to be able to see the buildings clearly, and the lake in the city. Jay leans forward and loudly asks Shyruk "can you let us off at the sea side please."

Shyruk takes a few hard flaps and turns to the left, so that they are heading directly toward the big building. Then he starts to glide. They are at about five times the height of any of the buildings as they start crossing the city below them. By the time they get to the big building they are about 3 times as high as the tallest towers. "Any favorite beach Jay?"

"By the pebble beach, near the amburst marina." Jay replies.

They start to dive slightly but toward the beach on the left, away from the marina. Then as they are coming over the water a slight turn, bringing them over the sea. Looking past the tall white crystals and the city behind them, and then turning more as they get closer to the water and the long building by the beach blocks the view of the city. As they approach the sea's surface Jay can see into it somewhat. He thinks he sees something moving inside the water, something big. He remembers Gremble and his time with him. Then they are meters from the surface crossing it fast, Shyruk starts flapping again. Towards the beach, even closer to the fluid so that Shyruks wing tips are splashing with each flap as the beach approaches. Up, and slowly down onto the shore they land. Shyruk gets down on the beach so they can get off easily. "It was good to meet you Jay, Sihiryan".

Jay turns and says "thank you" as Shyruk starts flapping to take off.

Leaving for the moon

Jay looks at the sea and the beach and the city then turns to Sihiryan "should we walk a bit or do you want to get home?"

She looks at Jay "do you miss Trentia?, I could see that you were getting to be good friends with her before you left."

Jay looks at the sea, "not yet. If I find things to keep myself busy on the moon I won't. But if I am bored there I will miss you too" turning back to her and giving her a solemn gaze. He takes a step towards the city, "should we walk to the street or do you want a taxi here?"

She smiles, "I will take a taxi here Jay but it will be best if you spend some time here at the beach I think." Taking out her tablet she works the screen with her fingers to arrange a taxi

for herself. A message from Herfermks opens when she
has got the taxi to come so she reads it. Then orders another
taxi for Jay 20 minutes later. "Your taxi will be here in 20
minutes Jay. My room will be ready for you when you arrive
and I will be working off world until you are on the ship to the
moon." Herfermks has something for me to do with the
vwortex at a new colony that the alliance is building for mixed
member species. I will have to leave this afternoon." She looks
at him and hears a taxi coming, walks to him and gives him a
tight hug. As the taxi stops and the door opens she lets go and
steps back towards the taxi door. "I will see you when I go to
the moon in six months. Bye Jay"

"Bye" Jay says as he watches her get into the taxi. He watches
as the taxi leaves. Jay looks at the city in front of him, at the tall
buildings, at the huge white rocks sticking out of the hills, at
the trees and the kiosks on the beach, and at all of the various
beings. He turns and looks at the sea and at the thin misty
haze above the fluid. He watches the vast splashes from the
waves as they break on the rocks in the distance and then he
looks at the sky. "Where is the moon" he says softly as he
looks up at the sky. Thinking about what it will be like not
being able to go outside for days at a time, maybe even weeks
or months Jay starts to wonder what he agreed to. He looks at
the aliens walking on the beach near by and at the ships flying
here and there over and through the city and starts to think
about earth. He thinks about what work he will have to do
when he gets back, about his tools, and about Heather. He
thinks about her being frozen in time while he is doing all of
these things, while he is living days and weeks and what will
be years. She is standing still in time he thinks, like Reggie is,
waiting for him to come out of the head on that fishing charter
boat. Then he starts to think that maybe it is just a dream, and
that he is so lucky to have such a vivid dream. That he will be

glad to enjoy the entire ten years of it no matter what it entails, and that he will be back to where he started and no one there will ever notice that he was away. Jay physically gives his head a shake and takes a deep breath. He looks at his hands and rubs them together then rubs his face. 'I am here, this is real' he thinks to himself and starts walking toward the street. He sees the taxi coming toward him and stopping at the edge of the street, directly in front of him about six meters away. The door opens and he sees Herfermks inside.

"Jay!" Herfermks calls and waves, he watches as Jay picks up his pace and climbs into the taxi. "Things are going to be different than you were told Jay." Gesturing with one hand for Jay to sit beside him. "Taxi continue protocol ryberian military privacy, Drive a slow tour of the beaches."

Jay watches the door close and the view of the beach as they start to move. He looks at Herfermks and sees an intensity of seriousness in his face. "What happened? You seemed so calm yesterday."

Herfermks looks surprised, "oh, that isn't my yesterday Jay. I'm working on your retrieval. Don't tell me anything about yesterday." Giving Jay a surprised and serious look "we have looked at several possibilities and the best way to get you to the moon is if you arrived there two weeks before the incident with the gowrlaks. So here is the thing Jay, when Sihiryan comes to visit you in six months you will have been there for almost five years and you can't let her figure it out. You will have to hide your new life there from her. I know it is odd but things are more difficult with the new security than we ever expected."

Jay looks at him, "So the new security is pretty good then?"

Herfermks looks at him for a moment, "well that is a good way to see it Jay I will work with that, I hope it helps my frustrations with getting things done." He reaches and grabs Jay's arm and the interior of the taxi starts to fade to clear "Jay we will arrive in your apartment with the lights off, you will wait until I leave before turning them on, the switch will be within the reach of your other arm."

Jay hesitates as everything turns to black, darkness. "Ok," he says. Feeling the floor softly beneath his feet.

"Stand before I integrate us fully Jay"

Jay does and feels the grip remove itself from his arm as he feels the weight of his body taken by the strength of his legs. "So what is going to happen now?"

Herfermks clears his throat, "Jay at the end of your time here, for the last week you were setting up this apartment for yourself and getting acquainted with the neighbors. You know the culture by then and develop a relationship where they are happy to smile and say high and not interact with you much unless you work at it. You have a simple map on the table to show you how to get to work and you have a routine to get there an hour before anyone else so you won't have to talk to anyone. Your workstation at your work place will have all the information that you should know about your work mates and the work you will be doing. You will have time to study it enough to get through the next few days and by then it will all be normal. Then you can just enjoy life and I will come get you when we have things to do. You have filled your meal room with things that you like and you won't have to go shopping until you have time to learn where to go shopping. Jay your work is simple. You look at ancient files of how the social structure was developed on the moon and when you find something interesting or curious you file it in my file in your tablet as a duplicate. Jay, don't go to the bar we went to until your day off. On your day off you do go there for an early lunch. Take a table with four chairs and occupy the whole table with your bag and jacket. At lunch I will show up and join you at your table. We will meet seemingly for the first time. You look a little younger now so it will all blend in well." He pauses for several second, "any questions?"

Jay thinks for a few seconds, So I am back in time to before I started work on Ramga" by about a week?"

Herfermks thinks and replies, "Yes."

"And I use my name Jay with the same story about my name and my past as I was going to use on Ramga?"

"Yes, good question Jay, Yes we put it all back deep enough that it has past scrutiny in all time scenarios that we have worked through."

"Ok, if there is nothing else I am ready." Jay says, "Oh can I contact Trentia from the moon?"

"Glad you asked Jay. No. No one can know that you are here. You are not in the records of ever being on ramga in association with anyone in our organization. You are actually not recorded as having been in Ramga during that time now. Your first interaction with me will be at lunch in a few days. You cannot contact anyone from Ramga, for any reason, not anyone from our group for five years. No mater what!" he says.

Jay thinks for a moment. "Ok, if there is anything that comes up I will let you know at lunch." Jay thinks for a moment, "Oh what about that girl in the bar, won't she know me?" he thinks about the time when they first went there and tries to remember if it was before he went to work for his first day. "Herfermks?" Jay waits a few seconds and starts reaching for the light switch. He feels a small panel and the lights come on slowly. It is a big room, with a wall screen on two walls and some comfy looking furniture on the other side of the room.

There is a wide doorway that goes to another room. Jay walks through it and sees that there are five doors. One with locks. Four without. He opened the one closest to the one with locks, a large closet. The next is a bathroom with a shower. The next opens to an area with two wall screens and a large dinning table with six chairs. The last door opens to his bedroom, large room, with a large bed in the middle of it. It has a shower in one corner and a door in another corner and one wall is cabinets that look like closet sizes. He looks in the corner door and it is a bathroom; small, a toilet, bidet like thing, a sink off the wall and the ceiling and walls and floor make the shower. He steps in and sees a robe and two towels on the back of the door as the lights come on.

Jay goes to the wall cabinets and opens them. Inside he sees three sets of clothes styles, casual from Ramga, the type he saw the locals wearing each time he went to the bar here on the moon with Herfermks, and some things much fancier. Examining them, he determines that the they are his size, soft but strong materials, some sheer and smooth like silk the others soft like fleece. The clothes in this style are in a variety of colors and shapes of shirts and slacks, some with pockets and some without. There are hats and socks and shorts also, all the same soft fabric. Jay pulls on one garment to test the strength and finds it to be far stronger than he expected. "Humm, nice fabric" he thinks aloud. Closing the cabinets he looks in the drawers and finds dressing accessories for him in one, two drawers of woman clothing in unopened packages and one of gadgets and bottles and boxes and packages of things. He opens another door and finds a machine, with quick inspection he figures it is to wash the clothes. Then the last door, a wet bar, with a murrk maker and a hookah or bong type thing, and a selection of bottles partially filled and some of various sizes yet un opened. Jay nods with a smile of approval. He goes back to the door with hanging garments and looks through closely. They all seem to be about his size. Jay asks himself 'what are the women's clothes for?'

"Room, turn on wall screens" Jay says. He watches as they change only in tone of color so slightly. "View of the corridor out side of my entrance." the wall beside his bed and adjacent to it beside him show a view as if he has just stepped out of his door and a Gyrekian walks right through him from the 3d image that they project. Several others are walking past his home's front door and none seem to notice him standing there. "Home, is this a present time image being shown on these wall screens?" he asks.

"Yes. Jay. It is a present time image of the corridor out side you home entrance" comes from the walls.

Jay looks down the images in both directions to see if he can see where the corners are to the joining corridors in either direction. He can see two intersections on the left out of his door and only one from the right side. On the right side the corridor has a slight curve to it. He walks into the dinning room / kitchen room and looks around. On the counter there is some wrapping paper. Jay looks at it and then turns over and sees the map. It is simple. Left out side the door, streight past the first intersection, right on the second, streight for three intersections then straight and the third door on the right. Up three sets of stairs left down the corridor and the second door on the right. Jay looks at the map tracing the path again and then takes a picture of it with his tablet. He asks his tablet how long until he next has to leave to go to work. It gives him a screen display of the clock showing a pie chart and then it shrinks into a corner of the screen as an itinerary shows a to-do list for him hour to hour. He looks at it and sees that he should be sleeping, and that in 7 hours he will hear the alarm. Then have 2 hours to make it to work. Jay thinks to himself 'What about breakfast?' Jay looks across the room and decides which door he thinks is the fridge. He checks, then another door, and then a third. In the third door is the fridge. Inside he finds what looks like duck eggs and several bottles of various fluids, what looks like cheese and something that has a note on it that says almost butter. There are two types of pastries in the fridge and many vegetables and some containers that he finds different types of meat inside of. He decides to try some of the fluids and likes his first choice, and has a second glass of it. Jay goes to his bedroom, undresses, has a shower and goes to bed. "Wall screens off, lights minimum" he says and listens to the silence. A few deep breaths and he is asleep.

The sound of Jays alarm, makes him laugh, it is his own voice telling him to get up and start a new life. It sings to him a little poem "Jay, Jay start your life today, it is morning on the moon Jay, Jay stop the dream I say, you've got work starting soon, your food is waiting your coffee too, you have a lot of earthly things to do Jay, Jay I say. It is time to get out of bed and play, wake up Jay do as I say, your life hear will soon begin. So go groom, shower and shave, cut your toenails too, you have important things to do." After a short pause it starts playing again so Jay gets up and walks to the shower. As soon as he is off the bed it stops and the room says, "security protocol Jay, one time alarm recording is erased."

After the shower Jay goes to the wardrobe doors and finds some normal clothing for the moon. He goes and makes himself an omelet. He fries some of the meat and vegetables, stirs the eggs with some milk and adds the cheese. Then he tastes the cheese. He hopes it is ok in the omelet. The flavor is smooth and smoky but not like cheese, more of a mango pudding type of flavor. He smirks, chuckles and shakes his head. Having a few spoons full of what he thought was cheese he watches his omelet cook. He likes the omelet, enjoys his mrruk, and cleans up before leaving for his work. When he gets outside he doesn't see anyone in the corridor he asks his home to lock itself and only let him in and gets a confirmation from the speaker in the door. Finding his way toward his work Jay notice that most of the doors are homes and a few are businesses of random types. When he gets to his work the door welcomes him and he opens it with the door handle. Walking through the office the lights start coming on ahead of him as he finds his desk. It has a nameplate facing his direction. He sits in the chair and puts his tablet on the desk. The workstation is dark so he says, "work station start". Nothing happens. He looks around the room. First taking a good look at all of the equipment on, under, and around his desk then checking that all the wires are plugged into something. He looks for a control panel but can't see one. He sits back in his chair and thinks then asks, "Tablet, how do I start my workstation?"

The tablet replies, "there is a security protocol, I can start it after you lift the switch behind the lower left corner of the screen and ask me to open it, and reset the security protocol to Jay one alpha at work and then think the thought open my workstation now. Jay, the first task will be to tell me to reset the workstation start sequence to Jay's arrival with 'security of Jay' as the verbal command to start it there after."

Jay thinks to himself 'Ok this is a little complicated'. He ponders the reason for a few seconds then shrugs and does it. The screen opens the hand panels open and the wall screens on his two cubical walls light up the wall screen on his floor light up and it looks like grass in a field, the ceiling wall screen lights up and it looks like as early evening sky. Jay nods, and gets an expression of approval on his face. He looks around the office and sees that there are other workstations similar to his and others with various configurations. Looking at the console and the hand screens he asks "work station, what is my first work to be done?" The screen in front of him starts slowly scrolling through lines of words that he can read, as they are in English. After about ten minutes he is finished reading the note. 'Well,' he thinks to himself, ' I always wanted to get off the tools and do something not so physical, so maybe working at this desk all day will be good for me'.

He moves his hands around on the various screens to see how they respond and then starts the searching in the Pre Records Achieves of Gyrekian History. Not knowing what he should be looking for Jay decides to look at ancient ruins on the surface. To him most of the pictures look like mountains with a few square or round or polygonal protrusions. As his coworkers start to arrive he notices there are similarity in the shapes of the polygonal protrusions on several parts of the moon, about the same size and in similar locations. Keeping to himself and focusing on his work as the others come in he notices that no one says a word to each other or to him. So he looks around the room, all casually dressed Gryekians, mostly men, calmly getting settled at their workstations. Jay starts reading about and looking at the details of one of the sites with polygonal shapes that is most remote from the others. He chose that one because it is the only one near the southern axis of the moon. Most of the other sites are around the equator. He

looks at the catalogued artifacts, the shapes of them the age
the purpose that they suspect they were used for and if they
are considered important as indicators of social or
technological development. "Important" Jay thinks aloud, in a
whisper. 'How can an artifact be important, if it was important
it wouldn't have become an artifact easily, it would have been
in use' he thinks and keeps going, looking at more images and
reading more information. He looks up, looks around at the
rest of the room, at the others working. He thinks 'how would
I know what was important and how would one thing be more
important than another for development?'. Pondering the
question he looks at many more items and reads many more
comparisons and descriptions and projections of what they
were used for, and how they influenced future items, and were
the result of previous items.

Jay is plodding through this work when he feels a grumble in
his tummy. He looked up from his screens and noticed that
others in the office have beverages on their desks and a few
even had some tasty looking snacks. He looks and notices that
there is a hall exiting from one corner of the large office space.
Keeping an eye on it he sees a female coming out with two
steaming cups, one in each hand. She puts one on a desk as she
walks by without saying a word and brings the other to her
own desk and sits, and takes a sip then looks at her screens
again. Jay thinks to himself 'this is the most quiet place I have
ever heard of.' Carefully lifting his chair to move it back he
gets up as quietly as possible. He steps deliberately softly
across the room and into that hallway to find doors to several
rooms, one with a door open. The one with the door open has
large printers and a few tables in it. The walls in this room
seem to be cabinets. The next two are labeled as toilets. The
fourth's doors open as he steps in front of them. It is a large
cafeteria and kitchen area. There are three Gyrekians working

in the kitchen. He sees the table with hot drinks serving equipment and goes directly there. One of the Gyrekians form the kitchen comes over to him as he is filling his cup with hot tea.

"Hello, your name is Jay correct?" taking a directly square stance to him, "my name is Ktrya. I am the chief in charge of the kitchen. If you want any special Kyranin dishes let me know and we will see what can be done. You know it has been a long time since I was on Ramga, I miss cooking some of the special dishes from the southern plains traditional cuisine. The fruits from there are so different from ours. I would have to send a helper to the market on the far side of town to get some fresh ones, but I think it is worth the trouble, if you want me to make one of those dishes for you."

Jay smiles "I would love to try one of them, or several over the next weeks or months." Jay lifts his full cup and turns to face the man directly. "It is good to meet you Ktrya, did I say it correctly?

"Yes Jay. Are you from the south of Ramga? It is such a beautiful place.?" Ktrya asks.

"Actual, no, I was born off world far away and have only spent a very little time on Ramga. I only know a few things to eat from there, kreptigs of course." Jay says.

"That is a shame," Ktrya says, "next time you are going if you have time go to some small farms in the south and try the grbesit berries. They are delectable but are only good for a short time after they are picked, they are always in season but not many are cultivated, most are picked wild. They are worth the journey I assure you."

Jay thinks about the salmon berries from where he grew up on earth, not available in stores but delicious when picked wild. "OK, Grbesit berries, grbesit. I will make the effort next time I am there, I don't suspect it will be soon though." Jay says.

"Oh, how long is your contract here for, Six months?" Ktrya asks.

Jay takes a sip of his tea then realizing it is a good temperature to drink; downs it and reaches to refill it as he starts to reply. "Well, I have agreed to spend the normal six months and am considering a much longer term. I have agreed to think about staying as long as five years."

Ktrya takes an actual step backward. "Did I hear you correctly?, You are considering staying here for five years, you know you don't get paid to stay here!" taking a long look at Jay as he turns with his filled cup of tea to face him again, "what compels you to consider this?"

"Well," Jay tries to think of something to say, "Well Ramga isn't really my home, and I don't want to return to the colonies that I was raised on so, to me, this moon is as good a place as any for me. It is safe and friendly, and I can easily have work here."

Ktrya looks at Jay for a few seconds, "welcome to our moon, if you make this your home you will be one of us." He smiles and adds, "I will make some of those special kyranin meals so that you can try them Jay. I am certain that you will like them." He starts to turn back to the kitchen then looks back into Jay's eyes, "anytime you want a break from your work come back to the kitchen and we can talk, anytime." and he nods and starts walking back to the kitchen.

Jay feels the kindness from him and is moved by it. Jay takes a sip of his tea and starts walking back to his desk. He sits down, sips his tea and starts his research again. 'I'm not well trained for this' he thinks as he looks at more images and reads about them. After some time he notices a Gyrekian standing beside him and looks up.

"Hello, my name is Kwantin, I will be your supervisor starting next week, I am in orientation now. You are new here correct?"

Jay takes a good look at him and stands up to face him to be polite, "yes, my name is Jay, I am new here and so far I like it." he smiles at the Gyrekian and can't help but to notice this guy's nose. It is longer than most, tapered toward the tip on the bridge and wide against the cheeks, larger than ever flaring nostrils and a big round tip. 'Almost comical' Jay thinks to himself.

Kwantin looks back at Jay and smiles, "yes, the nose. My grandmother was from another world. She died giving birth to my father and my Grandfather did the right thing. He claimed the child as his. He took some ridicule form several alliance species at the time but was welcome when he got back here on our moon." turning his head so Jay can see the nose from profile, "it is odd, the detail of it I mean, it works well but obviously not a typical nose. My father looked Gyrekian but his skin tone was darker and the texture of his skin, it was not so smooth. He made the joke that his mother gave him tough skin".

Jay takes a good look at the Gyrekian's nose and nods his head, "it is different. I have heard there is some who have strong feeling against inter species breeding. I don't. I wouldn't suggest it to anyone but I understand that it can happen and that no matter what, we will always love our children."

Kwantin smiles, "It is good to hear you opinion Jay. I have heard that you start early and that you also work late often. You are not likely to be promoted from your position but you are welcome to continue to work as you like, of course if you miss some time from work periodically it will be easier for me to over look it due to you regular long hours. I don't desire to sound harsh, but I am here as you supervisor not as your friend. If we meet outside of work I will be honored to develop friendship with you Jay, but here I can't."

"Thank you, it will be a pleasure working under your supervision."

Kwantin looks at Jay's desk then back at Jay as he stretches his arm pointing to the screen, "I noticed that the language is not from Ramga"

Jay smiles at him and nods "Yes, it is a dialect from one region of an alliance associated world that I was raised on for several years. My education was started there so I learned to read this first. It is easier for me in this language. I was lucky enough to have a Ryberian make me a special translator package to convert it," looking down at the screen filled with writing in English, "it makes my work go so much faster it is actually a joy to do it."

Kwantin stands there, almost toe to toe with Jay for a few seconds then he says, "Well then, I will see you again in a few weeks". Steps back and turns, then walks across the room and starts talking with another worker.

Jay sits down, looks around the room to see it only half full and gets back to work. After several more artifacts and articles about them he scrolls through some menus on his tablet and finds his personal history. He reviews it a little so that he remembers the names of a few planets and space bases from his youth. He looks at the ones where he was said to have spent his youth and some of them had been destroyed or badly damaged from regional conflicts. Never close to a time when he would have been at one, always some few years after he had moved away. 'Good strategy' he thinks to himself. He checks the planet that he was said to start his educational years on and it had been invaded three times since he left, the cultures that had been there are almost completely gone. Jay looks at a star chart to see where this planet is. He finds that it is a far distance away form other Alliance planets and even far form other associated planets. He checks the records and at no time have there been more than a few thousand Kyranins on that planet all at the same time, When he was there only a few hundred, non of them in his own area. Again he thinks to himself 'good cover'. Then he takes a look around the room as he changes his screen back to his research. There are only a few others still there at work. Jay stands up and looks towards the kitchen, then checks the time. It has been about 7 hours since he arrived. He goes into the dinning area, there are several gyrekians eating. Looking into the kitchen he sees that the one cook there is still making food. Jay goes to the buffet and fills a plate with things that he knows he likes and sits down for a meal. As he eats he listens to the conversations of the others in the room. Mostly about sports, some talk about artifacts and time lines of cultural development. After his meal he goes back to his work at his station and soon sees that all the others have left and that their work stations, all seem to be turned off. He takes the hint and turns his off to and goes home. He spends the evening looking at various places on the moon with his wall screens and looking around the corridors near his home and work and the pub where he will meet

Herfermks. The next day, and the next until the weekend are about the same. In the morning of the day he is to meet Herfermks Jay has his breakfast, showers and dresses and has a tea then remembers the long path to the bar. He checks the time and has another tea.

He sits and drinks his tea thinking about his work. How he is actually getting interested in what he is looking at. He still can't figure out how this research is going to help him or Herfermks' work, but he trusts Herfermks. 'I don't know what I don't know so I will keep going until something happens to change things again' Jay thinks to himself. It is time, so he gets up checks his appearance and goes to the door, out and locks it. Walking to the bar he says good morning to the familiar faces and the ones further from his home give him a friendly response. He starts to wonder what he said to his actual neighbors before he arrived. Smirking to himself about the situation and what he must have had to do or say to have all his close neighbors not talk to him. Jay looks to his left and sees Herfermks door as he passes it. A short distance and he enters the door to the bar. He finds a table with four chairs and sits down with his back to the corner. He sees that most of those already in the bar are off worlders of a species that he is not familiar with. There are three Amburst females eating lunch at one table across the room and a table of Vworktek officers having what looks like it could be beer. The waitress comes to his table and looks him over pretty good.

"Hello I will be serving you today, would you like some kreptigs to start?"

"Yes. Please" Jay says, as he looks into her eyes and losses his breath.

She stands still looking at him as he looks directly at her. "Something else?"

Jay composes himself, "I would like a mrruk. Sorry for my gaze but your eyes, they froze my thoughts as I look into them."

She smiles hard and blushes as she turns her body slightly from side to side and smiles at him. "And so what could I do for you, Sir," as she smiles.

Jay doesn't know what to say, he knows it is a flirt, he knows he will be introduced to her by Herfermks in a few weeks and he realizes that he is attracted to her. "anything you do will give me great pleasure and my interest could not be greater" he hears himself say.

She looks at him and blushes more. "Then with a look of epiphany on her face she turns to look at the bar, and then back to look at Jay. She winks at him and with a slightly loud voice she says "certainly our kitchen has the best equipment I assure you, come with me and I will show you sir" she nods her head and smiles at him then motions with her fingers for him to follow as she starts walking around the room toward the door at the far end.

Jay feels a little nervous but feels he better follow. As she takes him into the hallway from behind the bar to the kitchen she opens a door on the left and pulls him into the room closing the door behind them.

The light comes on as they enter and she looks at his face and eyes closely then grabs his shoulders and kisses him pressing her lips into his. After a few seconds she steps back form him and says "there is something about you too, my heart felt it when I looked at you." then feeling her lips with her fingers, I want to get to know you, wait until my father talks to you at least twice, then tell him you find me attractive. Nothing more. Don't say anything more than that." She looks at him for a second, "do you understand?"

Jay looks back at her still feeling something from the kiss, "yes, he talks to me twice, I say you are attractive, nothing more." as he starts to think about his situation.

She smiles and opens the door carefully looking both ways before going out. She motions Jay to go back towards the bar, "are you satisfied" She says loud enough that it could be heard if anyone was listening from the bar.

Jay say, "I am glad that you showed me, I have some fears when eating in new places" as he walks across the bar room, "Please, I will have the special and I apologize for my skepticism." Jay gets to his table and sits down. He re-thinks what just happened. 'I meet this girl in a few weeks and she flirts with me then too. She kissed me. I felt it.' Then he remembers what Herfermks said to him in a few weeks. He remembers what Herfermks said to him a few days earlier. He takes this vest off and puts it over the back of one chair. He takes out his tablet and turns it on so that it will look like it is in the middle of something and puts in front of another chair, then turns the fourth chair as if someone has pushed it back to go to the washroom.

She comes back with his mrruk placing it on the table in front of him, "you will have others join you?"

Jay looks a little confused as he answers, "Yes."

She smiles at him and gives him a wink as she walks away. She can feel Jay watching her walk and looks back after going past the bar toward the kitchen.

Jay gives his head a shake. Some Kuroberotes walk in and look around, they break into three groups and sit at tables close enough that they can see and hear each other. One walks directly toward Jay. Jay is curious, as he has never met one of these being before.

It stops and faces him from about a meter away, "excuse me, do you need these chairs, we have friends joining us and I would like to use these chairs".

Jay is not sure of the educate, so he stands, faces the alien and smiles. "I too have friends coming and I do need these chairs my friend, I am not able to let you take them."

The kuroberote smiles and tilts his head to Jay, "I am Sthatherom. It is good to meet a Kyranin today, I hope we can become friends one day." and smiles a sincere smile at Jay.

Jay smiles back "My name is Jay I will be here at random times, I will be happy to talk with you one day, but today I am meeting friends, I look forward to making friends with you one day Sthatherom." Jay nods and sits back down.

Sthatherom continues to smile watching Jay seat himself and nods then walks over and takes two chairs from a vacant table. He puts them around a table with four chairs already then seats himself facing the bar with his back to the door.

Jay notices that from where he seated himself he can see every one of his group that came in with. He can see their faces. Jay sips his mrruk as the bar fills up and various aliens fill the tables and finally more join Sthatherom and they seem to be watching the other Kuroberotes as they converse with various aliens at their tables. The bar is full and Jay watches as his new romantic interest bustles about serving all of the customers in the bar. She drops off his kreptigs with hast as she is passing by with four plates for another table, then back to the kitchen picking up from a group that just left on the way, then meals and drinks for another table, then another. When Herfermks arrives Jay is watching the girl with amazement and amusement enough that he doesn't notice Herfermks until he is at the table. Jay stands, "Welcome Sir, I was distracted by the waitress, she is serving all of these customers by herself, and doing a good job of it."

Herfermks sits down. He looks around the room and when he sees her turn her head toward him he gives a hand signal and turns back toward Jay. "Jay, it is good to see you looking so content. I am glad you are starting to like it here. Did you find something on the menu that you want?"

"Oh," Jay replies, "I didn't look, I just asked for the special."

Herfermks looks around the room, "I have two friends that might show up Jay. If they do you don't know them ok?" he looks at Jay for a second with a serious look, "it is always best to keep things simple you know." He takes the last kreptig, bites it in half and chews. "I was looking at Reggie's work on your world Jay. It is interesting but I don't know how to start yet. Have you done well with the research?" then looks at his tablet and starts to stand up.

"Well?" Jay asks, "Herfermks I don't know what I am looking for sir."

Herfermks waives at two Ryberians as they come in the door. "Patterns Jay, don't say my name. Cause and effect, if this then that, are there patterns, is progress predictable from events? I want to see how well you can derive from this data what we can expect to happen. It will be hard because things happen so slowly, I know. That is what you are looking for though Jay, cause and effect, patterns of cause and effect. It will take years I know. You won't age while you are here but work fast Jay." Stepping to greet his friends, "hello Teloion. Good to see you" and Herfermks leans to give him a hug, then looking at the other, "you must be Frestwy good to meet you." Motioning to the chairs so they will be seated beside each other with Herfermks able to see both of them and Jay at the same time. "I have ordered for us, I know the food here and I trust it will be Ok" Then looking to Jay and sitting down. This is my friend Delumjes from Ramga, I saw he had a table and the place was full so I asked if we could join him, he works in home coordination."

Jay recognizes them and is curious as to why they don't recognize him. "It is an honor to have lunch with you both, and with you too Sir as he faces Herfermks"

Teloion nods at Jay and smiles, "It is a pleasure to share a meal with a kyranin" and bumps Frestwy with his elbow.

Frestwy looks at Teloion then at Jay he hesitates a second, "Delumjes. It is good to meet a kyranin. I have only been off my world once before so you are the first Kyranin that I have ever met" He looks Jay over a little. "It is good to meet you I would like to visit Ramga one day I have heard that you have done a lot of great things there."

Jay smiles "Thank you, well actual I didn't do it all myself."

Teloion looks over and starts to laugh, "Yes, Kyranin humor."

The waitress brings four meals and six drinks. Two drinks for each Ryberian, with lids on one for each of them. Jay gets his meal last and she gives him a look of surprise and approval and a wink as she starts to turn to leave.

As the Ryberians start to talk Jay watches the girl fill the tray with empty dishes from other tables and head back into the kitchen. He starts listening to them talk about some political situation on a planet that he hadn't heard of yet. Jay listens as they come to questions about a situation of one regional government that they don't have much information on and then they look at Herfermks' expression. They look at each other then back at him. Jay looks at them and notices some minor shifts in Teloion's posture and arm placement on the table. He listens while Teloion talks at length about behind the scene secrets of several government officials, and the discreet progress that is taking place with various negotiations there. Jay realizes that Teloion has just spent some time there during there meal. He watches as their conversation slows down and comes to a conclusion. As there plates are becoming empty Herfermks slides his covered cup to in front of himself and looks at the other two.

"A celebration is due, what do you think?" Herfermks holds the cup up with one hand and holds the lid with the other.

The other two take there containers in a similar manner and Teloion says "success" and they all remove the lid and bolt the containers towards their mouths flicking and capturing the contents with a fast bite, and then immediate wide eyes chewing.

After ample chewing and expressions of satisfaction from the flavor Teloion turns toward Jay. "Delumjes," Teloion say "It was good meeting you but it is time for us to go." He stands and steps away from the table smiling at Herfermks, "until next time my friend, thank you for the chance to help."

Frestwy stands and nods at Jay and looks at Herfermks. "An honor and a pleasure sir I hope we can meet again," and takes a bow before turning to go.

Jay looks at Herfermks plate and then his own, "should we get some more food and maybe a beer?"

Herfermks looks at Jay long and hard, "Yes, we should." Herfermks looks at the bartender and does some hand signals. The bartender punches some keypad on the bar with his fingers then goes back to mixing drinks.

"Those are two of the three that met me at Crenshaw's" Jay says then is distracted as he sees the waitress walking towards them with a tray. Looking back at Herfermks, "they didn't recognize me."

Herfermks turns to look at what caught Jay's eye as the food and drinks arrive. "Hello, I hope you and your father are well!"

As she is putting everything on the table and her eyes keep turning to Jay she answers, "Yes Sir, we are good, I hope all is well with you, and that all your travels are safe and exciting" giving him a quick smile and taking the empty plates onto her tray. Turning to face him when her tray is full and saying with a smile, "it is good to see you." then turning and walking briskly back toward the kitchen.

Herfermks looks at Jay then starts to laugh. He leans forward and says softly "she has you already Jay, can you even remember where you are?" taking some finger food and sitting back in his chair and chuckling with a smirk.

Jay turns to him trying to look like everything is normal.

Herfermks laughs. "Oh Jay I was right about this. I think I may be in the wrong career" and he laughs.

Jay looks at him and takes a piece of one of the snacks and pops it into his mouth, then a sip of his beverage. "You find me predictable and amusing, is that why I am here?"

Herfermks laughs harder, "actual no Jay, but it sure helps me enjoy my work." Taking a pastry from the tray and looking it over before popping into his mouth he looks at Jay with a smile and takes a drink of his beer and nods. "Jay I am in high spirits. The work I was doing with those two that were here went well. You knew them didn't you?" After your telling me about them I looked into their lives. They do similar work to me but I was not sure if I could trust them. So I found an opportunity to work with them. It was in the past. It is complicated. But they won't remember you when they meet you because this was many decades ago for them." They don't respect the kyranins or most other species Jay but they enjoy doing good things to make it better for other life forms." It was a project that my father worked on with them with to alleviate tension on a world in order to prevent a major war between groups of that world's most technologically advance species. They think I'm my father. My father and I worked a disguise for him to look more like me, as that was the easy way to do it without changing any events. Then I watched them work with him and watched all the meetings and watched how they did things a lot. This is the only time I actually met with them, my father's disguise was effective, they still think that I am him, the tricky part was to have the home security office agree to adjust their time and placement of their travels for this meeting. They don't know the time and place we are now, they think it is decades ago on a different world where we met. My father is sitting in that pub alone now, we will join him, are you ready?"

Jay asks himself if he heard it correctly as he feels something hit his leg then sees the fading to black and then a slightly different looking bar. "Well, I guess I was ready" Jay says and turns his head slightly to looks at Birkjets. "Birkjets Sir, good to see you!"

Birkjets smiles and nods at Jay then turns to Herfermks and looks at him for a second, "well, how did it go?"

"It was good, he hesitated to go back and finish the task as we had expected but he did it, and he did it well. I went back and watched him just before the meeting and he didn't need any coaching just like you said. He simply changes a little data and shifted a few outcomes of conversations and moved some money around and the governments all felt that the negotiations were the path of best resolution to their differences," Herfermks pics up a glass of beer and takes a drink.

Jay looks at the glass in front of him and picks it up to take a drink.

"It's not beer Jay" Berkjets says, "It is good for you but it is stronger than beer."

Jay takes sip, nods his head and has another sip. "It is good, smooth and a taste that I can't describe." Jay smells the drink and has another sip.

Herfermks nods his head at Jay as he looks at his father, "he'll be ok" and puts a hand up and waves at the bar, "Bread"

Birkjets says "you are the only Ryberian that does that, shouting at the bartender. How do you think he feels, you know he can't say anything about it if he is offended!"

"hahah, Father, I was friends with his grandfather and father and he remembers me shouting at them when he was just a boy. I took him fishing on the sea of Cyreptrex once when he was almost grown, a secret we keep. He likes me yelling in the bar, it gets the regulars feeling like I am one of them and they feel closer to the alliance form it. If you did it he would be offended though I am certain of it." He smiles and has another drink, turning to look at Jay "Don't you yell at these guys Jay they will have to fight you to prove that you have no control over them, it is a cultural thing."

Jay smiles and has another sip, he looks around, 'It is a well groomed species' he thinks to himself. 'These guys do look ready to go though.' "I won't yell at them, is there anything else I should know?"

Birkjets says "Don't talk to the females Jay it can't end well." He looks at Herfermks, "remember that time the three amburst were in here and one flirted with the waitress. Hahahahaha,"

Herfermks looks at him and slowly puts down his drink, "I do remember, hahaha. She made him have sex with her right here in the bar and then told him he was the worst, most pathetic male she had ever had sex with, she went on about it until his friends were so tired from laughing at him that they left."

A female puts a loaf of bread on the table. Jay pulls a piece of it for himself and takes a bite.

Birkjets continues "then she felt sorry for him and made it up to him by forcing herself on him sexually several times as she got him more and more intoxicated on those herbal drinks that they won't let us try." He grabs a piece of the bread too, takes a bite and slowly shaking his head side to side, "he couldn't hardly walk in the morning and she was going at him still." nodding his head at Herfermks finally his friends came back in the morning and she told them that he got better with practice but he was still not as good as the Vworktek midget that she had a few times."

Herfermks laughs, "I remember they had to carry him out, his clothes all ripped apart and his genitals firm and swollen and so tender looking, I felt bad for him." grabs the rest of the bread and pulls it in half. "Hahaha, it was some show, Jay if you are smart you won't even look at these females." then stuffs a large section of the bread into his mouth.

Birkjets looks at Jay then at Herfermks "does he go for the interspecies thing?"

Jay starts to open his mouth and Herfermks talks first. "Dad he is a Kyranin now, he has little choice. He has to play the role, we talked about it and it was hard for him at first but he has gotten to accept it."

Birkjets turns to Jay, "I couldn't do it Jay. The thought of it just makes me feel sick, to degrade myself with another species. I am a happily mated Ryberrian." he shakes his head and his body quakes. Looks at Jay, "a kyranin, I hope you enjoy it Jay. I am ever grateful for your help with the gowrlacks. You have no idea how tricky they were. If they had known who we were they may have gotten some retaliations in before it was over." sipping his drink before another bite of the bread.

Jay looks at him for a moment. "Glad that I was a help." then looks at Herfermks "I haven't heard about this planet, did I miss it in the training about the alliance?"

Herfermks looks at Jay "no." watching Jay pluck some small thing out of the bread.

Birkjets says "Jay this is not an alliance planet, or an aligned planet. This place is independent. We trade here but we have no authority, or rights either actually. We are guests. These seemingly crude and primitive beings have world government and space travel but no treaties with other planets. No one bothers them because of their willingness to fight and their proximity to the three other planets in the region."

"Are those alliance planets?" Jay asks.

Herfermks puts his hand on Jays shoulder, "You don't want to meet them Jay, they are an insect species, they have very good technology and they think we all taste good. We don't interfere with them and they don't interfere with us. There is no communications or treaty but rather a mutual respect."

Berkjets interjects "At different times a few non alliance species tried to take some control of things here and it went badly for them."

Jay asks, "so these beings have a relations ship and communicate with the insect planets?"

Herfermks replies, "Sort of, they trade. This planet breads and grows large predator animals that the insects like to come and hunt for. They let them hunt in designated areas of various climatic regions around the planet. They watch the hunts and have gambling on the outcomes. The insects compete to kill the animals. The insect planets don't have wild space so this is a important planet for their cultural heritage."

"So what happened when the other species interfered here?" Jay asked

Birkjets shift in his chair. "That was interesting Jay." and stuffs the rest of his bread into his mouth.

Herfermks agrees, "it was, at first nothing, then there was an interruption in one of the hunts by the new rulers. They wanted to communicate with the bugs, hahahahaha."

"Don't think the wrong way Jay," swallowing the bread, "the insects monitor all communications in the region, even some of ours. But they choose not to interact." Berkjets says. "Their culture is very advanced and many thousands of years ago they tried to communicate with other species. It always turned out bad for both sides, so now they don't bother with it."

"So what happened?" Jay asks

Herfermks looks at Berkjets then at Jay, "they came into the hunt and stood between the insect and the animal so the animal got away and tried to converse with the insect using the local data of the insects language. The bug spoke to them in their language and told them that they had interfered with its' kill and it was going to have to kill one of them instead and gave them a choice of which one of them it would kill. It didn't reply to their questions at all."

Birkjets adds "the insect only waited a few seconds and without another word started killing them all. At the same time all of their ships in orbit were fired upon and all of their bases on the surface were destroyed. The event was so short that we almost missed it with our scans."

Herfermks looks at Jay "the insects went back to the hunt like nothing had happened. The survivors of the attack were left to fend for themselves here without any bases or ships or weapons. The locals let them live and work with them but they all died out after about three generations, mostly in fights over nothing important."

Birkjets eyebrows raise, "the next incident was a small fleet of aliens that had been expanding their realm that arrived and asked to talk with the leaders of this planet. In the meeting as soon as they admitted that they meant to stay whether welcome or not there ships were all attacked and destroyed. It was funny to watch as the generals called for a show of force and nothing happened. Then after being politely expelled from the government building they had to go out into the city and find work to buy their next meal. You see Jay, the local traders that come and go from this place would never host an enemy of the insects so they couldn't even get a ride off of the planet."

Herfermks starts "The last time a species got in trouble here they had a plan. They spent a few years becoming well liked on the planet and trading to it's benefit, it made arrangements for a large fleet to use this space as a port of call, a place to do repairs and refuel and acquire supplies. They fortified the

structures they had made for themselves on the surface
and had a grid system of shields to protect their ships and
their structures on the planet. When they thought they were
ready they demanded to renegotiate their trade under new
terms. The locals said no. They were immediately contacted by
the insects and told to leave this section of the galaxy within
three days. They didn't. They all died on the fourth day."

Birkjets says, "when we first started regular trading here we
considered inviting this planet to join the alliance. Before we
agreed on how and when to present the proposal an insect
ship uncloaked in orbit of one of our moons. We invited them
to visit our planet and to join our alliance. They said they
would consider our offers, and replied that since we were not
in any treaty with them now, how would we like it if many of
their ships were stationed around our moon. When we
decided not to invite this planet to join the alliance there ship
left. That was four thousand years ago. We can see through
their cloaks and know they can see through some of ours but
we have never had more conversations with them."

Herfermks adds "we know they had a few ships watching
some of the war with the Gowrlacks."

Jay looks at both of them and asks, "you aren't going to turn
me into a bug to spy on them are you?"

Herfermks laughs and shacks his head.

Birkjets looks at Jay then Herfermks and start to laugh too. "good idea Jay but no, we wouldn't want you to get caught and start a war."

Jay smiles and finishes his drink.

Birkjets looks in his flask seeing it is empty and looks at Herfermks "It was good to see you, are your concerns about Teloion and Frestwy satisfied?"

Herfermks looks at his father and smiles, "It is always good to see you. Yes, I expect there interest in Jay was only as a celebrity in time. They are good workers, I am proud to have served with them."

Looking to Jay Berkjets says "So my friend, will you be happy on the moon for five years?"

Jay smiles, "I think I will be."

He looks around the bar "well let's go then", and he fades to nothing. Herfermks puts his foot on Jay's leg again and they fade and Jay sees the bar in the moon again, as it was the second when they left.

Jay scratches his head, looks around the bar and picks up a snack. "What do you think those ones are up to?" as he nods his head towards the groups of Kuroberote sitting at the tables with various aliens across the room. He watches Herfermks turns to look. He chews on some dried meat watching as Herfermks picks up a pastry and has a sip of his drink before putting it into his mouth. He pulls out his tablet and starts working it. Jay notices him shift slightly and then keep working his tablet. He picks up another snack and swallows it then has a big drink emptying his glass. "They are swindling some traders that have it coming." He looks at Jay and smiles, "That's why there are so many of them I guess."

Herfermks looks around and gives the bartender a hand signal, then looks at Jay, "you aren't hungry are you Jay?"

Jay looks at him, "Me? no I ate the bead, and, I feel a little,,, woozy from the drink. I am enjoying these snacks though. I can see why you like to come here."

"The negotiations are for some goods that the other aliens, lets say, deceptively acquired from a friend of one of these Kuroberote. She is not here. These ones at the big table are her security team and the others making deals to buy the goods are her friends. They are making a deal to trade them for other goods that should be worth more so some cash is also being asked for but the goods they will trade to get her shipment back is actually heavily mortgaged to the Vworktek military. They will have to give it to them or pay the price, one way or another."

"Business can be so easy or so dangerous" Jay says and takes a drink. "I don't know if I would want to do business for a living."

Herfermks looks at him, "I thought that is what you did on your world Jay?" He picks up his food as the waitress puts it on the table, "thank you" and he takes a bite.

"What is that", Jay asks.

Chewing, "mm" nodding his head and taking another bite, turns it so Jay can see inside, swallows and has another bite.

"It looks like a meat pie", Jay says, looking at Herfermks as he takes another chomp of it. "How long were you there for?" Jay asks and only gets a smile as Herfermks takes another bite. "I did do business but I did fair service mostly to improve homes for the owners. I did find out I was working with swindlers a few times; but I would only work with them once and I didn't cover their tracks."

"Good to hear it Jay" Herfermks takes a drink, and takes something from a pocket and slides it across the table toward Jay "here is some currency, you will pay for our meal and say it was the first time we met and mention it being an honor to buy us a meal." Herfermks looks at Jay to see that he is listening. "That is a good drink you had there wasn't it"

Jay looks at him "I actually do notice a growing effect from it."

Herfermks says to him, "Eat more Jay, finish your beer and then pay and go home, you will sleep well. I am leaving now. I will see you in about a month. Don't forget that she will see you here in two days, and again on friday, so don't come in until next weekend."

Jay puts another snack into his mouth, takes the money, and stands as Herfermks does. "It was good to meet you sir, I hope to talk with you again."

Herfermks nods at him and walks out of the bar. Jay sits down and enjoys his beer and the snacks. He tries not to look at the waitress too much as he finishes the plate of snacks. Walks to the bar and offers to pay the bill.

The bartender looks at him, "It is on Herfermks tab."

Jay says, "It is an honor for me to pay for their food and drinks," he smiles at the bartender, "the food here is good."

The bartender smiles back at him. "Next time try one of those pies Herfermks likes, you may not think so anymore" and he smiles. He looks at the money takes some and gives some change.

Jay looks at the currency and has no idea of the value of it. He looks up and asks "is it appropriate to leave something for the waitress? I am new to the moon and don't know the customs yet."

The Bartender smiles and steps over to fill some beers from a tap. "Yes, the change will be enough." he smiles and watches what he is doing with the beers.

Jay walks back and leaves the change on the table and walks home.

He spends the next days working and in the evenings studying local customs from his tablet at home. He takes a new way home from work every evening so that he starts to learn his way around the area that he lives and works without directions from the tablet. The next weekend he ventures to the surface where he enjoys the view of the sky through the thin atmosphere. The next week is about the same. A few good conversation with the cook and he is starting to make a few friends in the cafeteria when he goes for his meals. The next weekend Jay thinks about going to the bar but feels that he should wait an extra few days so he does. He is starting to understand the process of searching for patterns he thinks but he hasn't found anything yet. He is falling into a routine of walking a new way home, stopping to get some food for his dinner, making it, and studying the moons maps and cultural norms before he goes to sleep.

Another week goes by and Jay decides to stop at the bar on his way home from the office. He walks in and sees the bartender and some other waitress behind the bar. It is a little crowded and there are only a few tables so he walks up to the bar and sits on a stool. The waitress comes and takes his order and brings him his beer. He sips it and enjoys the flavor. He looks around and does not see the girl. He listens to the chatter in the bar and watches some odd looking patrons have some questionable interaction. He sees that his glass is empty as he lifts it to have another sip. The bartender turns to look his way as he holds the glass looking at the bottom of it asking himself if he wants a second. Jay sees him putting down his towel and walking toward him, and turns to greet him with a smile as he puts down the empty glass. "Hello sir, how are you doing today?"

He smiles at Jay for a second then nods, "I am well. It is good to see that you came back, how are you doing?", as he leans comfortably on the bar to face Jay.

"I am well, I am getting settled into my work and starting to find a few friends there." Jay says.

"It is good to have friends at work, but friends away from work are not as easy to choose I suspect."

Jay ponders the thought for a few seconds "you are right about that, I hadn't heard it expressed before but there is truth in it. My work friends make me feel comfortable at work, but I haven't considered asking them to visit my home." Jay checks his feeling as his solemn face shows his deep thought.

"I suspected you were wise, Herfermks wouldn't have sat with you more than once if you weren't. Would you like another drink, or something to eat?"

Jay looks at him then his glass then back at him, "I would like some kreptigs and another beer. The waitress, the attractive one she isn't here now?"

The bartender looks at Jay for a second then starts to smile, "that is my daughter, so you think she is attractive?"

Jay thinks about what he said and what he should and shouldn't say. He straitens his posture and looks directly at her father then says "your daughter? Yes, I find your daughter to be attractive to me." He can feel the worry coming to his face as the bartender looks at him.

With a stone face and some seconds of reflective staring, "well, I will get you the beer and the kreptigs, Jay is it?"

"Yes, my name is Jay"

The bartender smiles and walks over to the taps and fills Jay a glass of beer, works on his screen with his fingers and then brings Jay the beer. "If you come back in a few hours she will be her. She had the day off but will be here to help me close tonight like always. Tell me Jay have you ever worked in a bar?"

"No" Jay says.

"If my daughter asked you to help here at the bar could you do it?"

Jay looks at him wondering what to do. She said not to say anything more, but he is asking a direct question. He looks at him for a few seconds as he thinks about the question, "I believe that I would."

The bartender looks at Jay's face and turns and walks to serve other customers.

After a few sips the waitress brings his kreptigs. He crunches them as he sips the rest of the beer then puts the correct amount of currency on the bar with a little extra for the service and walks home. His next few days are spent focusing on his work and enjoying his quiet home routine. On the second to last day of the week Jay hears some of the others at work talking about some festival and telling stories of the drinking and partying in previous years. By the end of the day Jay feels like a drink so he stops at the bar on the way home. When he walks through the bar he sees his waitress and she looks at him like he did something wrong. He looks back with a puzzled expression and walks to a table and sits down. Watching her server the other customers with hast until all of the tables are taken care of then she gives him a look and goes into the kitchen. Jay remembers her father saying she would be 'back later' that evening when they talked and realizes it was an invitation to talk with her. He starts to wonder about the Gyrekian mating protocols and pulls out his tablet as he sees her coming out from the kitchen with a tray. He watches as she rounds a few tables then heads directly for him. She stops just in front of him a meter away from his table and looks at him looking at her, "hello, it is good to see you."

She looks at him and then asks, "Will you be inviting me to join you?"

Jay stands up and asks, "please, will you join me I would truly enjoy to have you sit at my table."

She looks at him and smirks then puts down the tray and sits in a chair, "So Jay, you know nothing at all about our customs do you?"

Jay is surprised at her question. "I don't actually. Did I do something wrong?"

Taking a glass of the tray for her self, "not considering that you don't understand what to do."

"What should I do?" he asks.

"Take your glass and sit it in front of you." she says. Then watching him as he does it, she takes one plate of food with pieces of fruit on it and sits it in front of her and says "now take the plate of seeds and place it in front of you." She watches as he does it. "Jay" she says, "this is the important part. If you want to be my mate for a few years or longer you have to do this part well. Take the other plate and put it in the middle and then put a little of your seeds on it then a little of my fruit on it and then more seeds and then more fruit until all of the food is on the one plate. Then you have to mix the food and serve it back onto the two plates and ask me to take a drink with you, we will drink at the same time. My father will come over and top up our glasses unless one is empty. If one is empty he will take our two plates away. If we still have something in our glasses, it has to be a small but good amount. He will take away the empty plate and leave the picture for us to finish. Unless he doesn't like how you divided the food. So divide the food evenly. Then we will eat all the food and finish the picture and he will be happy, and so will we."

Jay thinks about all of what she said and nods.

"Well, what are you waiting for?" She looks at him like he is starting to annoy her.

"Oh" Jay says and looks to see that there is no utensils on the table, reaching for his seeds he asks "with my fingers?"

"Yes"

Jay puts some seeds on the plate, then some fruit, then some seed, then some fruit, then some seed then fruit until it is all moved. He mixes it all up and shares it as evenly as he can in his first try and looks at her to get a nod. "Will you have a drink with me?' as he lifts his glass.

Lifting her glass she smiles at him for a few seconds and starts to blush "yes".

They both drink down about two thirds of the fluid in the glasses. Jay feels the tingling in his mouth and throat then in his stomach. She puts down her glass and nervously looks at his as she sits back into her chair.

Jay watches her and sits back into his chair looking at her expression and wondering why she is nervous. He thinks about the feeling in his mouth throat and stomach that is turning to warmth and starts to wonder if there is a problem with the beverage and is about to ask.

"Jay, it is good to see you here" Her farther says from across the room as he walking towards them with a pitcher that looks heavy in his hands.

Jay watches as he pours from the pitcher into his daughters glass first, then looking down into Jays glass with a worried look on his face as he winks at Jay, hesitating before pouring Jay's. Jay sees his girls' face turning white, then pouring, Jay watches as her father gives her a good long look and puts the picture down as he smiles at her. Jay sees his smile pulling the skin of his face tight in several places before he lets go of the pitcher and picks up the plate, and nods at each of them. Jay watches him walk back to the bar. Then looks at her again.

She smiles and says, "We do have to eat it all Jay." and takes a handful and holds it in front of her mouth.

Jay takes a handful and brings it to his mouth as he watches her open her mouth and puts her hand to it he does the same. Wondering the significance of the ritual he starts to realize how good the mixed fruit and nuts tastes. He reaches for another handful as she does the same, then another and another until they finished the last little bit that was on the plates.

Jay sees her licking her fingers as she looks at him like he is the desert. He decides to lick his fingers off too as it is the first time he has been there and not had ample towels on the corner of the table. As Jay reaches for his drink she mimics his movements. He drinks half of his glass and she shows him that hers is empty. So he takes a breath and finishes his too. He sees her stand and come around the table to fill his glass form the pitcher then sit back down with out filling her own. He looks at her for a second as she looks at him, his hand goes toward the glass and he sees her head shake, so he stops.

"Come here Jay and fill my glass." She says.

Jay thinks then gets up and walks around the table and reaches for the pitcher, lifting it as he look and smiles at her, he starts to think about how pretty she is and how happy she looks and how he feels the warmth from the drink spreading through him. He looks into her eyes and then glances a little as the last of the fluid slides into her glass almost filling it to the rim. He sees the excitement in her eyes and goes back to sit in his seat.

She slides her hand to the glass and asks "ready", then watches him.

Jay looks at her, smiles back, and reaches to pick up his glass. She picks hers up at the same time as him he notices and he watches as she brings it to her lips at the same speed he does. He sees that she is waiting to start drinking it so he slowly lifts his glass, as he tilts back his head and watches her watching him. They both pour their drinks into their mouths and gulp it down until the glasses are empty.

She slams the glass down on the table and yells, "WOAnnSHEriiicK"

Jay Slams his glass down to and looks at her "do I say that too?"

She smiles at him and laughs, "maybe later Jay first come with me" and she comes around the table and grabs his hand. Tugging on him and turning toward the bar, she looks back at his eyes, "come with me".

Jay gets up feeling the beverage has already affected his vision and his dexterity he smiles, "ok, and starts walking, entangling his fingers with her's. "Where are we going?" he asks as he remembers the storage room near the kitchen.

She laughs, "You are coming to see one of our homes Jay."

A New Life

Jay thinks to himself as he follows her, hand in hand, into the back, through a door and up some stairs. 'Did I hear that right, she is talking about co ownership of homes,' working to keep his balance as they come to a door that opens as she gets close. Inside he sees wall screens showing forest views like in the forests on earth on all the walls. They stop inside the door and it closes behind them. She turns and starts undoing his shirt.

"Undress me Jay, that is your part" as she pulls his garments to loosen them and works at the buttons. "Mine opens from the back Jay, reach around" stepping closer to him and getting the last button undone on his shirt she glides her hands around on his smooth chest.

Jay feels the effects of the drink and hopes he can stay focused on what he is doing. He reaches around her and finds a zipper between the folds of her blouse. Once he gets it started it slides down easily. Opening the back of her blouse as she steps back and steps again and again pulling her arms out of it. Jay looks at her naked from her hips up in front of him. He feels the tension in his pants. He realizes that the drink is having another effect on him that he hadn't noticed until now. He sees her smiling at him looking at his face and glancing down every few seconds. Pulling off his shirt he steps forward and reaches for her.

She lets him come to her and allows him to brush her hair back with his hand then his other hand slides down her shoulder, over her breast and belly to follow the top of her pants around to the back looking for a button or clasp. "Oh Jay, you are new to our moon" she says and reaches to his pants quickly undoing them and working them so that they drop to the floor. "Can't you get mine off Jay?" she smirks at him.

Jay slides his fingers under the edge of her pants and tugs a little this way then that as she starts to laugh.

She grabs his cock and starts pulling it this way and then that, "is that how you get what you want from a female on Ramga Jay the Kyranin? You are a moon male now and you will have to learn new ways to get your pleasure." I am your maiden and you'er my lord. You will be good to me and please me well of your life will become boring and sad. So do as I say now Jay"

Jay looks at her looking into his eyes and he sees her playfulness and the sparkle in her eyes and he replies, "yes my maiden, what is you command, and he hears himself laughing and feels the floor against his back. He turns his head to see what made the "thud" sound but only sees the floor meeting the wall screen a few meters away. He realizes that he fell or was pushed over and asks her "what was in the drink"

"It is the bonding drink Jay. We are bonded now, it is safe, and you will be the same after it wears off, but now we will be together and nothing else will matter." as she climbs across him, pinching him here and there and rubbing and squeezing him in various places.

Jay looks at her on top of him playing with his arm and belly with her breasts full and firm in front of him, he looks down and sees his ridged cock as big and stiff as it has ever been and feels a glow through his entire body like the first flavor of the drink and the sensation it started in his mouth. He smiles to himself and feels a silly grin taking control of his face. Deciding to make the best of his new situation he starts caressing her. His hand follows his minds instructions but he finds he has to focus to feel the sensation of touch from his skin as he moves his hand across her. He can hear her breathing and his hand moving against her and her skin sweeping against his. Jay watches and sees her playfully stroking his chest and has to focus to feel it in his skin. He laughs and looks at her as she looks back into his eyes.

She grabs his cock and whispers "what should I do with this Jay?" and bends it side to side, smiling at him with a questioning expression.

Jay heard the whisper loud and clear. He looks down and sees that she still has her pants on and that she is working his ridged penis from side to side with more than a gentle force. He focuses to feel her hand's grip and motion on him as he watches. At first it isn't much but as he focuses he notices that he starts to feel it more and deeper through to inside of him. He feels the sensation on the skin and in his organ and in all that it connects to in his pelvis and in his belly too. "ooohwwwoo" and he looks at her as she watches it.

"well Jay, my lord!" She climbs over him so her face is nose to nose with his, " what will we do with that?" sliding her tongue across his nose in an annoying sloppy stroke, dripping slobber almost into his eye. Then sliding back down him so that his cock is in her crotch and she closes her legs so that her pants have a grip on his tower. "You can't do much with that until you find a way to get my pants off Jay"

Jay's mind still holding the sensitivity of the sensations in his hands and chest and cock, as he looks down at her smiling face looking up at him. "Oh, How can I get them off?" he asks her. She gets up and a straddles herself over him, one foot lateral to each shoulder so that her crotch is over the top of his chest. "The release starts by my left foot Jay, un slide them."

Jay looks at her left foot coming out of the pant leg and sees a small tab hanging there. He reaches over and pulls it slowly up her leg and over and down the other side and watches her unveiled as the pants dangle from her waist.

Stepping off of him she bends down and pulling another tab and the waist loosens and they fall to the floor. She walks around him watching him watch her and she starts to laugh. "Jay, do you like what you see?"

Jay smiles and looks at her, "I do" he says and starts to get up.

She climbs back onto him sitting on his chest with her feet beside his ribs, her shins on his arms and her thighs on his shoulders. "I like what I see too Jay, I am looking at you." stroking his hair and then his face, "Do you know what will make me happy my lord?"

Jay thinks for a second "no my lady, I am not sure, I could guess but I feel it will be best if I am told. So tell me. What I can do for you, how can I make you happy." he can smell her genitals and he can feel a wave of lust building in his organs and bones.

She slides a little forward spreading her legs a little and then a bit more so that her groin is touching his chin, then slides a little further forward as she lifts herself and spreads her knees a little wider resting her bulging full mounds around her opening against his lips. "Wet me up Jay."

Jay can feel the pulsing heat of her pussy on his lips as he focuses to feel what they are against. The aroma of her is sweet, filling his nostrils with an aroma like a mix of fresh strawberries and roses. As he stretches his tongue to meet it and feels the tender heat of her and the sweet tangy taste his focus magnifies the taste and sensation. He groans and reaches to grab her sides, but with his restrained arms limiting the reach of his hands his hand reach only the air beside her.

His attempt lifting her a little and she giggles and grabs his head with both hands. "Are you going to give me a good ride Jay?" and she pulls his head into her a little.

He likes the sensation on his tongue and as his focus is brought there, he momentarily forgets what he is doing. His tongue stroking, tasting, exploring her, while sliding here and there. He feels the texture of her, the flavor, and the scent and is lost in it all. His nostrils competing for a larger portion of his mind, the texture building memory as he finds each detail in and around her folds so thick and full they seem to be mountain ranges under his tongue as it covers them like clouds in the wind. Her flavor screaming into Jay's brain, as sweet as honey with a slow tangy edge scraping into him an addiction and a craving and a satisfaction all at the same time. His mouth and face so intensely occupied that he is lost in the experience and stretches to continue it as his new utopia is slowly withdrawn out of his tongues reach. Opening his eyes to see the bottom of her being lifted by those soft delicate legs and Jay start to remembered that there is more to the world than just his mouth's experience of her. He starts to get up but she steps across him turning around and is back down with her cunt snugly on his nose. Jay reaches the tip of his tongue to flick and lick at her where he can reach then notices his testicles being squeezed and forgets all else. His attention in that area, his body tense out of his control, and she slides her mouth over his rigid dick. He can feel that, it soothes the pain as she strokes it up and down with her lips. Holding his balls with one hand as she works her mouth over him as her vagina is being opened by the tip of his nose. With her other hand she starts to tickle his ribs. Within a few tries she finds the spot that works and Jay twitches. She waits and does it again and waits and again, still stretching and stroking with his tongue. Each time Jay twitches and torques his torso and arms and legs

his nose pokes a little deeper into her straddled crotch
until Jay is finding it hard to get air. Turning his head to take a
breath she lifts herself from him.

She rolls onto her back and moans, then a deep inhale, "oh,,,
Jay are you ok?". She roles onto her side and climbs up to be
face to face with him, then slides her leg over then down the
outside of his. Looking into his eyes she starts to smile, "you
couldn't breath?"

Jay smiles and takes another deep breath lifting her wait easily
as he inhales.

She starts gently kissing his face and mouth as she awkwardly
shimmies down him to find his hard-on with her genitals.
Reaching it she plays gracefully bumping and rubbing herself
against the tip of him.

As Jay enjoys the kisses awakening the senses in his skin he
brings his hands to her sides and fingers onto her back,
Relaxing his pelvis so she can have control of her playing as he
feels and caresses her back. He notices that she slows her
actions as be sensually explores her back's muscles and soft
skin. Her hair dangling onto his face tickles, and Jay relaxes to
feel the twinges of it start a murmur of euphoria spreading
through his skull. He notices that the skin on his belly is being
pulled downward by her movements and that her opening has
found his head and is gliding around and on and off of it. He

slowly starts to crunch, clenching his abdomen to bring his cock closer and slightly into her. He feels her teeth on his cheek and stops moving. Her tongue starts sliding swiftly across his face and into one eye socket, then the other, lapping at him like an ice cream cone. Jay's intellect questions this but he finds his mood controls his thoughts and he relaxes, and finds a perspective to enjoy it. Her tongue migrates to his nose, then to his lips. Then she stops. He can feel a tensing inside of her from the way he weight on him changes. Her slow deep breath is followed by another and then as she starts the third. She touches her lips to his, the tongue follows, as their lips gently feeling each other's her tongue start to explore his teeth. He brings his own forward as he lowers his chin to provide an opening for her to enter. She does finding his tongue just inside. Jay slowly slides it out further so she can have access to it. He feels her sweeping around it with hers as he notices her vagina starts to slide further past his penis's head. She starts coaxing his tongue out further buy sliding hers past his as far as she can reach and then stroking it hard towards her mouth. Jay surprised at the agility of her tongue grips her back as he lets his tongue extend further and further with each stroke until it is fully stretched into her mouth. All at once he feels her teeth grabbing his tongue and then pulling it as she lifts her head back and retrieves her lips from his. The stretch on his tongue startles him and he grips her back tighter while crunching his pelvis, somewhat. He sees her eyes open and her smile letting go of his tongue, realizing his involuntary thrust has made her smile he stretches it, slowly sliding into her until he is pressing on the end of her interior.

"Jay I like you, I think we that will be happy. Are you happy with your choice to bond with me?" as she shifts her pelvis side to side changing the angles of pressure on his cock and sliding her stretched vaginal end across his head.

Jay swallows as he considers what he has gotten himself into and says "Yes"

Her mouth is on his again and her excitement is clear. Jay tries to keep up as she torques herself around to bring various motions to shift the fit of her around his cock. "Help me Jay. Hold my back and don't let me off!" as she becomes more violent with her motion.

Jay feels his genitals sensations starting to glow. He is holding, squeezing her back, her lowest ribs and back with one hand over each kidney. He starts to slowly thrust his pelvis to extend and retract his cock as she bounces and torques against it. He feels the connection of energy from his eyes and brain to his genitals as the orgasm energy starts to grow in his balls, then his back, and cock too. He sees the sweat on her and feels it dripping onto him, her kisses are sloppy now and he hears a slight whining sound, he notices a stiffness starting in her movements and starts a little more pelvic movement and speeds his thrusting. He feels her gripping his face with her hands and then looking with stretched eyes into his as he kisses stops their motion. Her body still shifting and torque he feels her hot breath on his face as he feels the swelling in his cock and the pressing heat from his kidneys trying to reach it. The bellows of euphoria start in his guts and slide down his torso almost into his legs then change to a sparkling burst as it fills his balls and cock, he hears himself gulp a breath as the sensation heats his dick and the fluid starts to flow. Looking into her eyes and seeing her looking back, he feels her tenseness with his hands as she slides side to side one more time and a tear and a smile come on her face. The throbbing of his orgasm starts him to relax as she lowers her mouth to on his again, then he feels her hot around his cock, a new sort of heat, warmer, and deeper some how. His skin feels almost raw from it.

"wow,' he says 'your genitals are hot."

Whispering into his ear, "don't move Jay, not for a minute"

Jay lay there with her relaxing into him and playing with his ear on one side and whispering a song into the other ear. He feels his cock softening and the stretch of it as if it is being pulled on. Jay's sensations are calming so he reverts to caressing her back. Feeling the sweat from her, he notices that he is almost drenched in it. He starts thinking about his situation, already a month on the moon and on the trusted word of Herfermks he has entered a relationship with a young local female that he is attracted to, but has little understanding of her culture. 'So far so good' he tells himself and he lay under her and enjoys the intimacy. He feels her start to move her pelvis and with it a tugging on his cock. 'That's odd' he thinks and put all of his focus down there. Feeling it not hard at all but limp, and it feels attached inside of her. Fear starts to take him as he asks, "is my cock stuck inside of you some how?"

Grabbing his ears and gently stretching them to the sides as she smiles and giggles, looking into his eyes from a few centimeters away from his. Her left eye fixed looking into his right and her right eye looking into his left, "do you like it my Kyranin mate?" She torques her torso slightly to change the angles of the pulling as she kisses him again.

Jay feels the fear subside a little as he realizes that this is not an issue for her but he is still a lot concerned. "Is my cock going to be stuck in you for a long time?"

Her motions starting to take on a gentle rhythm, "that depends Jay, your juice can release it, if you have enough, If not we could be here for days. Does that worry you Jay? Or would you be happy holding me like this for days at a time, kissing and caressing me?" and she gives a few gentle tugs on his ears and squeezes his upper lip with hers then lifts herself with her hands on his shoulders.

Jay realizes that she is at least partly serious and the fear reduces a bit more. "I could cuddle you as long as you like" as he shifts his hands to the sides of her belly.

Sliding her knees forward on the floor she rocks gently as she finds comfort sitting on him and reaches behind herself and stretches to grasp his balls with one hand and moves the other one to his chest. Gripping his entire scrotum and its' contents softly in her palm and securing her grip with her fingers she smiles at his face. "I've got you now Jay as she gently grips his nipple between her finger and thumb.

Jay, still feeling the fear, fully aware of his limp cock being pulled inside of her as she moves and with her breath too, starts to laugh and replies, "Yes you do, don't you?" sliding his hands down her sides rounding her buttocks and down her thighs then back up. What will you do with me, my Gyrekian mate?"

Moving her fingers to his other nipple and massaging his testicles as she grinds her vagina onto him. She keeps looking into his eyes and says, "as soon as you get past the fear I will do things that you will want me to do to you often." and she raises her eyebrows.

Jay realizes that she can read the fear from his face. He relaxes and accepts that she won't hurt him, or do anything that could damage him. "This is a surprise for me, I truly have almost no knowledge of your culture or mating processes. Sex I know that, but the details I don't understand."

"Don't worry Jay, I am your mate now and your well being is as precious to me as my own. We are as one now, as I will be with you in our relationship for as long as it lasts. You can think of this ritual of the ceremony as a reminder of what it is to be as one. You have fear that some damage could come to your cock that would destroy you capacity for pleasure from it correct? Well if something bad happens to your genitals it will be the same to mine and then I too will loose my capacity to get pleasure from sex." she looks into his eyes and smiles. "We are one in this danger as we are one in all situations from now until we choose to end it. If you do something stupid it will affect me and if you hurt me you will find it also brings you pain. Maybe not directly but with my pain my ability to bring you health and pleasure decreases, so, slowly, it becomes a life with more pain in it." her rocking in a rhythmic manner is starting to bring some swelling to his cock.

Jay thinks about what she said as he enjoys the massage on his scrotum and the pressure of her on him. "I hadn't though of a relationship in that way, but it makes a lot of sense." Jay feeling the muscles of her thighs flexing slightly as she rocks and twists slightly to grind into him.

"You are coming back to life Jay", she says as she feels him swelling a little inside of her. "It feels better Jay. I know you have no understanding of it. From my side I feel a slight pain when you are not hard in this situation. It is like when in life you don't have my confidence pushing through you to succeed; and as a result you don't find it easy to manifest our goals. It harms my future. In this part of the ritual I have to find ways to bring you your masculine power so we can both succeed and have what we want together or I feel the pain. Just as it is your place to bring me joy and happiness it is my place to bring you happiness and joy. If I don't keep you happy you won't have the joy to make me happy from."

Jay feels the stretch on the skin of his penis changing to the other way, like he is pushing into something that is gripping his skin to prevent him from going further. He feels a pressure on the end of it pushing back into his perineum as she continues to grind into him. The massage on his balls is starting to cause urges for him to twitch and gyrate his pelvis.

Feeling him starting to move she holds his balls still and softly says, Let me do my part Jay, when we are done with my part you can do your part and I will be ready to love every bit of it. But if I can't do my part we will never be happy. Feeling Jay stop moving, she changes her hands, gripping his balls with the other, and shifting a little weight onto his chest. Feeling Jay full and firm inside of her she holds his stretched sack tight to her ass as she slowly rolls, torques, thrusts, and twists her pelvis in random direction just enough to constantly change the angles of pressure in her genitals and on his. "Relax Jay relax through all of it, focus hard at the end and stay relaxed, don't clench and don't move, don't hold it and don't force it out just relax, Let me do my part." as she continues.

Jay holding her thighs with a gentle grip focuses on relaxing his arms and keeping his and just tense enough to secure their positions on her shifting thighs. He relaxes his back and neck letting his head settle hard against the floor. His toes; he relaxes them, and his legs, and his pelvis, his abdomen, and then his breathing. Taking slow deep relaxing breaths as she grips, massages, and tugs gently on his balls. Feeling her manipulations and their sensations as her hands squeezes and shift one then the other, and then both. The surges of full almost ache like shifting sensations shooting and or gliding from her pressure into his guts. He feels the way she moves his wand and how it is connected deep inside of his torso, the way his gland pries inside of him as she slides from side to side and up and down on him, he feels it swelling and swaying empty warmth. He feels a tender thickening of it and an excitement in his blood. His hand feeling her thighs muscles shifting bring an excitement to his thoughts and he starts to realize his lust for her. Remembering her words he focuses and stays relaxed, watching her face as she stares into his eyes. He can see that her arousal is matching his as he feels the fullness of his orgasm slowly building. The warmth of the energy as it is accumulating in his belly, between his navel and his sacrum how it's fuzzy glow warmly spreads and increases in sensation, slowly spreading and building. He looks in her eyes and sees her smile relaxing, and her eyes starting to squint a little as she hastens her movements. He focuses to not follow his urges to move his pelvis and help her grinding. He focuses as the glow in his cock start to work it's way down and into his guts. He focuses on not moving as the sensation in his balls from her squeezing increases from her hasty movements and greater pressure and as he sees her biting her lip and feels his cock starting to pulse. Looking into her eyes he realizes it is her hot cunt that is pulsing and he feels his cock responding to it with a heat surge back down and around to his navel. The condensing of the sensation there swells and spreads to his anus. It starts to pulse and then his cock pulses too and the hot aching bolts from the pressure she is giving from the grip on his balls sets it all loose. He struggles to stay relaxed as he feels the alignment of all of the sensations from his kidneys, navel, sacrum, anus, balls and cock all surge as one and then as it peaks and he stays relaxed. He feels the gradual slow release of his fluids, filling his ducts and feeling good in them and the sensations sustain as the fluid slowly leaks up into her without pulsing at first. Just a few drips, he focuses to stay still and still feels the rush of his orgasm and now too feeling the fluid between his penis head and her grip on it inside of her vagina. He feels the friction on his skin and his focus is lost, his pumping begins, the energy sensations starts to decline as the friction sensations breaks his concentration and his pumping empties him into her.

She moans and squeezes herself onto him. Exasperating her motions to fill herself and feel the juices of him as they trigger her hormones to release her own moisture, and the friction changes the sensations from energetic to physical for her too.

She stops moving as Jay realizes that he is finished and getting soft again. She lays down on him and gives him a hard long kiss, relaxing into him, pressing her breasts against this chest.

Jay feels her pussy still pulsing slow around his cock and her heart beating the same rhythm on his chest. He notices he still feels the glow of his own orgasm too.

"Roll me over Jay. Before you get too soft. Roll me over and suck on my tits." as she start to roll herself off of him.

Jay responds, he does as she asks and helps her by pushing himself in the same direction. He roles with her so that he is on top and then getting up on all four he moves down, with his chest on her belly he starts with his nose bumping her nipple, then his tongue. He notices a sweet tangy flavor as he first licks it. Then he locks his lips to the other nipple. Tugging it with his grip, stretching it and letting it snap back. Gripping it again, wet this time and sucking on it. The flavor catches his attention, pungent and smooth. As he sucks he notices that as lightly sour liquid is coming into his mouth and the pungent is decreasing. His lips are affected by it in that they gain some agreeable sensation that lingers and has him wanting more. His hand on her other breast as his passion awakens. His minds focus splits from the nipple's intoxication flavors to the firm smooth beauty in his hand and then the scent of her wetness bellow shoots through his nose into the front of his mind. Lifting his head to look at her smiling back at him he switches to taste the other nipple. Feeling the fullness in his groin and the lifting of his erection he shifts his position making his neck uncomfortable but he wants those secretions in his mouth as much as he want to enter her again. Continuing to shift his position and crunching his body as best he can he still can't reach his cock to her, but her tries.

She watches what he is doing, wanting him to succeed and knowing he can't, and starts to giggle. Grabbing his ears and tugging gently "Jay", and then harder "Jay" lifting her legs to place her heals on his back, "Jay" as she pulls harder on his ears.

Jay looks up and feels her forceful towing on his ears and yields as she pulls him to her lips. Realizing the intoxication that he feels he focuses to be fully conscious of his body and thoughts. He feels his desire and the intensity of his emotions and understands that it is at least partly drug induced. But he wants her and now he can reach so in it goes. The smooth ripe sensation as he slides in stymies him. He stops every movement for a second, as the sensation is surreal and ringing through him like a siren. "oohHw" opening his eyes and seeing her face smiling at him. "Hi" he says lost in the moment of the feeling. He feels her vagina pulse a squeeze on him and he continues his movements, slowly thrusting to reach fully into her and then out slowly from another angle each time. Looking into her eyes and watching her expressions of joy he realizes that he is pretty high on whatever they drank; and it has some how affected his physical senses. He sees her face changing to an expression of unexpected intensity. Continuing his thrusts he feels her heals digging into his back and her torso crunching as her hands start gripping his back and her breathing becomes forced, full fast inhales and hard holding slow exhales with her mouth clenched and eyes wide open. He feels her pulsing vagina and sees her gulping for air so he stops moving. Her pulsing and convulsing crunches work his fully aroused rigid rod almost to climax before she settles her tensions and slows her breathing. He waits for her to say something, watching her eyes as they still look into his. Jay reaches his lips to hers with a gentle kiss.

She smiles so hard that her eyes squint and she whispers "again" and starts pulling on him and digging her heals into his back.

Jay starts to slowly grind into her causing a deep pressure inside of her as his length is too much for her position now. Seeing her surprise each time he crams it to the end he changes his position, lifting her up and crossing his legs beneath them. He holds her and she slides down sitting between and on his crossed legs facing him. Belly to belly and face to face. Jay starts kissing her and gyrating his pelvis to move his cock inside her as best he can. Allowing her to move as she chooses, he continues kissing passionately and gently, holding her back with his right hand and fondling her breast with his left.

Changing her position she finds an angle that she likes best and arranges her feet so that she has a little mobility with it. Looking into Jay's eye with hers as they kiss and grind on each other she feels her orgasm starting to build again, filling her belly with a secure pressure of light that slowly becomes viscous and physical. Her insides sensing him moving as if in an exaggerated slow motion, the stoking sending tiny zings to her belly, kidneys and womb. Her climax starting to build again, she changes her position to slow it down.

Jay feels the change pull his cock's root lower from his pubic bone and the pressure on its top and on his head increase his sensations of widening warm pressure in his entire abdomen. A pulsing in his anus starts to expand to his shaft and he feels her dig her nails into his back and shift her feet, slamming them into his back. It doesn't affect the flowing heat that swirls towards his genitals and the raw sucking feeling on his cock as her hot vagina starts to pulse. He feels the wet, as it is running down his balls and his own throbbing; sucking the wind from his lungs. He feels his chest and throat moving like he is making a groan but no sound come out. The throbbing in his pelvis and belly, and then the bursting of balls shooting there contents into her vacuuming cunt bringing his heart to a rate that build dizziness in his mind. He looks into her eyes to see them looking back into his. Her sweat and tears running down her face and over her smile. He feels her quaking a little and feels her tongue come out and lick his face.

"Jay." licking him some more, "lay down, I will lick you off first."

Jay dose as he is told, laying back, relaxing and letting her lick him like a dog licking an ice cream cone that its' favorite child dropped on the floor. Just laying there with no thoughts as she licks frantically in random places, moving him to get better access, then rolling him over to get his back. He can't believe she actual is licking him all over, he thinks about the way people say it in flirting on earth and starts wanting to laugh. "Are you doing it so completely for a reason?"

"Mmm,. Yes Jay,. It is the pheromones, they make me more physically connected to you" and she continues licking.

Jay thinks about it and remembers the way babies bond to their mothers from breastfeeding. "So this is part of our bonding ritual too?"

Looking at him as she finishes licking his hand, "Yes it is an important part, now your turn to do it to me."

Jay rolls over beside her and starts licking, her breast.

"Not just there Jay, you have to lick all of me," she lies down on her back and smiles at him.

Jay laughs and gets on his knees and is laughing to hard to get a good lick going, he gets his tongue on her then starts to laugh and his face is on her but his tongue comes back in. After a few tries she gets a little annoyed so he pokes his tongue against her stomach a few times and she starts laughing too. Tickling her gets her squirming and tickling him back then wrestling and rolling around and snuggling in each others' arm's.

"Jay, you do have to lick me, it is important to me," she says to him and looks into his eyes with a questioning expression.

Jay smiles, "Ok" and he takes a deep breath, "I will explain the humor one day. I will start from you head and go to your toes." He starts doing it thinking only of his task and trying not to miss any spots until he has sucked her last toe. He looks at her then snuggles up beside her. "How are you doing?"

"Mmm, I'm good Jay. Lets go shower and have some custard", she gets up and walks to the next room, then through a doorwayout of view.

Jay sits up on the floor looks around at their clothes and gets up to follow. Once standing he realizes that he is almost staggering to walk. Visually everything is normal he thinks as he follows where she went. He finds her in a large room with a wide vanity and three chairs on one side and a toilet, sink, a fountain and showers on the other side. Some heater racks in the middle similar to the one found on bathroom walls in Europe with towels on them. Jay walks directly into the shower and asks it to wash him. Then he looks at her sitting on the toilet and asks, "How do I start it."

She looks at him and smiles, "house, this is Jay, he has command authority now." looking him over pretty good as she continues to smile, "ask again Jay"

Jay asks, "house, shower me", the water starts flowing from the ceiling, and spraying from the floor. Jay sees a small spout on the wall and puts his hand under it expecting something to come out.

He hears a giggle behind him and turns.

"It must have been nice on Ramga," smirking at him. "Here you have to pull the spout to get your shampoo." she gets up and walks into the shower, pulls the spout taking some fluid and starts washing Jay's back.

Jay finds her careful washing of him to be very thorough and relaxing. He decides that he wants to do the same to her and is eager to start by the time that she is finished. Washing her he finds that as much as he is finding an odd sexual satisfaction in scrubbing her, he is feeling compelled to do a very good job of it. Once finished they towel them selves off and she gives him a robe that she brought home for him sevral days earlier. Then she gives him a tour of the apartment. Ending, Jay thought, with the bedroom. But after a tour in there She wants to show him the garden.

"Come on Jay, it is through this door," pointing to a door in the back of the bedroom that looks like just another closet door. Touching a panel on the door it swing into the hallway leading to the place she wants him to see. "You are going to like this Jay"

'I guess it is hydroponics, odd that it's not off the Kitchen' Jay thinks. "What is it, that I will like?" he asks as he follows her down a hallway about six meters. He looks around as going down the four steps into the space. It has a high ceiling with something that looks like roots or a vine with flowers and small long red fruit dangling from it. The stuff sparsely covers the entire ceiling. The roots also come out from the walls on one full side of the room and a small patch on one other side. "What is it" Jay asks.

"This is our gerupta garden Jay. This fruit gives us the juice for our bonding ceremony and it makes delicious spread for our breads too. These flowers make a delicious tea. It is what we drink here on the moon when we are at home. When we go out we try the foods and drinks from other worlds of course but at home Gyrekians drink tea from these flowers." walking to him and taking his hand, "come on I will make us some" and she starts walking with his hand in hers.

Jay keeps in step drawn by her pulling him toward the kitchen. "Is it tasty?" he asks.

"Well, It is an acquired flavor I am told" she says as they enter the kitchen. Letting go of him and opening a cupboard "sit down Jay I'll make it".

She bustles around the kitchen as Jay relaxes and notices how his body has an increased sensitivity to light and pressure, then he also notices that he has an increased capacity for sound. He listens to the sounds of her movements and then notices an insect crawling in the corner of the room. Watching it he starts to think that he is actually hearing it scratch and flap it's wings. He looks at her and asks, "what kind of bug is that?" Then hears her answer without seeing him or turning to look at the bug. "How can you know without looking? Jay asks.

Stopping what she is doing she turns to Jay, "Everyone knows what a berbit sounds like when it cleans its wings!" Looking down at it for a second, "don't step on it Jay. Not only is it bad luck to step on one, this one is going to make eggs. We don't have enough berbits in this region Jay, it is dry for them, this one with the eggs almost ready to be laid will stink if you squash it" she looks at him and smiles. "They eat smaller bugs Jay, you can put it out in the bar or the garden but please don't make me clean bug stains from our walls or floor. Berbits stain when you squash them."

Jay looks at her looking at him like she is worried that he would do it. "Ok I won't, I don't mind a bug on the floor or an the wall once in a while. Do you want to teach me how to make the tea?"

Smiling at him, "no, you can do it anytime, put the flowers in hot water and let it cool enough to drink, that is all" and she turns around to make them each a cup of it and brings them to the table. "Tell me what you think, but it is rude not to finish a cup of tea after you start it."

Jay smiles and feels a little pressured to try the tea. He smells it, the aroma is not much at first but after he exhales he finds he wants to sniff it again. He does, this time he comments, "It is an interesting scent. I can't describe it. Is it offered in the bar?"

"No Jay, we only have this on the moon, for us, we don't share it with off worlders, Herfermks has never had it and he was good friends with my great grandparents through my family to me. But we are together so you are one of us and you can have it now."

Jay takes a sip. 'Mild' he thinks to himself then taking another he notices how it slides along his tongue and builds it's flavor as he gets more into him. "Ah, yes, it is a little sweet just as it is, it doesn't need anything added does it?" taking another sip of it.

She sits across from him, "Are you hungry Jay?"

He thinks for a second, "No" Looking at her remembers his first thoughts of how attractive she is. He remembers how he felt that there was something special about her, the way she moves, her sparkling eyes, her smile. It was not any of them but the combination he realizes. Gestalt, the whole is greater than the sum of its' parts. He remembers the concept from arts classes in collage. He looks at her differently. Realizing that he is actually on his first date with her and has committed to something, 'long term?' he asks himself. So far she is fun and easy to get along with. "So what do you like to do when you are not working?" he asks.

Mostly I clean up our homes. I read and watch the wall screens. Five times a year I spend the weekend in other parts of the moon. But now I have you. So when I am not working I can have sex and visit with you after I clean the homes." Do you want to stay here tonight or will you leave and go back to your own place?"

Jay looks at her, he actually hadn't thought about it. He chuckles thinking how cliche it sounds in his thoughts but he actual hadn't thought about it because everything happened so fast. "Well, what would you prefer?"

She asks the house what time it is and after hearing the response smiles at him, " it is still early, we can have a snack and if you don't mind I would like to come and see your place and stay there on our first night."

Jay looks at her and her worried look like she asked for something that could easily be refused to her. He smiles at her and thinks about if he wants her there when he wakes up in the morning. He thinks about his situation and asks himself if he is ready to have a serious commitment to a female, here in this life. He looks at her and thinks about how certain Herfermks was that it was a good idea and what he had done with Herfermks. He thinks about how tenderly she licked him off and how delicately she washed and helped him towel himself after. He thinks about her expression now and takes a deep breath letting it out slowly and seeing the worried look starting to shift to a look of fear. "Yes, I would actually like that, sorry about the hesitation, I wanted to be sure, I wanted to search my thoughts now so that when we are there I won't be doing it then. Does that make sense to you?

Nodding at him, "yes it does, thank you, I made a good choice bonding to you. It is not easy becoming a couple. I have seen some fail at it. I am glad that you think before you talk Jay, I find it a most respectable trait." bumping his leg with her foot under the table, "what would you like me to cook for you?"

Jay likes her physical interaction and smiles at her as he thinks. Remembering the king and the witch story he answers, "anything you want to cook for me, I will be happy to eat." he watches her as her face changes and her smile seems to go inside for a moment. Then her eyes sparkle and she gets up and moves to the cabinets opening some and putting things on the counter, almost like a whirl wind she bustles around the kitchen opening and chopping and mixing and stirring and testing and heating various things as the room fills with various aromas. It isn't long before she is putting some large platters on the table, three of them. Jay is surprised at three. Then she brings glasses and cups and fills them all, three beverages above each platter, then the food. She serves up five separate piles of food on each platter. Then says, home tell father dinner is served.

"Your father will join us?" Jay asks

She stops what she is doing and looks at him with a puzzled expression. "What do you ask? My father is part of us, this is his home too and I am his family, how could he join us he is us."

Jay looks at her and thinks about her response, "I simply am curious. The third platter is for him I am guessing?"

Going back to what she is doing, "yes. Only our family eats here, when we visit other families, or friends, we meet in public places to share meals. It is the way we live here on the moon." She starts puting some utensils on the table, fork on each side of each platter, with a knife also on one side, and two differently shaped spoons on the other.

The door opens and her father comes in and smiles at Jay and sits down. "Jay welcome to our life! It is a joy to have you here with us." His smile stretching his face as he turns his eyes down toward the food then up to his daughter, "It is good to see your passion for cooking return." then looking at Jay with a more solemn expression. "When our daughters become a certain age they feel the need to have a mate. The longer it takes to find one the less they remember their joy in the daily things that need to be done. I am glad to see her happy again Jay. When you have children you will understand." Using a fork he puts a glob of one of the foods from his platter into his mouth and closes his eyes to slowly chew it.

Jay smiles and takes a fork of the food from his platter and tries it. He slowly savors the flavor too. Then he tries the next thing and the next. Not saying a word until he has finished his plate. His eyes half shut with the satisfaction and his body slowing down to digest, he asks "is it appropriate for me to help with the dishes?"

The Bartender winks at his daughter and turns to Jay, "didn't you read the contract? Jay you have to wash all the dishes for the rest of your life. It is a custom here. The newest male mate in the family does all the dishes."

Jay looks at him and knows it is a joke. He is not sure if he should go with it and try to wash them all or if he should just start laughing. He sees that they are playing it through. "Well, Ok then" he gets up and takes his plate to the kitchen and puts his plate into the sink. He waits a few seconds and hears nothing so he turns on the water and starts rinsing the plate. Then he looks for some dish soap, and a cloth or sponge but can't find one. He goes back into the other room and sees them slowly enjoying their food.

He walks over and puts his hand on her shoulder to get her attention but she keeps eating and ignores him. Jay sits down at his place and watches them savoring each bite. He starts to laugh and thinks about his situation. They watch him as he giggles and looks back at them.

Finally she starts laughing to. "You can take a joke too Jay, I am so glad. It is not all Gyrekians who can. Some get very upset Jay." She looks at him for a few seconds, "I have never heard you say my name! Do you know it?"

Jay looks at her, then at her father for a few seconds, and then at her again. He turns red. He swallows and looks her in the eyes and moves his mouth like he is going to say something but no sound comes out of it. He re thinks his response and takes a deep breath. "Actually I don't think any one has ever told me your name." Looking at her blank stare, "I don't know your name."

She looks at her father. "Did you ever tell Herfermks my name? Did you not tell Jay my name? Do you know my name?" then looks at Jay "I do have one, would you like to know my name?" Then she looks at her father with raised eyebrows.

He looks at her then turns to Jay. "I apologizes Jay," then looking at his daughter, "I am sorry dear, but the conversation never lead to names. I was so excited that the one you looked at so much was the one who was first interested that I didn't talk much. I am sorry." Turning back to Jay. "My daughter's name is Lekxzatrera. She has been an adult and able to start her own family in our culture for three years and you have my blessing to bond with her." Looking back into his daughter's eyes, "I thought I was going to have a chance to talk with him the other night before starting the ceremony. Then I was surprised that he came tonight and forgot to do it before you went to see him."

She smiles at her father then looks at Jay. "Call me Lex, or call me Trer. My Father has a name too, his name is Vrodst." Then she laughs, "you are an odd one Jay you bonded with me without knowing my name, What if you don't like my name, will you choose to leave our bond?" and she laughs louder.

Jay smiles. "I like Lex, and I like you so I will stay. I would stay even if I didn't like your name." He looks at her for a few seconds. "Lex, now that we are family, know that I do want to know the customs that I should follow in our home, or homes, and what is actually expected of me."

Smiling at her father, "see, I chose well", smiling at Jay and blushing a little. "It is your responsibility to do what ever work in the home that you notice needs to be done. Other than that you can do whatever you like. You do have one responsibility to me though. You must accept my sexual advances with excitement every time. Also, if I am in a sad or in a gloomy mood, or if I am sick or worried, you have to make me feel that I am desired by attempting to initiate intimacy with me. If I am willing you have to passionately follow through with your advances and make sure that I have whatever additional attention I need or want, or may want, or think that I need but don't actually want."

Jay looks at her for a few seconds seeing the seriousness in her eyes. "So my part in our relationship is to do as I choose and make certain that you are happy?"

Vrodst Looks at Jay "we are a simple culture, we keep our focus to bring happiness to our selves and each other to be happy and help each other with the basics. We do what we enjoy for the benefit of our selves, our families and our friends. Our lives are good and we have everything that we need." Lekxzatrera chose you, so I will do what ever I can to make you happy, so that she can be happy, so that I can be happy."

Jay nods his head.

Lekxzatrera takes the last bite of food from her platter and stands up chewing, and then swallows as she reaches for her fathers' plate with one hand and lifts her own with the other. "I will go wash these Jay then you can take your new mate home to our other home" as she starts toward the kitchen with the platters.

Jay thinks about his routine of going to work in the early mornings and turns to Vrodst. "I have work in the morning."

Vrodst slides his chair to face Jay more directly. " No Jay. You don't. You just bonded. You have some time off from work. If you go to work and you boss finds out you got bonded he will fire you and send you home. You have to spend some days at least going to new places and doing things that you don't always do. She won't tell you but I will. You should take at least a week and go to various parts of the moon that she has never been to. If you don't you will spend the rest of you life wishing that you had. It is a good moon, nothing like Ramga. But there is a lot to see here, you could never see it all but take as much time as you like and see as much as you want, and as she wants too." Nodding his head at Jay "This is the best advice I will ever give you Jay. I am an old Gyrekian and I have seen some sad bonds, and some good ones; and your work will always be waiting. You life is filled with one-time chances and this is a big one. Take it."

Jay looks at him in silence thinking about what he just heard then he sees his Lex coming back into the room and turns to face her. She has a tray with three tall glasses on it filled with a blue liquid. Putting it on the table she hands them both one glass and lifts the third for herself.

"Together as family, together we drink" and holds the glass down over her solar plexus for a second as her father does the same and she looks at Jay until he does it to, then says "we drink" and lifts her glass to drink it all. Looking at her farther then Jay, then giving him a nod and putting a hand out for her fathers empty glass. She watches Jay finish his and takes his glass too, putting them on the tray and then back into the kitchen.

Jay looks at Vrodst. "Do I call my work and tell them or just not show up?"

"Either way Jay; but don't leave my daughter alone and spent the day at work, don't do that. Missing work is never an issue now for you on our moon Jay, you are one of us."

Lex walks back into the room. "Ready Jay," going over to father and giving him a hug, "bye Dad, see you tomorrow" and starts walking towards the door.

Jay looks at Vrodst as he gets up. "Thank you for the advice, I will do as you say, and please, in the future, tell me things like this, that I have to know, and be sure that I understand."

Looking him in the eyes, "thank you sir". Jay follows Lex
out into the bar and then into the corridor about twenty meters
until Lex stops walking and he catches up.

She looks at him, with tears starting to form in her eyes, "Jay I
don't know where you live."

Jay walks right up against her and gives her a hug, "Lex, we
know, the half of us that is me will show the half of us that is
you and it is your home now too." He feels her arms grasping
around him tightly.

Stepping closer to him with one leg between his as she hold
him with her face against his chest. "I always knew I would
leave home with my mate one day, but now is that day and I
am afraid."

Jay holds her and thinks about his situation, he remembers
that Herfermks told him this was a good idea and he did and
does have a strong attraction for her. He remembers want she
said, that he was to always make her feel that he is attracted
and interested and to try to initiate intimacy. He slides his
arms to hold her in a more romantic fashion. "I like you
hugging me like this Lex. If you like I can carry you back to
our new place and you can snuggle me on the way." as he
reaches and bends down a little as if he is going to pick her up.

She jiggles a little, "no Jay."

He slides his face down her head putting his nose into her hair and sniffing, "mmm, you smell good, then putting his lips onto her ear, let me see how you taste."

"I don't want to make you tired from carrying me too far" she gives him a tight squeeze, "but I am please to hear the offer." Letting go of him and wiping her cheek, looking at his face and taking his hand, "show me where we live, at your place."

Jay starts walking with her hand in his, he notices how worm and tender her hand feels to him. His mind seems to be fixed on its' presents in his grip. He feels his legs gaining a new detail of sensation as he is walking and realizes it is part of the intoxication from the drinks they had. Feeling the security of her grip and how it is effecting his emotions soothes him in a knowing that he will be happy here in the moon. As they walk the quarter kilometer back to his place he asks her about where she would like to go and see with him the next day. He listens to her talk about some under ground water falls, and some mountains on the surface and a deep valley on the surface with enough atmosphere that they don't need masks and the desert on the south axis and the ruins of the ancient cities in the northern high plains. He realizes that taking the time to see them all will be a good idea, as her excitement to go to any one of them is spreading to him as he hears her talk about what they are said to be like. He stops walking and waits for her to finish her description of the underground plantations in the next city. "Here we are, this is your new home" as he gestures towards the door with his other arm.

Letting go of his hand so he can open the door "you can carry me in if you like Jay"

Jay snickers as he opens the door and picks her up, gives her a little kiss on the nose. Then he carries her through the door way and into the room. Holding her in his arms he asks the home to close and lock the door and to welcome its' new inhabitant. He gives it instructions to give her access to command controls, as she is his family now. Then he put her so that her feet can reach the floor and holds her until she is balanced on them.

Lex looks around and takes a long sniff of the air, "more oxygen and dim the lights 15%" She says then steps to Jay putting her hands on his chest and lifting herself on her toes and kisses him. "I'm tired Jay, show me our bed and she steps back and flirtatiously undoes a button on her clothes.

Jay smiles, turns and starts walking to the bedroom. Once there he takes off his clothes and lays down on the bed. Only half undressed she lays down beside him resting her head on his chest and sliding her hand to touch his genitals. For the next few minutes he feels her changing her grip on him several times, then it loosens and he hears her making some almost snore like sounds. "Lex" he calls to her softly. Then realizing that she is asleep he relaxes as much as he can and slows his breathing. He starts to think about his day. How it unexpectedly became his future. Jay thinks about his morning and starts to laugh. He had no idea when he left work that he would have a mate before going to bed. He realizes that he is not quite certain what it is to have a mate. Is it like a wife? Will he be with her for life? He thinks so, but he hadn't looked into the mating customs. All he has been doing since his arrival is to look at artifacts and the data and the speculated significance of the artifacts. He actually had not learned a single thing about the culture or what it is or how it developed. Jay starts to think that it is interesting. That after several weeks of study he is not actually looking at anything to give him a fair frame of reference to do the task he has been charged with. He starts to think about having a life with his Lex and slowly falls asleep.

Jay wakes up to a shaking sensation on his side. Opening his eyes he sees Lex holding a cup out toward him. He looks around the room and sees her dressed holding the cup and smiling. He looks and he is still naked. He sits up and accepts the cup, "good morning" and smiles at her, then smells the contents, "mmm, what is it?"

Lex sits on the bed beside him, so that she is facing him almost directly from the front. "Root tea, it will brighten your vision and raise your alertness. Shifting her eyes to his morning stiffy, I can see that you won't need any herbs for that!" Looking him over pretty good, "do you want me to do something for you before you get up Jay?"

Jay sips the tea and looks at her with a questioning expression. "uuum, what do you mean?"

"We are mates now, I don't know the customs of Kyranin couples but I have heard stories being told in the bar. I have heard a lot of stories Jay. But I have not had much experience. I want to please you and don't know what I should do. So for the first weeks I want you to tell me what you want me to do. I mean to please you sexually. Tell me when and what to do and how to do it best. I have to learn or I will never be the mate you want. I won't know unless you tell me."

Jay looks at her. Then he looks around the room to be sure he is not still dreaming he looks at his hands and turns them over. He looks back at her and takes a sip of the tea. "I would like to do some things with you in bed in the mornings. Not all the time, not every morning but many mornings. Just now we can share some tea and talk before we do anything sexual if that is comfortable for you?"

"I'll go get myself a tea," as she gets up, and turns to him, "would you like some biscuits with your tea?" she stands facing him waiting for a response.

Jay finishes taking his sip, then looks into her eyes and smiles, "yes my dear that will be perfect."

She returns shortly with a tray, some biscuits and her tea on it. Sits again facing him with the tray between them. She takes her tea, sips it then takes a biscuit and dips it into her tea, lifts it so the wet part is up and watches. "If you are not careful these biscuits crumble when they are wet." Then carefully brings it to her mouth and puts the wet part in, taking it off with her lips and looking at Jay with wide eyes. "mmmm"

Jay smiles and take up a biscuit and does the same thing with it. When he has some in his mouth he nods with a similar wide-eyed signal that it is good. They talk about snacks and what kind of biscuts these are and joke a little. After all the biscuits and tea are finished she swiftly clears the tray and cups to the kitchen and returns to take off her clothes, almost before the first of them hits the floor.

"Ok Jay! My kyranin male mate; tell me what to do." and she stands there looking a little nervous.

Jay looks at her and takes a deep breath, "come snuggle with me here, on the bed, and do what ever you want to do, we can start from that."

Jay's cock gets stiff as soon as she touches his side but Jay is still tired from not being awake yet and not having his mrruk and from the stress of getting boned the night before, so he just wants to snuggle first. He wants to relax and feel a little more familiar with her before he starts telling her to perform sexual acts with or for him. After snuggling and talking about what they like and sharing their fantasies, and places they would and wouldn't want to have sex. Finally they slowly start to get to it. Her hand slides across his belly and under his stiff cock as he lay on his back. She teases it, caressing his belly under it and then tickling his balls and then massaging them. The finally her hand slides up from his scrotum and onto his shaft. Jay is fully aware of her movements, as she grasps it, first with just a finger and her thumb, then with a gentle grip then with her whole hand, squeezing it tightly.

"Jay? Does that hurt?" she asks.

Jay turns his head to look at her expression, he sees surprise in her face, "no, it feels pretty good actually, did you want it to hurt, is that why you grip it so tightly?"

Letting go of it, "no, I don't want to hurt you!"

Jay smiles, "it is tougher than it looks isn't it?" he looks down at his firm pointing cock, I am often surprised at how durable it actually is. With the sensitivity that it has for pleasure one would expect that it would be very sensitive and easily hurt, right?" he looks at her with his eyes wide with expectation of a verbal response, "But no" and he shakes his head a little, It has a high threshold of acceptable roughness before anything is felt as pain from pressure or friction on or against it. You can squeeze it as hard as you wont and I'll like it" Looking into her eyes "what about your vagina, is it similar?"

She looks a little surprised at his question, hesitates and lets go of his cock. "I don't know Jay. Maybe you should show me what you mean?" She slides over a little and puts her leg across him so that her crotch is over his hand. "Try it, lets give it a test, start gentle and I'll say what is good and what is too hard."

Jay rubs her folds and ripples softly "you just had it in your hand, was it too hard? Tell me."

"...hahahaha, I get it" she giggles and kisses him. "It was just about right Jay hard enough, never too hard"

They spend the rest of the morning playfully exploring each others' likes, tolerances, and dislikes. After giving each other several orgasms and playing with the fluids they snuggle up and have a nap together. Jay wakes up hungry but has her stretched across him with her left hand under his shoulder and her left leg tangled with his right. His hunger a concern for him, but her comfort a priority he decides to massage her back and buttocks until it wakes her up. His right arm easily reaches her whole back so he starts with it by kneading her muscles beside her spine, his left hand can't get out from under her without becoming uncomfortable so he makes it as comfortable as he can. Finding the most comfortable spot for his hand is actually right against her pussy, he makes his hand as comfortable as possible. To his surprise she simply snuggles a little tighter to him. Continuing to knead the muscles of her back and massage her pussy he notices that she is mumbling something. It only takes a moment until her moisture dampens his hand enough to slip some fingers inside. He remembers the spots and what she liked so he starts with what he knows she likes thinking it will wake her up quickly. He hears her mumbling more and then lifting her knee giving him much more freedom and comfort for his left hand.

Thinking that she is waking up he continues and starts whispering sweet compliments to her. Adjusting his movements and pressure to match what she liked best the night before. She adjusts her head a little, half snoring and half mumbles some more. Jay smiles and keeps saying sweet things about her and hugs her firmly with his right hand.

She takes some deeper breaths then her pelvis starts to quake slightly and she lifts her head with wide eyes and looks at Jay, and turns her head to see his face as it smiles back at her. Feeling her hot throbbing vagina shooting ecstasy into her belly and filling her lower abdomen she is speechless as she awakens with the rush of it filling her thoughts. Her right hand slides over his chest as a drip of drool drops from her mouth and she blinks. Then takes a few panting breaths and squeezes herself into him pulling his chest's skin with her hand and moaning some soft sounds out of her mouth as she relaxes her pelvis and legs.

Jay feels the pain of her grip on his chest and the weight of her hips dropping onto him, and reducing the comfort of his wrist. He pulls out of her and asks, "Lex my dear, are you ok?"

Moving his head to see her face as it rests on his chest. He hears only her hot breath as it flows out over his shoulder.

"Jay? Will I wake to this every morning?"

Jay thinks about the way she is clinging to him and not moving at all. He can feel the pounding of her heart on his abdomen and the wet of her juices drying on his hand. "Not every morning Lex, every day will be different. Would you like to wake like this every morning?"

Changing her position and wiping the drool from her lips she looks up at his face and shift close enough to kiss his mouth. Laying herself limp on him she says, it is afternoon isn't it?"

Jay replies, "are you hungry enough for a lunch?"

"Can we go to the surface to eat Jay, I like the sky."

Jay moves his right arm to hold her back too and smiles at her as she climb on top of him better. He feels her shift so that his balls are between her legs and his cock is under her pubic bone. He feels the pressure on it as she slowly shifts one way then another. "We should shower and get dressed before we go to the surface. Jay. Is there something you want to do before we shower?" sliding her hand over his mouth, "don't tell me Jay show me, do what you want to do without saying a word, I want silence so I can hear your heart beating."

Jay slides one hand slowly down and over her buttocks to the top of her thigh then reaches inside her thigh all the way to the front lifting his shoulder a little and crunching his torso to grip the front of it with his finger tips and lifts her just enough so his hard cock can escape the clasp of her pubic bone against his belly. He arches his back to pull it down to below her bone and lets his hand slide up and grips her ass with it, stretching it across both cheeks, then sliding to firmly grip only her left one snugly and kisses her nose. Slowly crunching again his cock is sliding between her legs and into her folds. With the grip of his hand on her cheek he slides her side to side so that his dick bumps across her folds. Liking the sensation Jay holds her back, tightly squeezing her belly and breasts against him and moves his head to kiss her lips. Tenderly kissing her lips and he starts shifting his pelvis as he continues to slide her across himself. Feeling the sensitivity of his little head more intensely than in the past he notices that his arousal is gaining momentum faster than he had expected. "Lex" he says and he feels the thirst of his groin to feel the explosion, and he crunches, and again sliding into her and again harder, and pulling her down on him with his grip on her ass. The water in his throat prevent him from talking as pleasure turns hot and zings through his groin and into his belly, the fire in his cock and the ache in his balls all at once "eehhhehehhe". He drops limp beneath her.

She smiles as she lay relaxed on him feeling his throbbing cock still going and his heart in his chest pounding hard and slowing gradually. She looks at his face. His eyes wide open and his mouth just open enough to show his teeth. "Jay I think you need a shower, I will go first." She slides up to kiss him freeing his softening cock of the happy grip she had on it. Snuggling him and kissing him again before she gets up dripping his come out onto him as she does. "Oops, never thought about that." as she steps off of the bed and walks into the bathroom telling the shower what she wants it to do as she enters.

Jay lay there catching his breath, the feeling her lips still on his and on his face. He feels the coolness of the evaporation from his skin and the sounds of her showering. He feels his heart still beating/throbbing, but at a normal pace. Taking a slow deep breath he notices that there are new areas that he finds a new sensitivity in. Relaxing fully then taking another slow deep breath he feels them again but less. Stretching in some odd yoga positions he notices that he uses muscles that he didn't usually use, he could feel the same new sensation of awareness entering them too. 'That is odd' he thinks to himself as he hears Lex calling him from the shower.

"Jay, come join me so I can scrub you a little" she calls.

Jay roles off the bed putting his feet on the floor, then walks briskly into the next room and under the water dripping from the ceiling to her side. He smiles and kisses her face. She starts rubbing his back and diligently rubs all of him everywhere before asking the shower to stop. Silently they look each other over, smile and reach for each others hand, then she leads the way to the wardrobe doors.

"Jay do you have anything that might fit me?" she asks.

He point to the drawers with the women's clothing in them and says, "try in those two, you might find something that will be ok" then he lets go of her hand and smiles as he watches her open them and look at each piece carefully.

Lex examines each garment, takes some out of the packages and lays them on the bed. Folds them and hen the next, until the contents of both drawers have been searched and passed inspection. She turns to Jay with a blank look and looks at him with worry in her face. "I didn't get you anything"

Jay smiles at her "I don't need anything"

"You got all these clothes for Me Jay, they are all my size and they are all my style, how did you know?"

"All that maters is that you can find something to ware to the surface for lunch. I am happy with your love and attention, but you needed clothes for this home, that is all." Jay says; and thinks to him self 'I better remember to pay attention to what she likes and what she wears.' He opens the doors with his clothes in them and hopes that she won't ask more details about how he got or chose the clothes. He lifts out something he hasn't warn yet and asks, "Is this appropriate for the surface?"

"mm," she says and comes over to look through his clothes. She pulls out some other garments, looking at them, picking a few and handing them to him "these will be better." She then goes back to the bed and starts arranging the garments that she had spread out into outfit combinations. After she has them mostly sorted she turns to see Jay standing with the clothes she gave him still in his hands and him looking at her, "Well, are you going to get dressed?" then she picks up one garment from a pile and starts to put it on.

Jay gives his head a shack and starts to get dressed thinking about how he was staring at her sorting her clothes. 'I was mesmerized' he thinks to himself. 'I better call work and tell them that I am not coming for a few days' he tells himself. Looking at the clothes in his hands Jay stops thinking and starts dressing. Once dressed he goes and finds his tablet and sends a memo to his work. < I got bonded last evening and won't be at work for several days, maybe many days>. 'That should do it' he thinks and puts his tablet down. He walks back into the bedroom to see Lex fully dressed and looking great. "Are we ready?" he asks.

She smiles and looks at him, "just our foot ware Jay" and walks to him and kisses him and goes past to the door and slips on her shoes. "Come on, the lunch up there is great" and she opens the door, stepping out into the corridor. Stepping to the middle of the corridor she looks both ways then turns around and watches Jay come out. "Do you know how to get up to the top?"

Jay steps out clear of the door and closes it. "No, I found it once."

She looks both ways again then offers him her left hand as she turns to her right, "This way will be fastest" and starts walking. "So you have been on the surface?"

"Not really, I went up and took a look but didn't go anywhere yet" he says, "will I need to know anything, or have breathing apparatus or something?"

Steering him to turn at he first intersection she says, "I think you will be ok. We actually could live on the surface you know. There is enough air for us up there but we would be cold all night and hot all day. And we would get tired if we worked hard. That is why we build our cities under the surface. And if we have a war it is harder for them to hurt our cities. The ruins on the surface are from space wars you know. Some not directly, but after some of the ancient wars the culture was destroyed so we left the cities and they eventually crumbled." Stopping in front of a door that looks a lot like Jay's own door to Jay she says, "Lekxzatrera, security one, with

Kyranin seed Jay, my new bonded mate. Going to the surface for lunch and touristing."

He hears a soft beep like tone and the door slowly opens a little. She waits a few seconds and pulls it wide open. "Ok" taking his hand she goes into the room and stands in front of another door, a double door.

Jay hears a sound like an electric motor then the two doors open. 'An elevator he thinks' as they step into the small room and watches her punch some buttons on a keypad. The doors close, then feels the movement upwards. "How far under the surface is our city?" Jay asks.

"Not that deep, the top sections are only about 60 meters, where we live is about 90 meters, and the lowest part of our city is about 130 meters."

Jay can feel the shaking of the elevator as it speeds upwards. "How old is this elevator?"

Lex starts to laugh, "it sounds a little scary doesn't it Jay?" she tugs his hand and pastes on a scared look as he looks at her, then smiles. "It has been here for as long as my family has lived in the city. It is likely many hundreds of years old. But it is safe. It was made to work during earthquakes and survive space attacks. I think it will get us there. My grand father told me when I was a little girl that it rattled and shook the same when he was a little boy. My cousin is a builder. He worked on the maintenance of the lifts when he was young. He says that it is how the rails were made. They are a very hard material and the connecting of them was difficult with the technology that we had when it was made. It is even more difficult to correct so it won't get fixed, the rollers on the lift are also made of a very durable material and they won't wear out so it will shake for a long time, and we are ok with that here on the moon."

Jay feels it coming to a stop and asks "are we here?"

"Almost" she says as the doors open and the walk into the large room out side the elevator. "Do you see the other elevators Jay" as she turns him around. "See the symbol on the top and on the door and on the floor in front of the door? That is your elevator Jay. If you take another one it will put you in a different part of the city. It may be much lower or just far away, but you will be lost so best to always take the one back to you own area."

Jay looks at the symbol, then at the other symbols. He realizes that they are not even close to looking similar. "Good symbols, I will remember which one is ours." looking at all the other doors that look the same except for the symbols. "Wow, how many lifts are there?"

She looks at Jay "you want to count them?" looks at them all "is it important Jay?" as she counts them in bunches for a rough figure, "Maybe thirty." Then looks at him, there are other lift rooms on the surface from our city Jay, there are hundreds of lifts, maybe a thousand or more." turning to the exit, she starts walking with Jay in tow, "Lekxzatrera and new Kyranin bonded mate, Jay, up for lunch and touristing."

The surface

The door opens as they come up to it. When they are outside Jay looks back seeing the door close. He looks around and sees that they are in a deep valley with a variety of types of vegetation. He sees large openings on the side of the valley and many gyrekians doing various things. "It is busy up here"

Lex nods, pulling his hand, "this way, see the red wall behind the trees, that is where we are going." she pulls him for a few more steps until they reach the walk way to the entrance of the restaurant. "Ok Jay when we get to the door you must to do all the talking. As the male mate you have to take charge or they will not respect us, neither of us. I will do as you lead and eat what you order." looking at him as they are getting closer to the door, "Jay."

"Yes Lex" he says in a soft voice as they reach the doorman. "Hello, two for lunch, myself and my new bonded mate Lekxzatrera. Do you have a table with a good view of the sky?"

The doorman looks at Jay for several seconds with a puzzled expression. "Yes a table with a sky view, excuse me, but did say Lekxzatrera is you mate, did you two bond?"

Jay stand calmly but directly facing him, "Yes, we bonded to became mates yesterday, I am new to the moon but I plan to stay here for many years."

He looks Jay over then looks at Lex and smiles, then back at Jay, "Welcome Jay and Lex. Jay you are one of us now. It is good to be able to bless you on the next day after bonding. I will get your table arranged" nodding to Jay, "Jay," and then nodding to Lex, "Lekxzatrera." Stepping back and folding his arms behind him, "my name is Twemrict it is a good day for our moon Jay and Lex. I know some have issues with inter species mating but I am relieved we live in a culture that can respect the choices of individuals. Today, Jay, I feel will bring a new beginning for so many of us." He smiles and steps to his podium and works the screen with his fingers. "Please go right in, up the stairs to the third level and down to the middle of the room then out onto the balcony, the red table with three chairs, the server will take the empty one when you order. Jay may I suggest you order the platter of the day. With the extras."

"Thank You. Will it be too much for us to eat we are not that hungry?" Jay asks.

"Not a problem, the way it is served will assure your plates are not over filled." and he nods and winks at Lex then smiles at her then smiles and nods at Jay. Gesturing with one arm that they start walking in.

As they are going up the stairs Lex tells Jay that Twemrict and her were friends in their educational years and that he was a good friend too. That she didn't know that he was working here but was glad to see him, and asked if they could invite him for dinner in a few weeks. As they reach the third level she slides her arm under and around his coming close to his side. "Don't stop until we are there Jay."

Jay feels her stress and realizes that she must have taken a risk choosing to bond with a male from another world. He gets a smile on his face from the humor of his thought about her not knowing where he is really from, and a deep solemn feeling of respect and a little tinge of fear knowing that she could have some difficulties as a result of her choice. "I think I see the table" and he starts walking being sure to give her lots of room for her to stay beside him as they cross the room as they turn to go out onto the deck. Stopping beside a red table with three chairs and looking around he realizes that this table, more than any other, is visible from the entire place. He lifts the chair that will give the best view of the sky back, and gestures for Lex to sit in it and slides it closer to the table as she does. He moves the third chair out of the way of where he wants to sit to face her and sits himself down. Then smiles at her, "do you like the view Lex?"

Batting her eyes at him, then playfully she asks, "of the sky Jay? Or of you?"

Smiling back at her he asks "Would you like some tea or some kyranin wine before we order our meal?"

"No Jay, I am hungry" as she looks right at him.

Jay looks around, not seeing a waiter he gets out his tablet and tells it "Tablet we would like to have the special of the day with the extras." then he asks "tablet is it possible for you to have that order registered into the kitchen's systems so that we can have the meal right away?"

After a few seconds "Only using Herfermks special authorization codes and many secured subroutines is that possible Jay." The tablet displays on the screen <would you like a request sent to Herfermks for the authority to have your meal delivered right away Jay?>

Jay looks around the place and sees several tables looking at them and some staff peaking from behind some walls. He thinks about it for a second and nods to the tablet and thinks yes. Jay looks up to see two carts being pushed by servers coming out of the kitchen. "I think our meal will arrive soon", Jay says with a smile to Lex. Then he sees a third server looking his way as he comes out of the kitchen carrying some smaller trays.

"The views are both good", she says to him, then turning to look as the serving carts are wheeled up to their table by the servers. "That was fast" she says.

"Your friend must have told them for us" Jay says, as he points to something on one of the trays, "That looks interesting, can you tell me what it is?"

The server says, "a meat custard from the invertebrate surface species near the equator, a rare dish but delicately delicious and only available in this season. Would you like a portion sir?"

Jay looks at Lex to see only her eyes going up and down. "Yes, and a serving for my Lekxzatrera."

Jay looks at the various things on the two carts and doesn't know what to do. He looks down at his tablet and then up at Lex, "excuse me for a moment Lex, I have a confidential off world call, for work, I will be right back," then looking up at the servers, "It will only take a few seconds, please wait." Jay takes a few steps toward the railing and whispers to his tablet "scan me and Lex and tabulate what and how much of the food on the trays we will want to consume and order for me making it sound like I am saying the order as I wave my arm towards the trays and point in the direction of the trays. Can you do that so it will sound like I am actually ordering the options?"

He hears a "yes Jay" from the Tablet.

Jay walks back to the table and looks at Lex and smiles then at the servers and opens his mouth and starts pointing at the trays. The sound of his voice starts vibrating around the table and the servers start dishing the things as they are told onto his and her plates. The third server has three trays of various cakes that Jay looks at as he is still pointing at the trays. Once their plates are looking pretty well filled he nods at he server with the deserts putting his hands in his pockets, a small portion of each for us to share, but not until we finish what we have here now. Thank you" and he sits down putting his tablet on the table.

Lex looks at the food on her plate. "It is not what I would have chosen but it looks very good Jay, are you familiar with these foods?"

Jay looks at her plate and then his. Slowly turning his head side to side he looks up at her. "I hope we like it" and he starts laughing. He uses one of the utensils to put the brightest thing on his plate in his mouth and squashes it with his tongue. Then starts nodding his head, "it is good!" examining and savoring each bit without saying more than he has to until his plate is empty. He watches her enjoy her last few bites. Before her fork reaches the table the server with the deserts is on their way from the kitchen with their tray. As she puts her fork on the table he asks Jay "would you like some beverages after the deserts Sir?"

Jay looks at Lex and her eyes are going slowly from side to side. "No, thank you. This will be fine"

Smiling at the server. "The meal was superb".

The server nods and taking their empty plates heads back to the kitchen.

Jay offers Lex to take the first piece and sees her eyes going side to side again. So he picks up a fork and takes a bite of one of the cakes, then one from the next, and then the last. He looks at Lex and sees that she is waiting for something. He looks at her for a clue and realizes that she is nervous. He notices that the room is watching and he doesn't know what to do. His fingers slide over and he bumps the tablet without realizing it and looks over at it, and thinks 'what can I do now?'. All of a sudden he remembers in the pantry with the glass cages at Herfermks; Birkjets was telling him the first meal out ritual on the gyrekian moon. The male has to feed the desert to the female or the superstition is that he will never be able to keep her happy in bed.

Jay slides his chair closer to hers and takes a fork full of cake and slowly brings it to her mouth and smiles, looking into her eyes, until she opens her mouth and lets him put it in. She carefully closes her mouth and takes the cake off of it by pulling her head back. She smiles and winks at him as she chews and he fills the fork again, with the next desert. She slowly savors the first bite and spends some time shifting her tongue to clear all of the first bite from her mouth before opening for the next. Jay waits until her mouth opens wide and gently slides it in. He notices that almost half of the room is openly watching them and that most of the other half is watching too but working to not be noticed as they are. The last bite goes in and before the fork is on the table he sees the server bringing a tablet toward their table.

The server walks up to Jay and says quite loudly, "how will you be paying sir, and he puts the Tablet on the table face up to Jay with some figures showing."

Lex says to the server, and in a soft voice she says "we are bonded, he is one of us, how can you insult him by asking him to pay in this manner."

He turns to her and swallows, and looks at her replying in a soft tone to her "I understand, but our records show that he is an off worlder and thus the law states that he must pay. Not all of us are happy with the changes that could come of such bonds."

Jay looks at the server and realizes that he did not bring any currency with him. He thinks about the tablet, remembers the account that Herfermks opened for the two of them on Kuroggez. "Can your tablet derive the payment from my account in a bank on another world?

Only if you have malty world bank privileges and they are accessible through your tablet, most Kyranins carry currency, do you not have any currency to pay with sir, perhaps you could borrow some from you friend here. Jay stands and looks with a serious tone to the server, picks up his tablet and asks it "do you have access to my joint bank account on Kuroggez?"

The tablet answers "Yes"

Jay worries that he has no idea how to pay, he decides to wing it, "transfer my status and the funds to this servers systems and retain records of this transaction."

The server looks at him smugly and lifts his tablet to read the amount. He sees a new screen displayed. He looks at it closely, muttering as he looks it over. Then looks at Jay, "you are a Kyranin diplomat with shared accounts with a Ryberian high council member."

Jay looks at the shock in the young servers' face. "I was once a young server like you, with diligent effort and an open mind I have done many things." Now that my bill is paid, I feel compelled to say that the food was good and so was the service. Thank you and please pay my compliments to those working in the kitchen." He sits down reaches across the table and takes Lex's hand, "would you like anything else before we go?"

Lex looks at him, "were you on Kuroggez?" tightening her grip. "That is not a good place for a kyranin."

"Jay laughs" and looks up at the server, "is there anything else?"

The server turns and walks away.

Jay smiles at Lex, "don't worry I have no plans to go back there" he looks into her eyes and smiles, "lets go see the surface" and stands up.

Lex wipes her mouth with the napkin and slides her chair back then gets up. She looks around at the others enjoying their lunch and notices nods and smiles from a few and cold looks from a few others. "Well Jay,,, It was a good view, and a good lunch. Sorry you were asked to pay in such a rude manner. I will file the documents as soon as I go back to work in a few weeks." She looks around the room again to see what reactions if any from her words. Noticing bigger smiles, and colder looks from a few, she giggles and says softly to Jay "ok let's get out of here"

Once out side Jay goes to Twemrict and thanks him for the suggestion and tells him it was delicious. Lex stands back a few feet to watch and smiles at her old friend but not saying anything before they leave. They walk down the valley a few hundred meters in silence listening to the conversations of others and the sounds of the birds, insects and leaves blowing in the breeze.

Jay asks "do you think your friend suggested the special to make it difficult for me, I had no idea what to get them to serve us."

"I'm not sure" Lex replies, "if he comes to the bar to apologize for what happened with the bill then he didn't but if not then he did."

"How well did you know him?" Jay asks.

Lex takes a few steps before saying, "we studied together for several months, then we become friends away from studies as well. We dated a few times the next year but it didn't last long, a few years later we became good friends and that slowly ended when we started working. I haven't heard from him for almost a year."

"He was a good friend then" If he does come to apologize I will be happy to have him as our friend." then he puts his arm around her, "but I am not the kind of Kyranin that will want to have him join us in bed". Then watches in his peripheral vision for a response.

She looks up at his face and slaps his belly with her far arm and puts her close arm around his back. After a few steps, "is it true that Kyranins have group sex regularly. And that they don't get jealous about it no matter what happens during the group sex?"

Jay thinks about it for a few steps, "Well. It is part of our culture, and we are comfortable with sex just for pleasure, and we do it without becoming attached or expecting it to be more than just a good time, shared. It is true. However I can't say if some Kyranins get jealous or not. It is not socially respected to show jealousy but some may feel it. I haven't been on Ramga long enough to find myself close enough to any female there to grow deep enough feeling of build expectation so I can say I was never jealous myself. But then I didn't take part in much sex on Ramga either." then looking at her to watch for a reaction, "Why, do you want to try group sex?"

"No Jay, I'm not a kyranin, I am glad to be only with you. I just don't want to deprive you of it if you crave it or something" she says then looks up at him with a bit of worry on her face.

Jay smiles at her, "I have lived a full life Lex, I am glad to be bonded now and will be more than happy to only be with you." then pointing to a brightly colored bird near by in a tree, "What is that," pointing and looking harder at it, "is it a bird?"

Lex stops and looks at it as and Jay steps to turn with her, "yes Jay it is an odd bird, see it's face, the eyes on the front and the bright colors except on the legs."

'I don't see any legs"

"Yes, they change color to match what is around them. But the feathers are bright like flowers. They only eat flowers and fruits. All the other birds on the moon eat the insects. Also Jay these birds give live birth. The other birds lay eggs. Three types of the birds don't hatch their eggs they only hide them when they lay them. They do help the little birds of their kind

learn to survive and live but they take no preference
toward their own over the baby birds of others of their kind.
The rest of the birds are like birds on other worlds."

"Are there other animals on the moon?"

Lex takes a few steps then says, "only a few, there were many
once, most of them were killed in attacks from other world in a
war a very long time ago. Then after that we ate all the rest.
We ate the last of the rest of them. There was a terrible conflict
in our society at the time, some said we should stop eating
animals and others said they will die out anyway so why not.
Since the last one was gone our society has realized how it
effected or moon. The soils on the surface suffered as the
bacteria from the other animals was no longer present they
didn't grow crops as well and then the bigger trees started to
die and then the atmosphere started to change and then the
kinds of insects started to change too. Now we only have
insects and birds and mostly in the valleys. On the plains and
plateaus there is not much life. In the mountains there is some
cultivation of some herbs and worms that grow on the sunny
sides of the slopes where there is enough soil. But that is about
it. No animals except the ones we breed in the caverns and
most of them are form other worlds, some are genetically
modifies to survive in the places we grow them and again
genetically modified to make them nutritious for us. A lot of
the food we have here on the moon that we serve to guests is
traded for from other worlds."

Jay asks, "I heard that each home has grow rooms for the food that the family eats. Is it true?"

"Oh, Yes, we do have a room in each home where we grow the roots that you saw and another smaller one where we grow some other fruit and vegetables. Under the bar we have a grow room with a variety of rare specimens that we bread for the menu at the bar, most of these rooms are fully automated so basically we just go in and pick the food. Practically speaking we have little to do with it growing. That is done by our technology." she turns to look at him and stops walking. "I heard that on Ramga there are still aloud to hunt the wild animals sometimes. Is it true?"

Jay looks at her and thinks about the entire moons surface having been killed off by over hunting then answers. "Yes, the health of the wilderness is closely monitored and when there is enough extra of a food species in the wild a controlled hut is allowed." He thinks about how things are going on earth with the extinctions and the faulty regulations. "Fishing in the lakes of Ramga is also allowed within seasons and in the sea as well. But most of the food on Ramga is cultivated or raised on farms. Even in the lakes and sea most of our food is produced in controlled situations so that we can preserve our wild spaces to the levels that keep they healthy."

"One day I hope to see Ramga. Jay will you ever be able to take me there?"

Jay thinks about the question, "I don't see why not. I have heard that Gyrekian women don't travel from the moon but I don't know of any regulations on Ramga that would prevent you from visiting, or even living there for a time."

She starts walking again pulling him to come with her. After a few steps, "It is our culture Jay, we don't let out females leave. It is because of our high regard for their place in our social structure with the female being the center of the home. If we let our females leave then our culture could disseminate. It is not looked upon as a wise thing to do for a female, to leave the moon."

Jay says "I can see the wisdom in the theory of that but, if you want to see Ramga I am certain we can find a way for it to happen. Not right away but in a few years."

She looks at him and smiles, "do you want to climb to the ridge and look across the plains? It is a good climb and it will make us tired"

Jay looks across the valley, and up the slope that they are on and then at her, "yeah I would like that, I have been interested to see the surface since I first came to the moon. Can we travel across the plains? Are there vehicles for that?"

Lex starts walking up the slope and looks back to see if Jay is following. She goes a little further looking back again, "come on Jay, there are some transports that cross the plains, we can take one if you like. I'll race you to the top" and she starts climbing faster.

Jay gets a smile on his face as he starts to follow her up the slope. He notices after a few steps that he does not feel the strength that he did on Ramga when he was climbing the hills there. He starts to control his breathing, taking long deep breaths to get more oxygen into his blood and tries to keep up the pace so he can catch up with her. As he starts to get close he notices that he is getting dizzy and stops his climb to catch his breath and clear his head. He sits and looks down the slope into the valley. "I can't catch up to you Lex" he says and hears her stop climbing.

"Are you ok, Jay?" she asks.

"Yes, just need a little air, I will start climbing again in a minute, maybe not as fast." he replies.

"I will wait until you start again Jay, I don't want to loose my advantage in our race. It would be a humiliation if I lost to a male from Ramga."

Jay turns his head and looks up at her standing about four meters up the steep slope from him with a smile on her face. "Is it a point of pride to be healthier than your bonded mate?"

Looking at him for some seconds she replies, "No Jay, it is a humiliation to let a being from another world reach the top of the slope of a valley before us. We have races with the students that come here for educational exchanges from all of the alliance worlds. We always win. That is all. I would never want to try to show myself as being superior to you." She looks at him, "but it will feel good to beat you to the top Jay!" and she laughs.

"I trust that you will and I don't mind you liking it," getting up and starting to climb again "I am surprised how thin the air is compared to at the bottom of the valley."

She looks at him as he climbs towards her "It does get thinner at the top, and you are not accustomed to it. I will wait for you to get close before I run to the top and win" then she laughs and starts walking up the slope, "come on Jay, are all kyranins as slow as you?" Looking back at Jay snickering as he climbs, "so you think this tactic will get me to feel sorry for you and pamper you when we get back home?"

Jay starts laughing and stops walking, "Ok, so you want to make it interesting I will race you to the top. What will you bet that you will get there first?" then putting his hands on his hips "or are you scared to bet with a Kyranin?"

She stops climbing and turns to face him, "scared, I will bet, what would you be willing to loose?"

Jay looks down then back up again. "If I get there first you have to let me do anything I want to do with you when we go to bed tonight. And if you get there first I have to do anything you want me to do and only what you want me to do."

She looks at him for a minute as he slowly climbs closer to her. "Ok" and she turns and runs about thirty steps to reach the ridge at the top of the slope. As Jay keeps his slow pace only moving a couple of meters before she claims the win.

"Good" Jay says, "the race is over, now can you come and help me the rest of the way up?"

Lex looks down to Jay still climbing out of the valley and starts to walk back down to him. "Jay I am sorry, I didn't think it was serious for you."

"Oh, no Lex, it is all in fun, but I am having a challenge with the climb. I had no idea that I would get so little oxygen from climbing this high." He looks around the valley, "It is making me feel a little intoxicated."

Lex takes his hand, "it is just a little further Jay, don't strain yourself. I will have some demanding activities for you to accomplish later my slave."

Jay starts laughing and has to sit down to catch his breath. After a minute he gets up and with her hand for balance makes it to the top without stopping again. Looking across the plain Jay realizes that he has seen several photos of the same view. Pointing to a hill in the distance "is that where there was a surface city about 2800 yeas ago. And over there," pointing at some sharp peaks rising out of the horizon in the other direction. Is that where the Girestald ruins are?"

Lex looks at both things that he pointed at. "You are right Jay, why would you remember these places nothing has ever happened there?"

"Oh, it is my work, I have to look at all of the old artifacts and look for patterns in development from the cultures that developed from them. There are a lot of artifacts and speculations about what happened there in those places. I have been reading about them since I started working here and have not seen any patterns yet."

"Lex looks at one place then in the other direction at the other. Too bad you couldn't go back to the time when our ancestors lived there and see what it was like for them. I am sure that most of what was written is not that accurate. It is like the news about events that happen now, it you are there and read the news it always sounds like it happened at some other place or time. But when you did not attend an event the news is all that you know about it and it sounds to be so real."

Jay looks at the ruins and thinks about the truth in her words and thoughts. "Yeah. That would be better. If I went there, back then, I would learn the truth."

"The truth, the truth Jay, hahaha, now you sound like a researcher. You can only ever know your opinion, the truth is not the product of observation, what is recorded is only facts of events. It is not something that you can ever be sure of, the patterns can be understood but the truth will almost never actually be known. How can it be? The feelings of those involved are what makes things true or not, and usually the feelings are not ever shared and only sometimes shown. Like with our race, I won and I will take my prize. But the truth is I wanted you to win and was sad knowing that you couldn't. My hope is that your giving me my prize later will make my worry and sorrow about you having a difficult time with the thin air all seem worth while; and that it will help me overcome my fear of you living in a world that is not the best for you physical health; and my hope that all will be ok for you in time." She looks at him, "you see what I mean about the events not showing the truth?"

Jay nods, and thinks about it slowly as he finishes his other thought about her earlier words. "The truth, it is usually well hidden, isn't it?" He thinks silently for a few seconds. "You are very wise Lex, thank you. I will be considering your words for several months, maybe even longer. In fact it is going to totally change how I look at the information and what I look for in events and how I interpret what has been speculated about them. Hhmmm. Thank you" looking at the bumps in the distance that is the ruins, "how far is that from here."

Lex says to him, "half the day in a surface vehicle but only an hour total if we go to the deep level transport and come up there."

Jay looks at her, "really, lets go!" looking down the slope and starting to walk "which way to get there?"

Lex starts laughing "we will be there soon Jay, come this way first. I am thirsty and there is a teashop over there" pointing to a structure sticking out from between some rocks.

Jay adjusts his direction "good idea, I am too. I am surprised how fast I got tired. The gravity is less here than on Ramga and other worlds I have been too but with the thin air, my muscles have less strength. I didn't think it would be that much different than on the level where we live."

Lex looks back at him for a second and keeps walking "wait until we are in the deep levels Jay, you will notice something about the gravity there too." The air is thicker though, you will like that." Looking over her shoulder again to see that he is keeping up.

She slides with one foot in front of the other then steps quickly onto the flat ground walkway leading to the teashop, "Watch the edge Jay" as she steps closer to the entrance and looks inside. She sees the place is only about a quarter full and that there are three servers. No one is sitting out side on the deck and the sun is still hitting the entrance and shining into the room. She looks across the valley and likes the view as the shadows from the larger rocks stripe the far slope. Waving to get a server to look her way, "two, we will sit out here, we will both have tea and water please" Then walks to the table she likes and looks at Jay before she sits. "Is tea enough or are you hungry too?"

Jay pulls out his chair and sits down and takes a deep breath and looks at her then the view. "I think tea and water will be enough. I am a little tired from the climb but I don't think that I'm hungry. Great view", he looks at her for a second, she is looking back at him and he thinks 'did I miss something'. He stands up, "I am sorry Lex, is there some etiquette that I am unaware of, I am happy to learn all of the social norms right away if you could show me"

Lex looks at him, "oh, I'm just standing for now, I'll sit when I'm ready. I walk carrying things all day most days so I am not too in need of sitting down." she smiles at Jay. "Did I work you too hard Jay, or do you want to believe it was the climb that made you tired?"

Jay looks at her smirk and starts to laugh, he sits down snickering and smiles at her "I will be working hard a lot, it was the climb," and he laughs some more.

"By the time we are finished the tea Jay, the shadows will be almost gone on that side of the valley." She points up at the top of the side they are on, "when the sun starts to make shadows from those large rocks on this side you can see the light refraction off of the minerals and it sends colored stripes in the mist if there is any. It is not busy enough today to have mist from the teashop but sometimes the soil is damp enough to make some vapor and that does it too. Probably next time we will see it." Pulling the table back from Jay a little she slides herself onto his lap and puts her arms around him." She rests her head on his shoulder and slides one hand to his chest. "I am the luckiest girl on this moon Jay".

Putting his hand on her back and his other and her knees, "Why do you say that Lex?"

"Well Jay, it is different for us here on the moon than for the beings on other worlds. We like physical intimacy as much or more than other species but our aging process makes it crucial for us to find love early in life. When we are in the last years of youth we can't control our hormones and we have sex for fun with our friends and others too. But when we reach maturity it isn't enjoyable anymore without some deep emotional contact. It has been said by our scholars and scientists that it is due to our active intellect taking more control of our choices in the moment than our carnal drives. So what happens is it become boring for us if we don't have a strong emotional attraction." She kisses his nose, "I have looked at a lot of males coming into the bar and never once did I feel an attraction to any of them. But with you Jay, with you it was odd." sniffing his neck and gently holding his ear with her teeth as she softly exhales into it. "Jay," she whispers, "you make me want you so that my mind stops thinking" then forcefully feeling his chest with her hand, "my heart pulls me to you in a way that has me feeling the desire to bread with you Jay". Looking into his eyes "before I noticed you I was worried that I would find my attraction to a female."

Jay looks into her eyes seeing her seriousness, "I didn't know that was how things work here. Is it common for Gyrekian females to find attractions to each other?"

She smiles, "It does happen Jay, it is rare and it is accepted by most but there is not any chance of children so it is a different life after bonding with a female than we are raised to expect to live." Kissing his lips, "when we are small our mothers and grandmothers, and other females in our lives tell us about the joy they have raising their children and the pleasures and lessons from it and we grow up wanting to do the same. So when two of us bond with each other we feel the connection and the attractions and the passion but we will always feel like we missed out on raising our own children."

Jay looks at her for a moment. "You say it as 'we' when you talk about a situation of 'them'. How do you see it as we?"

The server brings the tea, puts it on the table beside them and puts a pitcher of water on the table too.

Lex gets up and goes to her chair sitting down and picking up her tea and has a sip. "It's good Jay, try it. For us as females on the moon we see our culture as a group that we all belong to. What affects any one of us effects us all. If we don't live our lives with our feelings totally involved in our choices then we are missing our chance to fully live this life. What one of us feels, we all eventually experience a tiny part of. Either from stories or from the effects it has on others who affect others who affect us. It is like the air. The air is not separate when you close the door to a room. What happens to that air in the room will spread through all of the rest of the air once the door to the room is opened again. It is the same with us Jay. What ever happens to one of us is forever influencing the rest of us. When the one we bond with is not happy, it will eventually affect all of us on our moon Jay. It effects the ones that live on other worlds too as they will eventually hear some sad news of one from the moon who was affected. So we have a responsibility to each other to feel our emotions and live in accordance with those feelings. Like the server at the restaurant, he feels it is wrong to breed with other species, so he had to try to break our bonding process. If he didn't try a part of him would sag inside and he would not be able to feel his joy. He failed but he tried, so he can feel he did live his truth and he did act to honor his feelings. He is living his emotions and he has my respect for doing it. I don't like what he did. But I do respect him for doing it." She has another sip. "Most off worlders can't understand why our female couples don't just take a male once or more times to make them both pregnant. Jay if one of us forced ourselves to have sex just to get pregnant it would make everything we do because of our true feelings questionable. The concept itself would become questionable. When we look at how our minds function, and analyze the long term effect that creating that questionable choice and activity into our constant thoughts it is clear that it could destroy all of us. Not just our culture, also our way of living in almost constant joy. If we wanted to live like drones we could do whatever others from outside our culture do but we are not drones, we are Gyrekian females. We will only bread when we feel the love and lust and passion for our bonded mate."

Jay asks, "what about in your late youth years when you have sex with friends? What happens when some females get pregnant from that?"

She looks at Jay for a minute, "Jay, don't you know anything about us, we can't get pregnant until we are mature. And even then it is a conscious choice. It can't happen by accident Jay."

Jay stops his thoughts and thinks about his words, remembering that she thinks he is kyranin and that kyranins can't get pregnant that easily either. Remembering Kyranin breading possibilities, "with us it is possible for an accident and an unexpected pregnancy can occur, it does happen on Ramga it is the same with the Amburst. It is very rare though. But it is only from a conscious choice here that it can occur?"

"If we don't feel the emotions our body won't produce the hormones to allow an egg to release and if we don't open our channels the egg can't reach the chamber of life. We have to strain the muscles of the channels to get them to allow the egg through. It is the choice to make that effort that in the end determines if we will have a child." She looks at Jay.

Jay looks back at her and starts to feel like he is a delicate desert behind a glass door that is being opened. He looks at her eyes sparkling and her lips somehow moistening themselves, and he feels the growing pace of his heart. Looking her over he realizes that he is strongly attracted to her.

Lex slowly licks her lips then breaks her gaze and has another sip of the tea, "how do you like the tea Jay?" watching him nod and pick up his cup she looks past it and into his eyes "I want to have a child with you Jay, are you ready for that or do you want me to wait?"

Jay takes too big of a drink and feels the heat in his throat from the tea. "fwoofh, hu, that is too hot."

Lex laughs, "so the thought turns you on then?"

Jay laughs, "a little, I would like to have a child with you and more than one if you want to. Can we wait a few weeks though until you are sure I know what it is to be a Gyrekian father. I am Kyranin but didn't grow up there so I am not sure what would be expected of me there, and here I have no idea what I must do to be a good father."

Lex looks at him with a cold look and slowly starts to nod. "So you do want me to risk my life to make your child?" and looks into his eyes with an intensity.

Jay looks back at her and thinks about what he said then about her question to him. "If you would be at risk Lekxzatrera, No. I don't need a child. If you would want to have a child I want to be a good father. I want to know how to be a good father to our child. That is all. I want you to make sure I will be a good father and then if you want a child I will be happy to have one with you." He picks up his tea looks at her face then takes a drink. "Do you want to have a child with me?"

Lex smiles, "I was joking with you Jay, I liked your response though, I am not at risk to have a child, I am young and it is safe. Thank you for your concern about it, it is expected after bonding to have children even if it is not safe. It feels good to know that I am that important to you already Jay. I like your idea of waiting to be sure you will be a good father. Some young Gyrekians don't think of that and their children have difficult lives." She finishes her tea and pores water into her cup and drinks it. Then fills it again and holds the pitcher toward Jay and nods to his cup.

Jay slides the cup toward her so she can reach it with the pitcher to fill it. "I like the tea but it is a little strong, I will see how it is watered down." Jay smiles at her as she put down the pitcher. "When we have a child will you stay home or will we have someone come and take care of the child while you work?"

Lex looks at Jay for a few seconds. "Jay, I will work when I want, but only if you or my father is with our child. When our child goes to education groups I can work again but for many years I will be home with our child. So will you Jay. You will not work every day when we have a child. You will stay home with us at least every second day. If you travel for work you will take us with you, and you will change your work plans if we need you at home. On holidays you will not work and when friends or family come to visit you will not work. You are bonded now and you will live with us in our world with our customs. If we go to make a home on Ramga then we can live by Ramga's customs."

"Will my work understand?" Jay takes his cup and tastes the watered down tea and drinks it. He looks at her. "If miss that much work will I be ok at work, will the accept it?"

Lex giggles, "they will expect it Jay, they will ask you to tell them how our child is often and they will invite us to family events if they have children near the same age. Not one of us will mind that you miss work to be with our child. Jay even that server that asked you to pay in such a rude manner would expect you to miss work to spend time with your child. For him it might be hard to accept the child as one of us and he will never accept you as one of us but he will respect you for missing work to raise our child." Lex starts to laugh, how did you get a job to study cultural development Jay, you can't understand our culture how it is, I see it in your face! How will you figure out how it developed?"

Jay smiles, "I agree, Herfermks told me it is a good job and that I must do it, and that I will be good at it. He got me the job." then Jay thinks 'I wasn't suppose to say that'. "Herfermks asked me not to say he was involved in arranging the job for me." looking at her he sees her understanding that he is asking her not to say anything about it.

"I am your bonded mate now Jay, nothing you say will be shared unless it is obviously meant to be shared." she points to the far side of the valley "See the shadows Jay see how short they are?" then she looks up at the crest of their side of the valley. "If you watch in a few moments the sparkle from the rocks will show." then looking around at the air in the valley, there isn't enough mist to see the colors refract but you will see the sparkles." then she looks at his face.

Jay looks up at the far side of the valley then at the large rocks on the crest of their side, then back at her. "I like the sparkle in your eyes, I don't think the sparkles on those rocks will make me as excited"

"hahahaha, Jay, keep talking like that and we will start my pregnancy before we leave this table!"

Jay looks at her and starts to smile then slowly pushes the pitcher and his cup to the side of the table.

"hahahaha," as she gets up, "lets go Jay, if we make hast we will get to the ruins while the sun is above them.

Finishing his tea he stands up thinking that he is starting to understand her humor. Jay smiles and they start walking down the path towards the bottom of the valley Jay feels the warmth of the tea in him and he feels his legs adjusting the change of walking down hill rather than up. He keeps pace with Lex and soon they are in the bottom, the doors open to the lobby like entrance room and they go past several shops to the first room with elevators. She points through a doorway to another room and as they enter it Jay sees three larger elevator doors, much wider and taller. She walks to the one on the left and says, "Lex, I am accompanied by Jay."

"This one takes us all the way to the lowest level. It is bigger so it can also take freight. It will feel like you are falling at first Jay. It is faster than the smaller ones and not as rough but it does take longer", she says.

"How deep is the deepest level?" Jay asks.

Lex hesitates, "about five times as deep as the lower parts of our city. It is our defense and emergency equipment and emergency supplies platforms on this level. That is why the connections to other areas were made so much faster."

Jay hears some air moving from between the elevator doors. "I think it is coming"

Lex smiles, "I hope so, we better step back so they can come out when it opens." She takes his hand and steps to the side of the door. Watching it open, then looking inside, "ok let's get in".

Jay looks around in it, about 5 meters wide, tall and deep. "It is big" Jay says. He notices that it also has doors on the back that are all the way to the top and wider than the ones they came through. The doors close and a chime sound is herd followed by a voice saying adjust your balance. Then it starts to go down, not so slowly at first. Jay almost feels weightless for some seconds. He looks at Lex as she smiles at him and nods, then he feels some weight on his feet, after a few seconds it feels normal. Then he feels more weight, and he feels heavier and heavier as it seems to be slowing down then it seems to stop, another second and then the gentle bump as it actually does stop. The same doors they came in opens, Jay follows Lex out. "It feels strange here, I feel, I don't know how to describe it, it is like a," Jay moves his arm as he watches it, "it is like there is something pulling and pushing on me at the same time."

Lex says "it is the gravity Jay, we are deep enough within the moon that it's force can be felt from the sides too, and not as much but also from above us, things here need less force to move and weigh a little less than on the surface" as she takes his hand again. "You will adjust to it in a few minutes. It is this way."

As they are walking Jay sees a window shop with a pot of tea and cups on the ledge, "would you like another cup of tea Lex?" as he slows down near the booth.

"Sure Jay lets have another cup." and she stops and lets Jay pour her and him self cups of tea. The attendant just smiles at them and doesn't say anything. She sips it and leans on the wall with Jay and he sips his. They silently watch a few Gyrekians walk by and some others stop to have tea as well. They exchange nods and smiles but don't say anything. When her cup is empty she waits for Jay to finish and takes his cup placing them both on the ledge of the shop. "It was strong, I don't often make it that strong myself. How do you feel Jay?"

Jay smiles at her, "I feel good, I am not sure if it is the tea or the gravity but I feel good all over my body. How are you feeling?"

Lex takes his hand and gives him a nod and a tug toward the direction she want to take him. "I feel good too Jay. Lets go to the transport. It is over here. It isn't far." she keeps increasing the pace until Jay is comfortably walking quickly beside her with a smile on his face. There it is Jay as she points to several wide sliding double doors evenly spaced along a much wider section of the corridor.

Jay sees several symbols above the doors light up but can't read them. "What does it say?" he asks as he walks over towards the doors.

"It is when the transport will come and the name of this station and the destinations on this line." She points to the top row. That one is here that end is where it comes from and that end is where it goes to" then turning to point across the corridor, "through there and down a level is the other direction. It will be here soon"

As she stops talking Jay hear a sound of rushing air and steel rolling on steel, then the doors open and the transports doors open a second later. Big wide tall doors, about 3 meters wide and 3 meters tall. Jay asks why such big doors?"

Lex replies, "Oh, the Ryberians helped with the planning so we made the doors and transports so that they will be comfortable if the Ryberians ever want to use them." then looking over at Jay, they probably never will want to use them but the size is good for moving equipment also." as they walk in and across the transport to sit on the far side.

Jay looks at the size of the car as it starts to move. The acceleration pushes him back in his seat for several second until it starts to approach its' full speed. Jay feels the vibration of the transport and looks at its' structural aspects, at the materials and the shape. He sees that the seats can be unclipped easily and that the handrails can also be unclipped. "So this can be convert to a freight transport quickly with very little effort?" Shifting his body a little to check the comfort of the seat. But nothing lacking in the comfort for travellers, it is well designed."

Lex kisses him on his jaw, "we are alone, kiss me" and as he turns his head to face her, her lips reach his. A soft gentle kiss as she feels him shift his body to face her more comfortably. Tasting the tea on his lips and feeling his breath on her lip from his nostrils. Stroking across the inside of his upper lip with her tongue as she feels his hand sliding up her side and across her back, then her tongue starts across his lower lip and feels his meeting it softly from above. Her thigh feels his other hand slowly moving and snuggly gripping it half way. Pulling back from the kiss as the train starts to decelerate and the inertia shifts them in their seats. Smiling at him, "we are here."

"Really" looking surprised, "one stop? And this is that far?" that was fast. He starts to try to get up and feels the increasing inertia as the transport continues to slow down. Jay grabs the seat and hangs on feeling himself almost sliding off onto the floor, "hohoholy shit, that is a lot of force!" he says as it lessens and then again once almost throws him before it slows more and then stops. He smirks at Lex, "can I get up now?"

Lex snickers, "yes, you will be safe now Jay" She gets up as the doors open and they walk out onto the platform. She points to a large set of doors on the side, "there is the elevator Jay." and starts walking.

Jay looks around the room, "this looks like a work or storage room."

Lex says "come Jay and she calls out to the elevator "Lekxzatrera and bonded mate kyranin male Jay going to surface, scan for security clearance." and keeps walking towards the doors, looking back at Jay as he starts to follow. She hears the engine starting to whine from the direction of the doors and as she gets close feels the force of the air blowing from the crack between the doors. As Jay steps beside her they feel the sound of the deceleration and the settling of the lift car into its dock. The doors open and the lift doors open at the same time. Gesturing with her hand for Jay to enter she steps forward and says, it will take us right into the ruins Jay. Because of the structural features of the ruins they were chosen as a sight for surface defense in case of an attack on our moon. You will see why when we get there as they stop at the side of the lift and hold the hand rail it starts to close it's doors.

From the walls, "welcome to lift to the trukshat ruins, will you be needing the lift to return down to the tunnels?"

"Yes, request for return access for both of us only" and she turns to Jay, "the security protocols are always ready Jay, if you want to come here alone you better learn them correctly or you could find yourself in a bit of a situation." she looks at him. "First we have to file the documents for you to be one of us or else we will have to use the Kyranin diplomatic protocols and they are much more complicated."

"Oh," Jay says, "why is that?' as the lift starts going. Jays' knees almost buckle as they start moving, he feels the heaviness continuing for several seconds as they accelerate. As he starts to feel stable he hears her telling him that with the foreign diplomat security protocols there are many variables due to the delicate regulations around the sharing of technologies and the multitude of categories of security clearances from all the other worlds. He watches her face as she explains the process but is missing the details as he is enjoying watching her passion to explain the information. He feels himself almost leaving the floor as the lift starts it's deceleration process, the weightless sensation feels like it is reducing his weight by about half for many seconds before it starts to reduce and he feels the reduction in speed. "It is fast" he says as it seems to stop, then the docking bump and the door open. Jay walks out with lex by his side, "it looks like we are in a pyramid Lex."

"We are Jay. These older ruins were under the ones that we have legends and some bits of history of." She walks to the wall that is angling up about three hundred feet to the apex of the room. She rubs her hands on the wall. "feel it Jay, It is as smooth as polished Chrystal. It has not tarnished or been broken in the wars that destroyed the cities built on top of them. But there are old scares in the surface on the out side, not deep though. It was scuffed by some kind of beams but only one of the pyramids was penetrated." Pointing to a corner, "an exit at each corner with tubes leading to balconies half way up, those balconies have shield generators that were fixed by the ryberians so they share that technology with us." we don't understand how it works and the ryberians haven't made any effort to help or hinder our research about it. But they have taught us how to use it and come regularly to check it and do maintenance." She looks at Jay, "what do you do with Herfermks when you work with him?"

Jay looks at her and walks to her taking both of her hand in his and looking directly into her eyes. "I can't talk about that Lex. I can tell you that I will always be safe when I work with him but I can't talk about anything we do for work or related to work or about the technology that I have seen working with him." he holds her hands tighter for a second then, "If I do we can be made to forget it and that will make his work harder and it will end our friendship with him."

Lex looks at Jay and swallows, "did you feel the surface Jay?" then nodding with her head at the doorway in the corner, Lets go up to a balcony." and she starts walking holding his hand, "I understand, security protocols Jay. I will never ask what you can't answer." pointing to the line on the floor, without me you need to pass security for off worlders to cross this line Jay. If you did it wrong you would be detained for hours or days until you were past every sort of scrutiny that the alliance has got. Once your certificates of bonding are filed and accepted you will have security freedom for the entire moon."

Jay looks at her, "it is that easy?" to gain security access, all a spy has to do is bond,,, I guess it wouldn't be easy to get bonded if it wasn't real, would it?"

Lex looks at him "no, it is rare for one of us to choose and off worlder. And sometimes the bond is accepted but the security is restricted. But you are a Kyranin. And that is different. You will be accepted and your diplomatic status will be sustained also." Looking both ways into the corridors as she takes him across the line on the floor. Which one Jay?"

"Is there a difference?"

"Not to me"

"Lets go your way then" Jay steps against her, kissing her face then puts his arm around her and starts them walking. He looks and sees that the floor is in steps about 5cm high and 30 cm long. He can easily take them two or even three at a time but they don't. He sees it is the same material as the walls. Some sort of an alloy, and the floor is rough like 200 grit sand paper, "it is still rough he says."

Lex looks at him, "yes Jay, we don't include the pyramids in the history because we have no proof that they are from our history. "The ryberians have told us that there research dates then back much further than any proof that our species lived here." Letting go of his hand, "lets run up there Jay" and she starts running, Jay follows catching up to her as she enters the balcony. Jay looks at it and remembers the balcony at Herfermks world. This is different, much bigger with walls that he can see through when he gets close, and that light comes through somewhat. It has a podium near each corner and as he gets close to look at one it lights up.

"Jay, don't touch it ok," Lex says to him "it will turn on the balcony and draw energy to ready the shields."

Jay steps back a little. "I won't do anything to get us in trouble".

"It won't be trouble Jay there is lots of energy available." she walks right tight up against the wall and presses her face to it, come take a look outside.

Jay does like she did and is shocked. He sees out through the wall like it isn't there. He can feel it on his forehead and hands but it is like he is looking through an open window. He looks at the ruins around them. He sees that the buildings have been built then partly knocked down as far as he can see. He can see the hint of shapes of pyramids under the taller buildings and asks, how many pyramids are there?"

"Jay, there are thousands of them. We don't know for sure because we find more in new locations every few years. They all have the balconies and some still partially work before the ryberians fix them fully. She walks to the corner of the room on the pyramid side of the room. "Do you want to go outside?"

Jay turns and starts toward her, "yeah, I would, how is the air out there?"

She smiles, "like at the top of the valley." waiting until Jay is beside her, "two to go outside, recognize us to come back in latter" and the wall retract on the balcony for them to walk out onto the surface with it's rubble and debris. Jay steps out and slides one foot down the slope about 25cm. He looks at the slope and the debris on it. Looking up the slope he realizes that part of the pyramid is covered with what looks like dead trees. There are various small buildings covering part of it. Then with more scrutiny he realizes that almost all of the pyramids are covered. From the size he expects that only about the top third of each of then is them are above ground."

"What do you think Jay?, is it interesting?" Lex asks as she steps right beside him, sliding a little on the rubble too.

Jay looks at the view of the ruins all around him and says, "I don't remember it looking like this in any of the images."

Lex bumps him on the side with her shoulder, "well, lucky for you your woman knows a few things then, you probably thought she was only good for serving drinks and having great sex, well now you know she is smart too."

Jay laughs, "and she has a good sense of humour" He snuggles close to her then slides his wet fat tongue across her face from ear bottom to eyebrow.

"mmm Jay that is not the place to rub your tongue like that."

Jay kisses her mouth and starts down the hill, "come on Lex. I want to see those structures over there" Stretching his arm out at some two level white stone buildings. He hears her steps moving the rubble and gravel as he starts down the slope. After a few steps he looks over his shoulder to see her following and keeps going. As they approach the two level structures Lex comes beside him and holds his hand. "Have you been to see these before Lex?"

"No"

"How old are these buildings," Jay asks. "They look quite different than the stone work in the tunnels bellow."

Lex stops walking and looks at the buildings. They are about thirty feet in front of the closest one. She looks at it closely then to her side at the others. "Ya, Jay they are well built. But I have no idea how old they are. As a youth we study construction design and got hands on training with it. I can see that the way they build these is not how we do it now. It looks like they took random shaped stones and put them together with some other substance." they both walk right up to the wall and look at it closely, "lets go inside"

452

"Is it safe?' Jay asks.

Lex looks at him. They have been here since before we built the cities under ground Jay. I don't think today they will fall." and she steps toward an open doorway, looks back at him and winks then goes in.

Jay follows to not see her when he enters the room. "Lex?" he looks around and sees her top in a doorway at the far end of the room. He picks it up as he gets to the doorway and looks at it to be sure. "Lex" he calls again, listening then looking around he sees fresh footprints in the dust at the entrance to the next room. Following through he sees stairs with a shoe on the top step. Jay smiles and starts quickly up the stairs taking the shoe and looking for the next clue. He feels the lightheadedness from the thin air but still has his strength so he continues but slowly. Through the next room, another shoe, then the next room. "Lex" he smiles.

"Jay, what are you doing with my clothes?" she laughs. "I thought Kyranins like to be naked but here I am wearing only a smile and you have your clothes and mine on you" and she laughs again.

Jay drops her clothes and starts to take off his own. "This is a great space" he is looking up at the opening in the ceiling, four sided and rectangular. Feeling dizzy as he drops his pants and undoes his shirt. Looking at her eyes look back into his as his shirt hits the floor. Still light headed he steps towards her and starts to feel the fuzzy sensation in his head, nother step and the embrace.

Lex can feel Jay's balance starting to decline and pulls him slightly indicating to get on the floor. Jay responds. As he bends his knees she guides him, kissing him on the way down onto the floor. She gets a smirk on her face and asks "Jay can you make like a four legged with your feet and hands on the floor and your belly up? I have a fantasy".

Jay strokes her side with his hand and looks at her sitting on his belly, her firm breast in front of him. "OK" and he puts his hands on the floor beside him and lifts his knees to pull his feet closer to his body. Seeing her shifting her weight to let him up he presses and lifts himself against her as she raises onto her feet. He shifts one hand then the other until he is comfy then says. "I don't know how long I can hold myself up like this"

Lex smiles and lifts her left leg across and stands beside him, "it will be long enough Jay, just take long slow deep breaths and feel me in your heart." then looking down at his genitals, she takes them in her hands and starts to massage them, rolling his limp cock and squeezing and tugging his testicles softly but firmly. Looking at his face then at his junk, and at his stretched chest and belly as his cock starts to grow. She feels herself getting aroused as she plays with him and enjoys the view of his firm body and smile. As his cock stiffens to stand on it's own she winks at him and bends down to give it a stroke with her nose, then a nibble on the bottom of it with her lips, as it bounces back up at her she catches it in her mouth, lifting it higher and looking over at him stretching to see what she is doing. She winks again then with a slobbery turbulent melody of movements her mouth pulls and bends and pushes his cock in every direction as she pulses his balls not so gently with both hands. Hearing Jays breath effected she holds them still slightly stretched from him and looks in Jay's eyes with just his hard head in her mouth. Holding it firm with her lips locked on it's neck and her tongue firmly stroking it one way then the other as she barely touches the sides of it with her teeth. She can feel his stiffening and see the strain in his face as he keep holding himself up in his arching posture. Feeling her own arousal, she opens her mouth and stands to face him, shifting her hands to hold his cock. Feeling the warmth of herself she swings her left leg back across him sliding her self into position. Then stuffs him into herself as she watches Jay's reaction, his eyes, the colors of his face changing and the widening of his eyes and smile. She hears his breath deepen and slow and feels his surge of strength for a second. She leans forward changing the angle of their joining to touch her breast to his chest. Slowly moving her pelvis and reaching under to slide her hands over his clenched back and buttocks.

"I'm getting dizzy Lex"

She looks at him, and "not yet Jay, I need a minute".

Jay takes a slower deeper breath as he tries to relax out the strain in his arms and shoulders "ok" and he presses up slightly against her to change the angle on his joints.

Lex squeezes and pulls on his back as she delicately strokes her nipples against his chest. Turning herself to bend his cock a little, and then grinding against him to enjoy his length fills her insides. She feels her orgasm approaching and focuses on her feelings of desire and trust for him bringing the sensations toward her heart. The tingle, hot from her nipples, and the glowing pressure in her cunt building a connection to her heart as she looks into his eyes. She sees his eyes partly closing one at a time and feels him starting to give a little and says "Jay, lower your shoulders to the floor Jay" and she grips his back and follows him down grinding herself on him as best she can as he does. With a thud his back drops the last four inches and he moans as she slides her knees to the sides of his ribs and tucks her feet beneath him. Starting to passionately kiss him and grabbing his neck as she slides up against him grinding as he still holds himself up with the strain of his legs. Her climax is starting, almost at a peak, creating a fervor in her as her mouth melds with his and she feels the fresh raw sensations of security and lust from her breast into her heart and feels Jay starting to lower his pelvis. Sliding her feet apart to his hips as his butt reaches the floor her orgasm bursts and the waves connect all of her feelings, physical and emotional for him to her sense of self awareness as she tastes him, his lips in her mouth and relaxes onto him as he lay there, unmoving beneath her. Seconds pass as her bliss holds her savoring his flavor, then her focus on the feeling of him still in her, softening, and still. She looks at Jay as the pulsing in her genitals starts to subside. "Jay". She looks at him with his eyes partly open. "Jay?" Then she notices him inhale and the fear ends. The relief brings her back to the sensation of glowing still through all of her and she clings to him. Thanking the gods for bringing her such a mate, a lover and friend and one willing to do what she asks and to trust her so fully, and to listen to her desires. She feels him beneath her and as she feels his ear with her lips she notices him move his pelvis, a slight shift to one side. The motion it causes sliding on his cock and gliding it slightly exciting the still excited skin in her vagina with its half hard mass. Liking it she waits. Feeling his breath she decides to wake him. 'But how should I wake him' she thinks. Her desire and lust offer her the first choice and she starts to sit up on his cock, half hard inside of her. Then taking his hands in hers and holding them with hers. Leaning one way then the other to slide her legs wider to give her better control of her movement she starts to grind into him so that his phallus strokes inside of her. Rocking and twisting and shifting and starting to feel her own climax approaching again she looks at his still sleeping face and calls "Jay" her climax is approaching fast, "Jay" and she feels the lust compelling her as the sensation builds quickly spreading through, up to her navel and filling her buttocks "JAy" gripping her teeth and squeezing her hands as the flood of sensation takes her, one more sliding grinding thrust and the pulsing fills her the grip on his hands as the waves reach her face. Feeling him fully hard inside of her now as her orgasm settles back to a simmering glow she lets his hands down and lowers her belly to his and kisses his face and whispers his name. As her orgasm retreats she starts moving again and sees his eyes open. Kissing him and continuing to move she feels a warm bellowing flood of emotions coming from her heart and feels Jays arms on her back. He whispers into her ear and her heart pounds.

"I love you Lex" Jay starts crunching his pelvis as he tries to remember how he got there and where he is.

Lex feels her orgasm starting to return, the anticipation of it larger than the sensation this time. But it is building and taking her thoughts as it's own. Her lust for the orgasm is guiding her physical to pull here focus form her feeling for Jay to the physical desire for pleasure of pulsing flaring glittering heat and throbbing soothing euphoria. It focuses her thoughts to the sensation of him sliding against her inside as he licks her ear and holds her back. Then her heart feels his pounding against her, and her breast pressed into him flowing the sensations as her orgasm start to glow again "uuuuuumm jaay". She kisses his mouth and he grips harder and crunches again, harder and harder as he starts to quake her hot cunt. She feels the flooding of his fluids as the shock of it stalls her senses for a split second, them the tidal wave of emotions and her climax explode all at once as he is till pumping and she convulses involuntarily as they feel each others' energy surges.

Jay lay still holding her. His Lex. Looking up at the stares, in the daylight of the moon through the opening in the roof, with the thin air it looks as clear as a night sky from earth. The after glow still filling his thighs and torso, her on him and hugging his thighs with her feet, her breasts on his chest, their bellies together and her breath on his neck, "Lex" he stokes her head with his fingers finding there way slowly though her hair. "I am so glad we found each other." Taking a deep breath realizing how thin the air is. Feeling her on him first and smiling then feeling how his body feels inside. Then noticing that he has a craving for some of the root tea of the moon.

"Jay, Thank you for taking me out here." as she plays, stroking his chest with her fingers watching as the pressure leaves a change in the skin color for a second. "You know most of my life I have spent in the bar. Except for my educational years I never left our homes. Well I went shopping and visited family. I have been to the surface only for special lunches with family and friends." lifting herself with her arms and sitting up on his pelvis again. "Do you want to do it again?"

Jay looks at her and feels his willingness to do anything she wants. "If you want, or we can go home and have some tea first and a meal and a shower and relax first"

She feels his cock limp under her as she slides on it and smiles to him. "The tea sounds good, and I am getting hungry." as she stands up and looks around for her close. "The climb back up to the balcony will be longer than the walk down."

After getting dressed, enjoying the view of the stars together, and talking about the design and construction of the structure they start back up the hill to the balcony. Only part way up Jay notices how he feels the weakness in his legs and how he is panting to get enough air.

"Lex how is it that I feel so strong in the city underground and so week here, I know that the air is thin but if I don't have to strain I am ok." Jay asks, as he notices that his thinking is also not as sharp as it usually is.

Lex looks at him and keeps walking slowing down a little. "Take longer deeper breaths Jay" then watching him to see that he responds. "The air is thin but there is more oxygen in it than on Ramga. We have 4% higher oxygen but much less air pressure. At the deeper levels out air pressure is greater than on Ramga though. In the city it is about the same pressure, so in our home you get more oxygen in to your blood than on Ramga with the same breathing. Here at the surface you get a little less and because the pressure is lower it exchanges slower in your lungs. Jay, if you breath better you can get more. Try it" she stops and waits for him to catch up to her then takes his hand smiling into his face. "Focus on your breathing Jay not just now but all of the time. It will take a few months to change but you will start to breath like us." Then you can do more on the surface too."

Letting go and turning back up the slope, "come on" and she starts walking again.

Jay thinks about her words and starts taking slow deep breaths and holding them in for a second before slowly letting them out again. He slows his steps slightly and after about a hundred yards he notices that he is feeling better. He catches up to Lex at the entrance to the balcony and they go in together, then down to the elevator, down it, and back into the deep tunnels. They stop for a tea from the dispenser before taking the transport back to their city. Jay notices how much he likes the tea now. Examining it in his mind he compares it to his coffee addiction from earth. He likes the tea, he thinks about the flavor and the feeling in his mouth and the smell; but his like for it has nothing to do with any of that. It is an inner craving. That subtle craving is satisfied now that he has had a drink. 'That's not like coffee' he smirks 'with coffee I still wanted more when I had to pee so bad I couldn't wait'. He looks at Lex as they walk toward the doors to the transport. "The tea is a little addictive isn't it?"

Lex smiles, "Yeah, I suspect it is like the mrruk, we drink it all the time and never think about it." She takes his hand in hers and after a few steps stops in front of the transport door and turns to Jay, "do you like the tea? Is it as pleasant as the mrruk?"

"Yeah" Jay responds thinking more about how cute her smile looks more than about the question. "Do we have to call the transport?"

Lex looks up at the top of the door. "No" and looks at Jay again. "The light indicates that it is aware of us and is going to stop for us when it gets here. If there is no light you have to call for a transport and if the light is red or blue you should introduce yourself and your security clearance."

Jay looks up and sees a slight green glow coming from the surface of the wall above the door. He looks closer and realizes that it is more accurately glowing green just in front of the wall above the door. "Interesting how the light appears" he says without thinking.

She looks up at it. "It is. It is part of the old technology from the pyramid that the ryberians got working. They adapted it to our communications systems that control the transports. It is the same for all security for the pyramids."

Jay hears the rushing of air from the cracks in the transport doors. "It sounds like it is coming"

Lex looks across the room to where the tea dispenser is, "Do you want more tea for the ride?"

"mmm, no we can make some when we get home." Jay says, kisses her and looks at the doors. He can hear the transport stopping on the other side then the click and the doors start to open. He finds a seat and holds on to the handle and to Lex as the doors close.

"haha, so. You are ready for the ride Jay?" Lex smirks at him and hangs onto the handle too.

Jay feels the inertia as it starts to go, he feels her elbow gently in his ribs and looks at her smile as he gives her a bit of a hug with his arm. Still feeling the acceleration and her snuggling into him he starts to think about the transport with only them on it both coming to the pyramids and now going back. 'She seems to act like it is normal, "Lex, if I wanted to take a small space craft to look at the pyramids from space what would I have to do?"

Going into Space

As she snuggles into him a little closer and tighter "tomorrow Jay, I want to eat dinner and go to bed with you tonight".

Jay leans his head against hers, kisses her scalp and snuggles with her, still gripping the handle with one hand. "Tomorrow we can fly into orbit in a space ship to look at he ruins from space?"

"I like it when you say we Jay. If that is what we are going to do I will register you as my bonded mate after dinner tonight, then we can have sex for the last time before we sleep."

Jay thinks about how she said it. "OK"

The next morning Jay wakes up alone in his bed. He lay there for a minute stretching and enjoying the life coming back into his mind and the dreams fading away out of memory. He looks around the room and remembers his life there on the moon, his work and Lex. He looks around the room. Relaxing, he listens and only hears silence. Remembering the night before and the day, and the bonding the day before that, "good morning Lex". Hearing nothing, "house, is Lex here?" he asks. He listens, as the house responds that she has gone out. Jay sits up on the side of the bed and looks around the room. No sign of her, her clothes are gone, or put away. He walks to the sanitary room and showers, dresses and goes to the kitchen. No sign that she ate. He looks in the cooler and sees nothing has moved since the night before. He sits at the table and feels a craving for some tea, turns to see the dispensers on the counter. Gets up and takes a cup from a cupboard and fills it with tea. Thinks to himself 'I'm glad there is a tea dispenser, I wonder if all homes here have one,' and sits back down. "House, can you locate Lex for me?"

The walls reply, "Yes, she is at the market collecting supplies for your cupboards and cooler."

Jay looks at the wall and sips his tea. "House, can you show me a view of her in the market where she is now?"

The wall screen lights up with colors and images of a plaza with several shops and some tables with products on them in the wide corridor between the shops. Jay looks at it and sees Lex in one of the shops with a bag in one hand and picking through some produce with the other. He watches as she puts several items in her bag and starts walking out of the side of the wall screen's image. As she does the image changes and he sees her walking to ward him in the new view, then past him, then away, out of view. The image changes again as she again steps into view, with a content smile on her face as she walks with a bounce in her step.

Jay sips his tea and thinks out loud "Lex you do look good".

He sees her stop with a surprised expression, and she looks around, "Jay? Are you watching me?" and she gets a silly grin. She starts to do a little dance, showing off her agility and curves. Then starts walking again.

"Can you hear me?" Jay asks.

Lex looks around as she walks "I can't see the cameras, but I know how they work. I'll be home in a minute, unless there is anything you want me to go back and get for you?"

Jay looks at her as she walks past him on the wall again. "No, I'm good, I'm having a tea. Can you see me too?" and he waves and puts one foot up on one of the other chairs.

Lex keeps walking and smiling then stops and looks at a wall in the corridor "corridor, show me my bonded mate."

Jay sees the wall she is looking at in the corridor light up and it shows a real time image of him sipping his tea with one foot up on a chair. His surprise shows as he straightens his posture and turns to wave at her from the screen in front of her. "I did not know about this".

Playfully looking him up and down Lex responds, "mmm, my mate does look good, Jay stand up"

Jay stands up, and looks in the direction that the camera seems to be shooting him from. As he looks at the wall screen of her looking at him, he hears her say to take off his clothes. "What?"

"You heard me Jay, you are my kyranin bonded mate, you are suppose to be naked at home! Take your clothes off now!" and she starts laughing "corridor, screen off" and she giggles as she starts walking again.

"House, screen off" Jay says, then after a second he starts hastily taking his clothes off. He sits down and sips his tea some more. Looking down at his hairless naked body he starts to laugh. 'In my time on my world I'm a over the hill, dead end job pauper; and here in this life I am a spy living as a newlywed diplomat, with a job that I can do whatever I want and live like a king. Thank you God!' he thinks, then another sip of tea, a gulp, and looks at the dispenser considering another cup. He looks at his cloths on the floor and decides to put them in the bedroom, in the cupboards, he does. Then gets another cup of tea and sits back down. "Wall screen, show me the news events of the past few days and upcoming entertainment events that Lex might want to attend", he sips his tea.

The wall screen starts showing government announcements about trade agreements with new associated planets and various alliance planets, and then sports highlights of various worlds.

Lex comes in the door "Jay I found some fresh crystem in the market, should we eat in now or save it for tonight?" She looks him up and down and goes into the kitchen, puts the food away and comes back stopping in front of him and smiling; watching him sipping his tea. "You are the obedient one aren't you. I will be a happy female. You look good naked Jay". She goes back into the kitchen takes a cup from the cupboard and fills it with tea, takes a sip, and returns to in front of Jay. She looks at him for a few seconds then steps up bumping his knees apart with her leg and sits on his right thigh, then kisses his cheek. "Jay, I have a ship arranged for us; for the afternoon. It will be waiting for us as soon as we can get there. Should I tell them we will be delayed?"

Jay looks at her, puts down his cup and puts his arm around her and smiles. "What ever you want Lex, I am happy to get dressed and go now, or we can stay here for a while and enjoy ourselves."

Lex slides her hand down and grabs his whole package and gives it a little tug and a soft shake. Still holding it she smiles at Jay, "Lets go to space first we can play later, I think you will be more ready after you have been in orbit for a while!" She lets go and gets up, looks at his groin and walks into the bedroom. "Jay do you have space clothes for me?"

Jay thinks about the question, he has no idea what she means, "do we need special clothes for the space craft?"

"hahe, no dear, something sexy and exciting, I haven't been in space with you before, I want to look more exciting than the ruins." as she walks into the doorway, holding the edge of it and showing enough of her naked self to indicate her interests.

Jay smiles at her as he gives her a good close look, "well, if you can't find anything in the drawers we can stop at the store on the way and you can get whatever you like".

Stepping into the doorway to fully expose herself, "Jay, You are the best mate I could have ever hoped for." and she steps out of view toward the drawers.

Jay sits in his chair feeling like he did something right with a smile on his face. 'I think I am going to like it here on the moon' he thinks to himself as he finishes the tea and looks at the kitchen deciding if he should have some more. As he starts to get up he hears Lex.

"Well, how do you like it, do I look good enough to get some attention or will the ruins be all you see today?".

Jay turns to look, and he sees her smiling in one pose then another several times. "I don't think I will notice the ruins", Jay says. Then puts the cup on the table and walks over putting his arms around her and smiling. He moves closer, closer and kissing her lips, then again, and then more passionately, then dancing with a sway, one way, then the other and stepping together in a circle, and stopping. "I love you Lex" Jay smiles as he looks at her looking back at him. She just stands looking at him with the smile and a second passes. He leans to kiss her again and she gives him a quick kiss that feels a little stiff to him.

Lex starts towards the door, "lets go Jay the ship will be ready."

Jay thinks about her reaction as he starts toward the door and stops, "Lex?" hesitating a second, "Are we OK?" he watches her stop and look back at him and notices a tear in her eye and a pale look on her skin. "What is it Lex, you can tell me anything, I am here for you 100%."

She steps close to him and hugs him with her head on his chest. "I am sorry Jay, I have to confess. I was so happy when I felt attracted to you because you are kyranin and I had a fantasy to have an orgy like we hear you do on Ramga, but you love me and now it can't happen and I feel guilty that I still want it." her hand clasping his cloths and clenching as she hugs into him. "I do love you too Jay. I really do. I am Gyrekian and I will never stray form our bond. But I did want that fantasy I really did. I am sorry. Now that I think about it I, I don't know what to do."

Jay hears a whimper and feels her muscles twitch. He thinks about her, how she was so excited that he was Kyranin and what she said about their bonding. He thinks about what his values are around sex and how happy he is with there new situation, and how his past few months have been on Ramga, and how he may have to go back to earth one day. "Lex, it is ok, I am Kyranin. I don't mind, we can find a juice that we both like and we can do it the kyranin way any time you like." as he holds her tightly and kisses the top of her head. "Lex if you want that fantasy I want you to have it, I want it too. I want it so that as we grow old you will feel glad that you bonded with me. I want you to get to do all of the things that you want, and all of the things that you think you want so that you are sure you got a life with everything included." He feels the stillness of her hugging him. Listening for a response Jay searches his feelings to see how it will be for him to live up to his words. He feels an inner calm, he feels her still motionlessly hugging him. He feels a deep satisfied feeling, and the warmth of kind love and contentment. Kissing her head again then saying, "Are you ok?" he starts to think about how different it is for her on her world that it was on earth.

Lex loosens her grip and turns her face up to look at Jay. Seeing him smiling down at her she lifts herself on her toes to kiss him as she shifts one hand to grip his shoulder to help with the height to reach his lips. Looking into his eyes as he bends his neck bringing his lips to meet hers'. A soft kiss, "Jay, you really would let us do that?"

Jay looks at her. "Why not?" Smiling and holding her back with his hands gently cupping behind her kidneys, "it is common in my culture. We don't talk about it too much but it is normal, we all do it."

Lex looks at him, "we can't let the Gyrekians know about it Jay, they will shun us, me especially. It is against our culture. It was my fantasy but I didn't think I would want it so bad as to mention it. But it has been growing in my mind every day since I first kissed you in the storeroom of the bar. I was hoping that we could just talk about it and I could forget about it."

Jay looks at her and smiles, "if you want Lex, but it will probably be easier if we go to ramga for a vacation and live out your fantasies there. We can dress you like a kyranin woman, and with a little cosmetics everyone will think you are a kyranin woman. No one will say a thing."

Lex looks at him. "Ramga is far Jay, there is a space station that we can get to in a few hours of space travel. There are lots of kyranins there and only a few of us gyrekians. We can go there without being missed here on the moon. It would be safer for us to do that."

Jay shrugs, "Today?"

Lex's eyes grow big, "Nn, no, if you want," she starts to feel the fear of living her fantasy. "Maybe another day, soon, or in a few months?" Feeling her excitement and fear too, "I don't know Jay, can we think about it and talk about it more too then make a plan to do it?" as she fidgets with Jay's clothes in her hands.

Jay looks at the mixed expression on her face and asks "will there be anyone else in the space craft with us today?"

"No"

"Ok lets go, we can talk about this latter?" leaning to kiss her, waiting for her to respond, the kiss and then he starts walking to the door, "lets go".

As they start down the corridor Jay asks "do we go to the surface to get to the ship?"

"No Jay they are on the deep level, we have to go to the out side of the city then down. There is a tunnel connecting the close elevators but it is mostly used for business and defense work. This way is best." She reaches and grasps his hand. "You surprise me every day Jay, I am not sure what tomorrow will bring but I am getting to like thinking about my future with you a lot."

Jay looks at her and keeps walking.

"Until you came in the bar the first time I had no idea that my life could be so exciting. I never imagined I would do anything more than be a server in our place. Now I am going to help you with your work, travel off the moon, have a family, and wake up with you every morning."

Jay looks at her, thinking about her words. He realizes the life they are starting together and questions why Herfermks pushed him to it. He feels his happiness, and his satisfaction with his choices. He thinks about the future she is talking about there on the moon with a family and wonders when he is slated to go back to earth with Herfermks' ten-year plan. Herfermks likes this woman as a friend and now he is going to have to leave as she has a young family, it doesn't make any sense. He thinks about his feelings for her and what choice he has on if he will stay or leave to go back. 'More than ten years' he thinks to himself. 'Maybe forty years, I bet they can do that, if I do good work for them, it won't make any difference from the other side, in the time on earth I will still be in the bathroom only a minute. It can be longer, forty years is what I will ask for next time I see Herfermks'. He looks at her, starts gripping her hand a little tighter and looking at the details of the designs in the walls and the elegance of the floors, and the way the lights are all set into the walls and floors and ceilings so that they never shine into your eyes no matter where you look. He looks at the way the others smile and nod as they pass; and at the variety of shops and businesses and offices. He thinks about how they don't use money and he looks at Lex again. "So who maintains the space crafts?"

Lex looks at him for a second. "The technicians Jay who do you think?" As she stops by a door that opens as they step in front of it. Looking in Lex nods her head to the left, "that blue elevator goes down to the personal ship bays" and starts walking towards it.

Jay walks beside her, hand in hand. "Do you have a personal ship for your family?"

"No Jay, all the ships belong to all of us. These ones are for personal use, so we have them available in the personal ship bays. Our business ships are in a different types of bays and our defense ships are in secured defense ships silos." The elevator door opens and several Gyrekians step out and they walk in. "Lekxzatrera and Jay to the day trip bay, level three." and she looks at Jay. "I put you into the security with your common name, I hope you don't mind" as she smirks.

Jay laughs, "I am glad, I even have a hard time pronouncing my full name correctly." The door closes and Jay asks, "Have you flown one before?"

She looks at him, "we learn to fly them when we are children. In simulators of course, but in our last three educational years we learn to fly all the ships and use all the defense weapons and communication equipment."

"I am curious about how you choose what work you will do during your educational years, how is it decided what you will study?"

Lex looks at him. "What ever we are interested in. Is it different on Ramga?"

Jay remembers the information that he was told in his training, "there are the basic skills and information then they get to chose what to specialize their learning in. Also if there is an special talent that become apparent then special training in the areas of the talent is added."

Lex looks at Jay, "what about you, you say they, how were you educated?"

Jay watches the door open and looks at Lex. She starts walking, letting her lead him with her hand. "I was educated on other worlds, it was varied, my parents did some of it, and a lot was self directed, some mandatory training on some worlds. I got to make some choices, and some times I had to study things that were of no interest to me at all."

"That one, the red and yellow one" Lex points, "so it was very different for you than for me. Here we can learn whatever we are interested in from our first curiosity. Only the technical use of tools is taught to every gyrekian the same way. I was interested to be a space technologist for several years. I learned to make and repair spacecraft engines form most of the designs and styles used in the alliance. But by the time I was half way through my educational years I was not interested anymore. I started to like art and music; a year and a half at that and it was history, then, intergalactic politics, then weapons, then cooking and dance. Then it was child rearing. Did you know that there are over 200 developmental stages for intellectual growth of a Gyrekian child before they are of the age to start their educational years?" looking at Jay for a response and seeing his surprised look. "Many of them over lap and they can effect each other if they are disrupted or stymied by trauma. Either physical or emotional trauma will slow and possibly retard the intellectual and emotional development of a child. The first five years of correct child rearing is crucial for the development and safety of our culture. Without fully stable minds in our next generation we could fall as a culture and become as destructive as the worlds that are unable to control their own governments." Stopping a few meters in front of the red and yellow ship. "It is hard to imagine that we could digress but we have seen all of the signs of the thinking patterns that could lead to it in the children of Gyrekians who live off world when their children were young and had some hardships in their situations. If they didn't give their children the proper care the symptoms show all through their lives." she looks at Jay then tugs his hand and nods her head, "that is Krewn, He was my study partner when I was learning to maintain space craft engines. Krewn".

Jay looks as the guy stands up from the pile of parts on the floor some distance away as he turns around to face them.

He looks at them, "Lekxzatrera" he comes walking towards them. "I saw that you were coming to take a ship," looking straight into Jay's eyes and lifting his hands for a shake as he approaches, "and you are Jay. The new kyranin bonded mate?"

Jay smiles and shakes his hands, "Yes, good to met you Krewn."

Krewn holds Jay's hands for a few second as he smiles at him. "Lekxzatrera was always the fastest learner and the best friend in our groups. I am glad she found a mate. I am happy for you. I hope I can become friends with your new family as it grows."

Jay looks at Lex's smile and feels the grip on his hand from her, "I will be happy to have you as a friend"

Krewn turns to Lex "I went over everything in person on this craft, it is ready to go anywhere in the alliance. Don't travel to fast, I remember how you like to fly!"

Jay looks around the room. The ceiling is about 50 feet up and the walls are a good distance away. He looks at the ship. It seems to be sitting on the floor like a big odd shaped container, like a shipping container from earth but an odd shape. About 50 feet long, he can see a similar one across the room the same shape it is about 30 feet wide and they are both about 30 feet high.

Krewn says "k1762, Lekxzatrera and Jay have control, open entry", a section of the outer surface seems to fade into nothing. "Ok, you two have a great time, where are you going?"

Lex looks back as she is walking toward the opening, "just into orbit to look at some ruins".

"Sure, just bring it back in one piece. If you don't want to tell me I'm ok with that." Krewn gives a disappointed look.

Jay looks back at him, "I am studying archeological sites as part of my work and I wanted to see them from space. It will be my first time seeing the moon from space, I missed it on the way here."

Krewn waves, "ok, I was hoping you had some secrets Jay, have fun!" and he turns back towards his work.

Lex and Jay walk into the ship and the door reappears behind them. Jay looks back and can't see where the opening was. It is just all walls now. Lex looks around and starts up the stairs, "come on Jay lets go to the front so we can watch the view as we launch." She hurries up the stairs and to the room ahead, then sitting in the middle of three seats.

Jay looks at her sitting in the seat, it is far too big for her, it looks like a love seat, he looks around, and all of the chairs do. He looks for it and does not see a control panel, Or a view screen. Or any nobs or buttons, "so where to you drive from."

She looks at Jay. "You haven't been in Gyrekian space craft before, have you Jay?"

Jay looks at the surface in front of the three seats. Then asks, "Where should I sit?"

"Here with me, this is the best seat" and she gives him a wink. "View open. Control access. Launch ready."

"Launch ready" the ship repeats back to her as the surface in front of the seat that Jay is sitting down on with Lex turns transparent and and a 3D translucent panel appears in front of Lex.

"mmm, nice ship" Jay says. "no one ever talks about Gyrekian ships. From what I had come to believe they were not this advanced." sitting down on the seat beside her he looks for a seat belt or something to hold onto.

Lex slides tightly beside Jay and the translucent panel in front of her stays in front of her as she moves. "We don't talk about our technology Jay. We don't give off worlder's rides in our personal transports, and we don't sell travel to our allies. Our business ships are of two types. One for only us and the other ones that we use to do off moon business that are often entered by others. Those off moon business ships are of average technological appearance so the other species don't want to learn about them. They don't go fast and they can't cloak themselves. They don't go too fast and they can't go too far without getting more fuel. That way we don't have to worry about them being stolen."

Jay looks at her, he takes another look around the room they are in. It has some in wall cabinets, two doors on one side of the room and one on the other, the floor is smooth but it felt soft like carpet to walk on. The ceiling has murals of landscape like in the canyon they were the day before. "Where do we go out to the surface from?"

She smiles at him. "Jay this is your moon too now so you have to respect our privacy about our technology. You know this is true. So I can tell you Jay, we have more technology that you expect. We travel through the moon by dimensional flux variation. We don't need an opening. Outside of the moon we stay cloaked so that except for the Ryberians top secret reconnaissance orbs, nothing that we know of can trace us."

"Wow, that is beyond what we have for technology that I know about." Jay looks at the surface in front of them. "So what will I see when we take off, the inside of the rock that we are going through?" as he looks at the screen seeing the room out side of them then looking at her beside him.

She slowly turns toward him with a silly smirk on her smile, "it will be dark then you will see space" looking at him with tight lips and squinty eyes for a second, "It is like you don't know much about space ships Jay have you ever flown one?"

Jay feels himself turning red "actually, I have only done it in a simulator. I have never had to fly one. I have always been a passenger." he watches her for a reaction.

She puts her hand on his leg, "This time I'll do it, but watch, next time I will teach you." She rubs his leg up and down. I like your honesty Jay. I have seen some others from other worlds lie about such things in the bar so often. It is not a big deal. My father has never driven a space ship. My mother was a pilot when she was young. It kind of flies itself if you ask it to anyway." Giving his leg a squeeze and then bringing her hands to the translucent panel in front of her, "Ready" then turning some of the colored lights and moving some others then taking a deep breath and looking at the surface in front of them and putting her fingers into ten lights on the lower edge of the translucent panel. As she starts to move her fingers the surface in front of them turns black and then it looks like a window looking into space.

"Are we in space?" leaning forward to see better "I didn't feel a thing". He looks at her fingers still in the lights on the panel.

Lex moves her fingers and the view from the surface in front of them changes until they are looking down at some pyramids with building on and around them on the surface below them. "There Jay, that is where we were yesterday. Ship stay" she takes her fingers out of the lights and points at the image on the surface in front of them "that one in the side with the round thing on that side of it, there, on the other side the line down to those buildings, we made that when we went down there.

"Oh, hhhm." Jay says looking at the area. "There are a lot of pyramids there. Do they all have balconies and defense technology?"

Lex looks at them and then at Jay "why?"

"Oh" Jay turns to her, "I am curious, it just seems strange that such and advanced technology would have been left intact to be built over by a later civilization that didn't learn how to use it or even enter it. It is such an interesting situation, that structures that much older were built with such advanced technology in them, and that still can be made to work. Especially when you consider that the buildings built on top of them have fallen into ruins from time."

"Yes" Lex says. "It is odd. They all work. Some of them can still fly too." she looks at them. "It is not know to all of us, but when I studied space craft work one teacher showed us one that did still fly and we examined how it worked. It was intact. It functioned perfectly and it is a good system for fast travel over vast distance. We keep it a secret even from the others of our moon. We don't know the origins of the technology or why it was left. The technology was and still is studied by our moon security science teams. They don't share what they know but once in a while we get upgrades of various technology as a result of their work." Lex looks at Jay's eyes. "You are with me now Jay, you are one of us. You can't tell Herfermks of our secrets, it is his rule too. It is our technology now so it is only to be shared if our moon decides. You can't be a spy Jay! Do you understand?"

Jay looks at her. I understand but it is my job to do research for Herfemks on anthropology from artifacts and history and cultural effects thought to be derived from various influences." Jay looks at her. "He never asked me about any technology questions though, I think I do understand. I can be loyal with the work but can't mention any of the technology that he does not mention to me first. Is that it?"

"Kind of Jay. If he asks you can't answer. If he describes you can't comment or compare or agree or deny. If he suggest you can't confirm. If he mentions you can't have an opinion. If he persists all you need to say is that it is a topic of technology and you one of us now so you have nothing to say about technology." then she looks down for some seconds before looking back at Jay, "He is a good Ryberian Jay be would never ask, but if it comes up in conversation you must be carful. You can't betray us, it is worst for you, as you will not be trusted by anyone ever. If the ryberians want some technology they can get it without asking you about it, that you must know."

"That is true Lex" Jay remembers some of the things he had done with Herfermks. "It is about me keeping my honor and being a trusted mate and member of the moon, I understand" then looking at the pyramids. "Lets go look at the next set"

Lex looks at him, "do you want some tea Jay? I am getting thirsty".

"Ok, Yeah, some tea, and maybe a snack. Is there a kitchen on this ship?"

Lex says "ship, move to above the nearest other pyramids like the set below us now, put the view of them on the dinning area viewing surface." Then she starts walking toward the door, "come Jay it is up stairs."

Jay follows. As he reaches the top of the stairs he sees the entire top level is one room. It has sloped ceiling in the corners and a few pillars and has a kitchen in one corner and a bar in another. The rest of the room is like a lounge and dinning room. There are sofas and tables and chairs. The kitchen has everything that any kitchen on ramga has plus a tea dispenser. Lex opens a cabinet and takes out some containers and dumps the contents onto a platter. Jay looks at it seeing various biscuits, and cookies. They go together and get their teas. Then sit on the sofa and start sipping the tea. After a few sips Jay asks, "how soon will we be there" Then he picks up a cookie and stuffs it into his mouth.

"Ship, show image of pyramids below us"

The wall across from the sofa lights up with the image of the surface showing some forest and some ruins. Jay looks at it and has another sip of his tea then he stands up and walks over to it. He looks closely at the surface with the images on it. "These ones are totally covered with forest and the other ruins are mostly covered too. I can see the shapes of the pyramids though. They seem to be about the same size as the other ones. Three big ones and five small ones, the other set had six small ones."

Lex looks at the image. "Yes it is true." she looks at the image from the sofa and sprawls across it making herself comfortable. "Ship move to another set of pyramids and show the view from the same distance and angle." she watches the screen blur and become clear. "This is different Jay"

Jay looks at it. He sees two intact large pyramids and one that looks like it is cut in half with one half turned over and pushed into the moon. One of the small ones on it's side and a lot of big rocks and sand over all of them. But no ruins on them, "why no ruins"

Lex looks at the image. "Ship, move back to get a wider view." the pyramids slowly shrink and the view slowly shows more and more of the moon until it is clear that the pyramids are on a high altitude plain. "No air"

Jay looks at the terrain. "Mmm, yeah that makes sense."

Lex has another sip of her tea. "Jay come sit with me"

He looks at her and smiles and walks back to the sofa as she calls for the ship to move to the next one. "Lex, Thank you for this day in orbit." Putting down his empty cup he stretches out beside her. "Is there any research on how that big one was cut in half?"

Lex snuggles into him. "It was talked about in our military training. The Ryberians have knowledge of weapons that can do that type of damage." kissing his cheek and stroking his belly. "It was determined that it was a time distortion weapon by some of our scientists and that it was a radio activity beam by others. It is so old that it is hard to determine. The edges of where the weapon had hit has been worn from friction over time. The radioactive or time distorted energy signatures have

also been distorted by time. Our scientists say time hides
all secrets if you let it."

Jay thinks about that statement. 'I won't let it', he thinks to
himself. Liking the way she is stroking his abdomen he starts
fondling her back and legs, kissing her face and rolls her on
top of him to massage her back. "Lex?" he asks, "how soon
would you want to start a family, children".

Lex smiles and looks into his eyes, smiling harder as the
seconds join together and Jay realizes that he is on his second
breath waiting for the answer, "any time Jay. I feel it in my
heart that I want your children to be with us, our children."
kissing him hard, passionately for several seconds then
stopping and pulling back with a questioning look. "When do
you want to have our children?"

Jay smiles, still feeling the action and pressure in his lips from
her kiss. "Anytime you like Lex. Now is good for me, but if
you want to wait a few years we can do that too."

Lex looks at him with seriousness in her eyes. She slowly gets
up and stands beside the sofa and looks him over pretty good.
"Now" and she starts undressing, "take your clothes off Jay!"
as she pulls her garments down and undoes her foot ware.

Jay sits up undoing his shirt as he watches her carefully taking off all of her clothes and then starting to help him with his. He feels the excitement and his cock is full. He feels his heart pounding as his last sock comes off. He feels his mind consumed with his surprise of her enthusiasm as her mouth covers his cock, wetting it well. He watches her face as she pushes his chest back and down, then climbs across his legs, straddling him and lowering herself onto his pulsing rod. Her hands: one on his chest, one grabbing his cock to direct it into herself. Her mouth reaching toward his as he feels the sweetness of her vagina swallowing his penis. Her lips on his and the passionate kissing resumes. Almost instantly he feels ready to come, the warmth within him and the tingle in his balls, the intensity on the skin of his cock. Lifting her as he rolls and still inside as he lays her down and settles on top of her. Again her mouth meeting his and he feels her heels on his back as the feelings in his belly start to blur. His hands go to her breasts as he squashes her belly with his more with each thrust, her hot breath and her nails in his back, the heels, one on his spine, and one on his thigh. The flavor of her saliva filling his mouth and he gasps it in feeling the burst from below and her moan, and whine and moan again, his throbbing as his legs and back and arms loose their strength, his heart pattering fast as he feels her gripping him tightly.

"Jay, lets go to the station this week and find a juice, so we can start a family this week".

Jay feeling dizzy and smoothly satisfied, still bubbling with bliss, "ok, but you can get pregnant with just me, without the juice" relaxing his weight on her as she continues to clasp him with her arms and legs, in silence.

Lex can feel the fluid from Jay inside of her. She can feel his cock getting soft and smaller. She likes the way he feels on top of her and the taste of his kisses still in her mouth. Feeling him with her legs and arms clamped to him and smelling his skin. He smells kyranin, sort of, she thinks. His smell is unique to her and she likes it. She licks his collarbone and looks up to find his eyes. " Jay, we can get pregnant with out another kyranin? How?"

Jay lifts himself onto his elbows taking some pressure off of her, "It is rare, but some of us have both, juice and seed. I do produce a little juice so it is possible."

"Are you willing to find a juice with me to be sure?" she asks as she is still holding him and looking into his eyes.

Jay smiles, "I am certain that we will get pregnant without one. I am willing to find a juice so that you can live your fantasy with me as soon as you are ready to. I want you to have everything that you ever wanted, and I want you to have it as soon as possible."

"But won't you be jealous?"

Jay looks at her and smiles. "Lex, I am Kyranin. It is normal for us to have sex with three. I am happy to do it. I am part of the moon now but I am still me, I won't be jealous. I will be loving and open and kind to you, and if you want to do it several times to be sure that it works I am happy to do that too." Jay gets off of her and snuggles her from the side. "It may be hard to understand from a Gyrekian way of thinking but for me, a Kyranin. I am with you for love and to raise children. We are one, one family, we are two parts of the same team, we, will love each other and do what we have to do make each other happy. If you don't get to do whatever you want it is my loss. If I fail to make you happy I will be miserable. To have sex so that you can be happy, any time, any situation, with any number of others that you want." kissing her face. "Lex, Kyranins see sex differently, It is not so important, it is fun. It is special when you feel love as I do for you, and I am not interested to look elsewhere for it. But to give you the experience of being a Kyranin woman, it is my honor to please you like this."

Lex looks at him as he is saying it. She looks at him thinking of what he says. After a second her lips move, then they close and she slides her hand up his ribs and down over his heart. "You love me, so you are happy to do this with me. It is different than the Gyrekian ways. I do want to do it Jay. It is scary for me but I do want to. I am scared that it will be his child and not yours." she takes a deep breath. I understand the reality that we can scan him to be sure he is only a juice, but, I have the fear anyway."

Jay looks at her. "It is fear, don't let it control you. Do what you want to do, live your dreams, live your fantasy, live with me and have a family." Looking at her expression "Lex if you don't live this fantasy what will you feel like when our children are running around and filling all of our time with watching them, what will you feel like when you send our children to educational classes and your time to do your own activities starts again. How will you feel about this desire for this fantasy then? Will it still be holding a wanting in you to try it? Or will time make it into a lost secret?" Jay kisses her softly. "I understand that if you do this now you will be free of it. If you don't it will always be there, a sliver of darkness between us. Something you wanted that you didn't get, something that can't come back, a void that can't be filled. Lets do the right thing, together, as one, let's live your fantasy, lets make you a Kyranin bride and get you the juice we need, Lets move past your fear and let you live your fantasy."

Lex looks at Jay and nods, she looks more intensely at his eyes, "so we are going to do this?"

Jay asks, "Is it going to make you feel better when our children are grown up?"

Lex looks at Jay then moves to sit on the edge of the sofa for a few seconds, then a few more, and she begins to nod. "You are right Jay when I create the image of us with growing our children and the fantasy still un-lived I want it more and more as years pass. It is like you say, a black sliver that grows into a wedge. I am a little bit afraid to do it though Jay."

Jay shifts and puts his arm around her. "Me too," then as their eyes meet, "lets think of the fear as just being a little nervous, and keep doing whatever the next part is until it is over." He watches her face until he sees her stress start to leave. He sees her nodding.

"I like the way you think Jay. It is best to think about the results before taking the actions, and to take the actions that will bring the results that you want." She turns with a smile and kisses his cheek, stands up and looks at her clothes. "I'll get dressed and we can go to the station." she reaches down and picks up her garments and starts walking for the stairs.

Jay looks at the image on the wall of the pyramids below them. He sees the three large ones and the point of two small ones. They are all covered with newer ruins and with earth and it looks like some kind of vegetation too. "Ship, why is there vegetation on these ruins?"

The voice comes from the room, "the altitude here at this site is lower, it is in a large low land near where equator. The vegetation that grows in this lowland is the most diverse on the moon."

"Ship, Can you show the other pyramids location on the viewer with red lines, the ones not visible in the shape of the surface." Four red squares show up and all of the visible pyramids also have the squares around them where their bases would be if they weren't partly buried. Jay looks at the screen noticing the arrangement of the pyramids. He asks "ship, can you message my tablet with the location of the previous site, the one with the broken large pyramid, and the approximate time of its destruction." Jay gets up and puts on his clothes. He goes to the first room they were in and gets his tablet. He looks through the door and sees that Lex is not there. He finds the time travel program that Herfermks put into his tablet and sets in the data from the ships message into the program. He asks the tablet to help him set up the details of the time and space travel and waits, he looks again to see that Lex is still not coming to the room. He asks his tablet about the air at that time when the pyramid was cut in half and if he can breathe there at that time. His table indicates that he can. He asks the tablet to set the faze-shift and time acceleration to be ready to slide him past the events that happened near that time at that location. He watches as the screen changes one set of controls after another until it stops. He ask to set up a return time to a few seconds before he leaves and to return him across the room from where he is now. Then he thinks the command and sees himself appear across the room, then sees the fading and unfading to a short distance from the pyramids. He feels the coolness in the thin air and can see the pyramids tops about 600 meters away. He sees the time starting to speed up, a lot. The sparse vegetation changes, then faster like waves, and faster like a strobe of colors. He sees the pyramid broken. He says "tablet, back up through time at 10% of the speed." The scrolling of days stops and then starts again slower. He sees the pyramid back in one piece. "Tablet, again move forward in time at 10 % of this speed." he watches the scrolling slower as sees some flashes and the pyramid broken in half again. " Tablet, again move back in time at 5% of this speed and be ready to stop on my thought."

He sees the colors of the vegetation changing and the changes in the sky, lots of movements of light and flashes on and around the pyramids. Jay sees a very bright flash and sees the ground move beneath him like from an earthquake. Then the beam and the pyramid crack and explode open. Next he sees several other beams from the other pyramids and some flashes in the sky as bright as the sun in many places. Then he sees the fire starting all around him and burning the vegetation. "Tablet stop me in this time, keep me out of faze, and tell me if I am in danger from the time distortion or radiation." He hears his tablet tell him he will only have a few minutes before the radiation will effect his separate faze of reality and that the time distortion will start to effect him in two minutes as well. Jay asks his tablet to take readings of the pyramid and the beings in them; and of the radiation and energy, and type of dynamics of both from the weapons from the ships in space hitting the pyramids and from the pyramids shooting at the ships in space." Jay says "tablet, slowly back up from this time at 50% speed of the time we were going and record all the data as requested." He watches as the battle slowly goes in reverse. He sees that life forms are moving through the area around him very fast still and that they are a mix of various species that he has never seen. When he gets to a time before the battle he asks "tablet, move forward in time at the actual pace of the passing of time here now on this moon. Tablet how long will I be safe breathing this air and how well will I be hidden from their technology by being out of faze from them?" The table replies that he is safe for a few minutes after the explosion of the pyramid and that it cannot detect any scans that would reveal him or it.

Jay starts walking towards the pyramids then thinks about his situation, "tablet, how close can I be to the battle and be safe from the beams and debris while I am in this different faze,

and can I go back to the predetermined location directly
from any spot I choose to from here at this relative time?"
There is a hesitation from the tablet as Jay takes several more
steps toward the pyramids. The tablet tells him he is safe
anywhere there until two minutes after the pyramid brakes
and he can be sent back to the predetermined location and
time from anywhere near here until them. Jay puts the tablet
into it's pouch and starts looking at the pyramids, and at the
beings that he is getting closer to. They vary in size like
humans, from about 4.5 feet tall to almost 7 feet tall. Some are
more hairy, some are more hunched and round, some have
scales, and some have only three fingers and feet like birds.
The faces on them are different too. Jay notices that there are
some small animals sitting in the shade that seem to look at
him as he passes them. Then he sees the streaks in the sky and
the dots that appear where the streaks stop. He notices that he
is not the only one to notice them. Soon many of the beings
have hurried off in various directions and the others are
looking up and pointing and talking to each other about what
ever they are seeing. Jay keeps walking and some vehicles
come to pick up most of the beings in the area. Then as it starts
to get dark some of the smaller pyramids lift off and disappear
either into space or move across out of view over the horizon.
Jay keeps walking and looking at things. "Tablet, I haven't
seen any technology other than the vehicles so far, where is the
technology of these beings?" The tablet replies that it is only
detectable in the pyramids and in the vehicles that have
returned to the pyramids. It replies that all of the pyramids
have initiated some kind of a cloak and shield that it cannot
scan through.

Jay looks up at the sky, " tablet, what can you determine of the
ships in orbit above this moon?" after a few seconds the tablet
replies to Jay that they have good shield technology and they

are very large ships. It tells him that is all it can tell from it's ability to scan them. Jay thinks 'I am not getting much information here, maybe I can go inside a pyramid.' Jay starts to walk toward the closest one, and looks to the side at the one that will be cut in half soon then asks his tablet if he can get inside one of the pyramids. He walks almost up to it before he gets his reply.

The tablet says "the only way to get inside of the pyramid is to enter it before the first threat arrives from the ships in orbit. It is two days ago in this time."

Jay stands looking at the pyramid a few hundred feet in front of him, brightly painted with murals of various aliens doing various things. "Tablet can we travel back a few days to enter the pyramid ship, move me into the ship still out of faze, and then move forward in time to now once inside the ship? Once in there will I still be able to make the transfer back to our own time in our own ship after the explosion and destruction of the other pyramid and the bright flashes in the sky after that?" After a few seconds Jay gets his positive answer and asks the tablet to set it all up and put him into the ship, and move him to the time a minute before the orbiting ships show up on their sensors. The tablet indicates that it is ready and Jay thinks the command.

It and Jay fades to the inside of the pyramid; Jay is in a large room with many tables and beings jollily eating and conversing. He sees that they are the same mix that he saw outside. He looks around and sees some serious looking ones near a door to a large structure in the middle of the pyramid. He walks past them and into one of the rooms inside. There are four beings sitting around a table on one side of the room and seven beings siting in front of control panels with displays and instruments in front of each of them. Jay walks and looks at the displays and looks at the instruments, "Tablet, learn what you can from this technology about the ship, the weapons and then about the cultures that developed and control it." Jay turns his attention to the four conversing at the table. He looks at them as they're looking at a display of stars and planets on the table between them. One with what seems to be a high level of concern is pointing at several stars and making sounds that to Jay indicate a high emotional charge in his message. The others look concerned but skeptical to Jay. The one of them waves his arms and points at some other stars and sounds less concerned. Jay asks, "Tablet, this star chart on the display that these four beings are sitting around, record these stars and planets as shown, and the conversation of these beings about them." Jay looks down as he feels the tablet shift it's position in his pocket slightly. Then he hears the sound of yelling from the next room and runs over to see three beings seated in front of consoles with a large wall screen showing the ships arriving around the planet. He watches as some yelling takes place and the ones on consoles start working on their consoles very quickly. The others either rush to use other consoles or move to watch the ones being worked on. A few other beings come from a door in the back and yell out some short phrases. Then Jay hears the hum of energy starting to build up after a few seconds he can feel the vibration of it at the same amplitude as the sound of it. His tablet says" one minute until the other pyramid is broken, and three minutes before you will be damaged if you are still here." Jay turns to the big screen and watches as the view shows the other ships arriving from three directions into the orbit of the moon and then the building of a glow around each one of them. He watches as the beings in the room work diligently on their consoles and talk back and forth between them selves. Jay sees lines extend on the screen from the ships in orbit, and notices a silence in the room. The first beam comes down from the ships and Jay thinks it must be hitting them as he sees and feels the ship shaking from something. Jay says to his tablet, "Tablet, give me a ten second warning that it is time to leave before there is danger to me." He watches on another screen as some beams go from the planet to some of the ships in orbit and the glow around them is decreased, then more beams, and more beams, and more yelling and more sound from outside the room, Jay looks out of the room into the large area in the pyramid and sees many beings scrambling to make room for others. He looks back at the ones working on the consoles and sees the worried expressions on their faces, and more yelling, he looks at the ones that came in from the other room looking at each other in silence. Then the room shakes and they all look at the big screen to see the image of the pyramid beside them broken and half of it pushed down into the ground a bit. Jay looks back at the three that were looking at each other, they all take a small device out of their clothes and say something into it and then look at each other. The others in the room with worried looks look up at them and say nothing at all. Then Jay hears it and looks at the big screen. He sees beams instantly reaching all of the ships around the moon all at once and then he sees them all light up and disappear off the screens. Then the display adjusts its' brightness several times and the room is so quiet that Jay can hear his own breathing. One of the three says something and the large screen shows a view of outside. The brightness is getting brighter and then the smoke of a few things then all flames for several seconds. Then darkness. Jay listens and not one being says anything. His tablet does. "ten seconds,,,,,nine,,,,,,,eight,,,,,,seven,,,,". Jay puts his hand in grabbing the tablet and thinks the command, and fades back into the ship to see himself fading away from the other side of the room.

Jay stands there for a second thinking about what he just saw. "Tablet, security, Jay's own file. For all data for the past event." Then he puts the tablet back where it was and sits in the wide chair waiting for Lex. He takes a breath and looks out into the next room and watches in that direction as he thinks about it more. He sees her coming.

Lex sees Jay sitting in the drivers seat and thinks he must be waiting for her so they can go. "Jay, I am concerned, you seem too willing to do this, is there something that you want to tell me about the sexual preferences of Kyranin males?"

Jay looks at her, "what," he thinks about her words and what they were doing, "oh, no my love, I was thinking about work." he looks at her. "I am glad that I am not working now, I think maybe I work too much. After our bonding time I will work less." He watches as she sits beside him and realizes how lucky he is to be in love, and to be loved back and to not be in fear for his life and the lives of his family. "You look great Lex. I want to have a shower too before we get to the, the place, where are we going?"

Lex looks at him. "Jay we don't have to do this now. I thought we were going to. I thought that is what you meant."

Jay kisses her face as he sees she looks a little worried. "I just don't know what this space station is called, I am happy to go there now." furrowing his brows, how will we get there without them finding out about your personal ships?"

Lex smiles "we will dock in a Gyrekian cargo transporter near the station and take a shuttle. We always have a few cargo transports near such stations for storage of equipment and trade cargo. If you hurry you can shower and get dressed before we arrive at the cargo vessel."

"So it is close?"

"hahaha, Jay, it is not that close, hurry, the shower is on the middle floor at the far end of this craft." I will have your tea ready when you get back." She kisses his cheek and smiles as he gets up. She asks the ship to show the control console and puts her fingers into the lights again. Then she looks at the screen and sees the face of another Gyrekian female. It looks back at her. Lex smiles and says "Lekxzatrera and bonded mate Jay, Kyranin male, requesting permission to arrive on inner dock."

The female looks at her for a second then looks down on her console and then up at her then down again. She reads the information there and looks up and smiles. "Congratulations, I would not be so brave as to mate inter race, how is it so far?"

"It is much better than I expected" a growing smile takes control of Lexs' face, I was scared when I first felt the bonding urge, but I couldn't stop it. It was real," slowly turning her head side to side, "I tried to stop it several times but it just felt stronger. It is better than I ever imagined."

With a perplexed face the other female asks "did you get any trouble from others?"

"Actually, one server tried to embarrass him into deportation for not having currency for a meal but he did have it." Lex smiles a proud smile, "It was after we bonded but before I recorded it so I have no right to complain, the server had the right to ask. Even though he was my mate already he could have been expelled from our moon permanently. So to prevent further problems I am going to disguise myself as a Kyranin while at the station."

Nodding at Lex in the view screen she says "a good idea, there have been some harsh statements made here about inter species relations." I will enter you arrival to the station as Jay – kyranin male and female friend. The security here is private and only surveyed by our teams, and over looked by the ryberian high council if there are any difficulties. The records will show the truth but no announcements will be made at the station about you being a Gyrekian bonded couple of mixed race." she smiles. " Have fun there, it is an exciting place compared to the moon."

"I haven't been since I was a cadet, more than a few years ago now" Lex smiles at her, " thank you, I see the codes and coordinates now. Any advice in appearing to be Kyranin?"

She laughs. "Drink lots and don't have a really good conversation."

Lex laughs and moves her fingers in the lights and says some commands to the ship and then gets up to make tea for Jay and her self. She puts his tea on a ledge by the entrance to the room and sits back down at the controls. Lex watches the big image and looks to see that the details on a side screen are correct as well and asks the ship if everything is on track for arrival. After a few seconds it gives her a detailed update of the docking codes and trajectory and temporal shift data and arrival time. Then a few seconds later it gives her the details of the shuttle that they will have access to, the coordinates to go to and from the station and the rooms to choose from for their time at the station. She chooses a typical Kyranin style room without a tea dispenser to help with her disguise. As Jay enters she confirms all the arrangements and asks him if she looks Kyranin enough.

Jay walks around to in front of her and looks her over pretty good. "Mmm, yeah, you look good enough to attract any Kyranin male."

"No Jay do I look Kyranin enough that they will believe I am Kyranin?" she looks at his smile and points to his tea. "Your tea is there."

Jay looks at her a little more. I think you should do some make up, some face color like they do on Ramga, tint your eyes and chin like they do there. The chin to match your clothes, I think that is the idea, and a bit of color around your eyes, not to be notice unless someone looks closely." Then he looks a little more and walks over to get his tea.

"I have a room for us on the station Jay. We will arrive under your name and will not be mentioned to be from the moon." I want to see the room first, so I feel comfortable when we get there with our juice. I want to know you are ok with this Jay." she looks at him as she stands to face him, "I am nervous".

Jay sips his tea and turns to her. He steps towards her and takes another sip then walks to her, has another sip and sits the tea down on the seat and puts his arms around her. "It is ok Lex."

"I do want to do it Jay. I am scared, and I want to do it. Is it odd that I want to do it even though I am scared?"

Jay thinks about it comparing it with many of the things he was scared to do and forced himself to do anyway. Then he thinks about Reggie asking him if he wanted to travel in time and space. "hahahah, no Lex, hahaha, it is normal to have doubts and fears and still want to do something that just does not seem possible because we have learned that it is not possible. It is normal to have fear in such a situation. If you want to do it I want you to do it. No matter what happens I will be glad we tried it. I will be with you all the way and I will never let you think it was a bad idea. I want it as much as you do." Jay feels a pull from the side like the ship they are in started moving. "Did you feel that?"

"Yes" Lex says, "it was the inertia of the cargo vessel. We are docked in it now. I will go do the face color like you say in the transport to the station." starting to walk she says, "common Jay lets go."

They go down and out of the vessel and Jay looks back to see the doorway reappear as a wall behind them after they step though it. They walk a short distance through a few doorways then into a hanger with several small spacecraft in it. One has a door open on the back and she leads him into it. They make there way to the front and strap themselves into it. She looks over the console and the screens and asks for permission to power up. The answer comes over a speaker and she flicks some switches on the console. Jay hears some sounds like the humming of a high speed electric motor and then hears the closing of the doors from the back of the craft to their control rooms door. Jay looks back and can see through the windows in the interior doors that the large exterior door is closed as well. Jay looks at all of the switches and knobs on the control panel. "It is not the same as the other ship."

Lex looks at him and starts to laugh, "no Jay it is different, a lot different, but don't worry it is just as safe. Not as fast and it has no shields or weapons. You better put your head back on the headrest or your neck could get a strain when we go out the door.

Jay looks around then at the screen in front of Lex that shows a set of lines like a target with the image of a door behind it. "Is it going to open first?"

Lex laughs again. "Jay when that door opens we will be sucked into space and the engines will start to push us toward the station at the same time." She looks at him. "You don't know much about this do you?"

Jay looks at her, "no, mostly only a passenger" turning his head side to side slightly, "not a pilot".

Lex flicks a few more switches and says "Lekxzatrera to control, Jay and Lex ready to depart".

Jay watches the screen as the door on the image opens then he feels himself sinking back into the padding on the seat and the screen change to show a light dot with a circle around it and the target on the screen pointing toward it. The shape of the target and the lines from it start to change as the dot with the circle moves to the middle of the target and starts to get bigger. Then the dot in the middle starts to take the shape of a wheel with a hub in the middle then more shape. Jay hears the speaker. "Welcome Jay, Kyranin male and guest. You may turn off your drive engines any time. We will guide you into bay six. You accommodations are ready, and we are happy to have you with us for your visit. Your ship will be refueled and ready for you any time you want it."

Lex looks at Jay and gives him the nod to say something.

"Thank you, we may only be here for a short visit." Jay looks at Lex wondering if he has to say more. She seems to be happy with the situation so he smiles, "your face color?"

"Oh" Lex says and opens a door on the console pulling out a bag that looks like a purse to Jay. She opens it and finds some make up like containers inside. As she opens them Jay looks and it is like make up, just like make up on earth he thinks to himself and watches as Lex used the tools in there to spread some color on her skin, just slightly tinting it toward the shade of her top and then changing tools putting some clear fluid around her eyes. She leans toward Jay, " Jay, can you see it enough around my eyes. Jay leans towards her, looks at her eyelids, lashes and then her chin. "So what part of Ramga are you from?"

Lex smiles at Jay, "guess"

Jay laughs and says "Ok, when we get there we will check out the room, then the bars and restaurants, and stores until we find a male that we both like. Then when we choose we bluntly ask him to help us. Unless he has a really good reason like an incurable disease that we could catch he will say yes. Then we go directly and have sex with him until the fluids change to the correct color. Ok. I don't know if we can make that happen."

Lex looks at Jay, "what about if we don't tell him I am trying to get pregnant?"

Jay looks at her, "then he might want to continue relations with one or both of us afterwards. It may become a problem."

Lex looks at Jay, "can we get your tablet to project the color or can I use some make up and put it on me so it looks close enough?"

"I think we can" Jay says as he feels the ship being pulled sideways. "Is that normal?"

Lex checks her view screen "yeah, it is their energy fields taking control of our craft for docking. We will be inside in a minute." She looks at Jay, ask your tablet to see what will work best.

Jay takes out the tablet and looks at it. He asks, "Tablet, we are going to invite a Kyranin juice to help us get pregnant as if Lekxzatrera is a Kyranin female. We want the Kyranin juice to believe we are successful in achieving a kyranin style impregnation with the three of us. Can we produce a change to the color of the combined fluids after our sexual activity to indicate that she is fertilized and pregnant from our activities?" the table replies that from the substances that is used to color her skin this can be achieved. It suggests adding the correct color and smearing it with the mixed fluids and showing the resulted color should satisfy him. In Kyranin tradition the success of breading is not ever questioned by the juice. So as long as you give any reasonable indication of success he should accept his part is complete."

Jay remembers the greenish tint that the fluid turned when it worked and he says "green, and slightly bluish green"

Lex looks in the face colors and nods, she plucks out the soft block of color from the holder and puts it into her pocket. They feel the vessel clunking down onto the dock floor and hears, "you are docked. You may disembark as you choose." Lex looks at Jay and undoes her safety straps "should we go?" Then bites her lip signaling her excitement and apprehension.

Jay smiles and puts his hand on her leg. "Yes my Kyranin mate, lets go get pregnant."

Making their way to the room they agree on a signal to give each other when they want to talk to and scan one to see if he is a juice – a nod toward him with a wink, and confirmed with a wink back and a nod at him from the other. A turning of the head if it is the wrong one or if the other doesn't like him, crossing of arms if the scan shows him to be a healthy juice. A thumb up at each stage of conversation with him to determine the interest is still continuing. Three thumbs up from both and then they ask. As they get to the room they look at each other nod and wink, cross their arms and put their thumbs up three times. They laugh, hug and open the door to the room.

Lex looks around, goes to the kitchen, the shower area, the bed, the table and chairs, and sits in a chair. "Wow, I can't believe I am so excited Jay, I,,, I am so glad you are sportive of this. I can't tell you how right you are about me needing it to happen. The more I think about it the freer I feel. The closer I feel to you and the more certain that I will be happy in the future." she takes a deep breath and looks at him. I don't know if I would be as willing if it were the other way around"

Jay looks at her, "If I was from the moon and you had lived my life and were the Kyranin male you would be willing. You would be me and I would be you. But I am me and you are you." He takes a deep breath. "I am ready" he starts thinking about all of the Kyranin males that he has talked to. He liked them all actually. He hadn't thought much about having sex with them but he did like them. Then reminded him self that it isn't about him having sex with a male but about his mate living her fantasy so that she could feel complete and be happy. Then he thinks about how it was when he was the seed, for the other couple and how it was with them. It was a team effort and it was not competitive but a group effort to succeed. Jay decides to remember this concept as he follows through with his efforts. Jay walks to the door and opens it looking at Lex. She looks back at him and gets up, walks into the doorway and gives him a very passionate kiss.

They walk together through the halls not saying much. They enter an area with shops and cafe's. They look at the aliens there and don't see many Kyranins. They go into a bar and see a table of Kyranin females, but only one male, sitting with some Korobs. They both look him over and look at each other turning their heads side to side. Next they find a gym. They sit at the juice bar and watch the patrons coming in and leaving for longer than it took to each drink two beverages of some things they had never tried before. Next, to another bar, then more shops, and finally Jay says, "lets go get something to eat, I'm hungry."

Lex looks across the hall and down seeing a sign in Amburst. "Do you like sea food?"

Jay looks at her, "Yeah."

She nods her head, Jay looks and smiles at her then they start walking holding hands.

As they enter the place the Amburst sever waves them to a table near the kitchen and brings them each some tea. "I am sorry but we haven't been able to get any decent Murruk here for several weeks". Jay starts to laugh and the server looks at him. "What" the server replies to his laugh.

"Sorry, I spent a weekend under the sea once with friends and the way you say mrruk reminded me of a joke I was told while I was there." Could you surprise us with whatever your scans show is safe for us to eat. Can I pay from my account on Kuroggez for our meals and drinks, and the drinks of anyone who we ask to join us?"

The server looks at them and smiles as Jay hands him his tablet. He taps Jay's tablet onto his own and looks at he screen, "It looks like your account is good, I will be sure everything you are served is safe for both of you and for any guests you acquire." he looks at both of them and then hesitates and asks, "are you expecting guests"

Lex smiles at the server, "we are hoping to meet someone here, It is not certain."

The server smiles at her and bows as he steps backward, "the quality of our food is" and he turns and goes into the kitchen.

Lex looks at Jay and whispers, "what was the Joke?"

"They Hate Mrruk", Jay looks behind him to be sure that the Amburst can't hear him, "to them it is the worst flavor in the galaxy, if a cup of mrruk won every award for flavor ever given for any food or drink they would still rather spit it out than swallow it. Hahaha"

Lex looks at Jay, "so it was his joke about not wanting to serve mrruk that you found funny?"

"And that he makes it to us as an apology" Jay looks behind himself again then smiles at her and nods. His eyes are adjusting to the light and he looks around the room. He notices that there are two kyranin males sitting at tables alone. They both look relatively fit and healthy. Jay looks at the one closest to them and determines that he looks well groomed and intelligent, and looks at Lex to give the nod and wink. She looks back at him with furrowed brows and nods at his table. Jay looks again to see two amburst women sit down with him.

He looks back at lex as she looks back from the other one sitting on his other side in the corner. He sees her looking at him for a second then nodding toward this one in the corner and giving him the wink. Jay smiles at Lex and looks into the corner at he guy. He can't see all of his face but he looks ok, not too young, clean cut, well dressed, health. Jay looks back at Lex and gives the nod and wink. They both smile as Jay brings out the tablet again. He works it with his fingers and gets it to scan the guy. It comes back that he is a juice, that he is healthy, and that he is alone here on the station. Jay slides the tablet with the screen showing the results to Lex as he feels his heart beating harder. He sees her getting nervous as she reads it and looks up at him. With worry and excitement in her eyes she slowly nods at Jay. Jay takes a deep breath and gets up. He walks over to the other table and stands beside the Kyranin.

"Hello, My name is Jay. My mate and I are having dinner over there and noticed you are alone, would you like to join us for dinner?"

The guy looks up at Jay, he looks across the room at Lex, and then at Jay, "Ok". He stands facing directly at Jay "My name is Drowin, I am on my way back to Ramga after being away for several years. My business venture was not as I expected so I am having to return home empty handed."

Jay smiles at him and puts his hands on the Kyranins' shoulders and says to him, "Life is long and there is always another opportunity. Ramga is your home and you will always have a good life there." Then turning and gesturing toward

Lex at their table "come sit with us I would love to hear about your adventure."

Jay takes a chair from a nearby empty table and places it for Drowin. Lex this is Drowin, a business man on his way back to Ramga after several years away."

Lex stands and takes one of his hands with both of hers. "It is good to meet you. I have been on the Gyrekian moon for a very long time and can't give you any news from Ramga."

Drowin smiles at her. "Thank you for inviting me to share a meal. It is good to see a Kyranin woman with her mate. On the worlds I have been working there are few Kyranins and they are mostly single. It was fun but I will be glad to get home. I miss our culture and our food. I haven't had a good Amburst meal in years."

Jay sits, "I have a feeling the food tonight will be good, the server seems very Amburst in his ways."

Lex and Drowin both sit at once as the server arrives with two plates. He hovers over the table, putting them down he looks at Jay and Lex and turns back to the kitchen. Jay looks at the kreptigs on one plate and the pastries on the other. The pastries are nothing he had ever seen before so he takes one of them first. Lex takes a pastry and nods at Jay as she chews it.

Drowin picks up a kreptig and looks it over, then pops it in his mouth and chews. "mmm" he takes another. Closing his eyes as he chews it. Then smiles at Jay, "what are those?"

Jay looks at him, "I have never had one before. I don't know what they are called."

Lex says "they are good." and she takes one of the kreptigs popping it in her mouth like Drowin did.

Jay picks up one of the kreptigs and holds it up in the air and says, (as Lex's eyes are getting big) "we all love these kreptigs, thank god that we can find them everywhere!" He watches as Lex looks at him like she wants to scream.

Drowin looks at Jay "Not where I was". He chews the rest of his pastry "We didn't get any Kyranin food there unless we had it shipped directly to us."

Lex waves at the server and hand signals for a beverage.

Jay looks over at the server looking back at them then pulling out his scanner and going back into the kitchen. Jay takes another kreptig and asks, "Where were you?"

"About six months travel out of the alliance toward the outer edge of the galaxy. There are some planets there with climates similar to Ramga's but not much life on them. I was going to build some agricultural industries."

"How did it go?" Jay asks

"Well", Drowin says, "I had it built and the crops grew, but getting them to market was difficult. I could arrange the space in ships but the trade laws required some paper work that could never get completed before the ship had to leave. Over three years I lost 2/3 of my harvests due to administrative hold ups. There was no administrative avenue to rearrange the rules or to get the administrations to preapprove anything. I tried everything."

The server puts two beverages on the table for each of them and asks "is there anything that you want to order?"

Drowin says, "I'll have a grandillia-sours please." And smiles up at the amburst.

Jay says "me two"

Lex asks, "do you have tea, any tea, maybe some of that tea that the gyrekians like."

Jay looks at the server, "and one of those for me too"

Drowin says "I haven't had a sour for four years, I can still feel the taste in my mouth sometimes. I have wanted one for a long time, it reminds me of my educational days with the amburst. We played sports in all our spare time, it was a lot of fun."

"How long ago were your educational years?" Lex asks and puts down the empty water glass.

"It was before my farming work on Ramga, I ran farms for fifty years before I left to do this business. I was good at it, I liked it."

Jay looks at him "are the farms you built on that planet still functional, do you still control them?"

"Yes but I can't make them earn enough to stay there." Drowin looks at Jay "why?"

"Well", Jay says "not all species are direct and honest like us, some build their culture on corruptions. Did you offer them bribes to get you product's to clear their regulations faster?"

Drowin looks at Jay "Are you serious? I could loose my honor and license on Ramga for bribing an official for something like that."

Lex looks at him. "That is true, I have looked at the laws and regulations of several worlds. It is not tolerated in the alliance." but you were not actually in an alliance world were you?"

Drowin looks at her then at Jay then drinks his water and has another kreptig. He looks at both of them again. "They did often look at me like they were expecting me to say something and they did always look sad when the ship actual left without taking my products. Could it be that simple?"

Jay starts to laugh loudly. "This is why we are loved by so many of our alliance partners and hated by others. We don't ever think of corruption. The corrupt are all around us and we never suspect because we would never consider doing it."

Our laws are not enforceable against us out side of the alliance so if you did offer them bribes there it wouldn't be against the law. But I would bet anything, they would be happy to get your things wherever you want them to go for a small bribe."

The server comes back with the sours and the teas. He dumps the rest of the pastries onto the kreptigs' plate and says "your meals will be here in a minute," then turns and walk back toward the kitchen.

Drowin looks at Lex, "what is he bringing?"

"I don't know" Lex says, "Jay talked to him, I don't think he said what it will be."

Jay smiles "he didn't say". Jay looks at Lex and waits for a sign. He watches as Lex looks at Drowin and then takes another pastry, dips into her tea and bites it. He watches her chewing slowly as she looks back at him. Jay smiles, "Well I hope the meal is good", he raises his glass of grandillia-sours and nods at her then him and takes a drink of it. "Oho, that is a strong one."

Drowin takes a sip of his and nods and drinks it all down. "howf, yeah it is. He turns toward the kitchen and holds up the empty glass."

The server comes out with three plates and puts Lex's down first. Then looks at Jay and Drowin and puts their plates down too. "I am glad that you liked the sour, I'll get you another, and he looks at Lex would you like one as well?"

Lex looks at Jay and her eyes ask him for an answer. She sees him not too excited about her having the sour. The server looks at Jay, and nods, smiles and I will bring some wine, and other sour for each of you, and anything else?"

Jay looks at the server with a bit of hesitation in his expression and gets a smile and a nod from the Amburst. Jay asks Drowin "what do you think of the new security measures the alliance is embarking on?"

He looks at Jay then takes a bite of his food and nods chews swallows "if it is needed I hope it works."

Lex asks "Do you have family back on Ramga?"

"I have a brother and my parents and grand parents all living on our farms. I have a sister who was working in an amburst city under the sea when I left. I think she is still there" and has another bite.

The drinks come and they continue with the meal, Lex only has a few sips of her wine. Jay notices that his second sour is much weaker than the first and that the wine is good but he can't drink it as fast as Drowin.

Jay looks at the food on his plate and thinks it looks like curry and wild rice. He smells it and it has a subtle sent that he likes but has never smelt before. He looks up at the amburst "What is it?"

The server looks at Jay, then at the others, and changes his posture putting his hands together and smiling slowly at them until all three are watching his face. "It is a family recipe that my grand mother taught me when I was a child. She told me that only our family ever made this dish and that she had learned it from her grand mother. The seeds are soaked in the oil from a special kind of life form that only grows in caves deep under the sea. Then they are warmed but not cooked in wine made from the fruit of the long weeds that grow near the rocks at the edge of the sea. The fish is a common fish that is usually eaten alive by us under the sea but it is slow cooked in the ink from the shelled crebudet creatures. They are friendly, shelled things with many boneless legs. They don't taste good but their ink is delicious if cooked correctly. I have to get all of the ingredients shipped live from the sea and it came in today. So you are lucky. I hope you like it!" and he turns around and walks to another table.

Jay looks at Lex then at his plate, smiles and looks up at Drowin who is looking back at him. He nods, looks at Lex again "well, let's eat it". Jay takes up a forkful of the chunks of the fish, bits it and chews, the flavor changes as he chews it. First it is mildly sweet and smooth, but as he chews it more and it mixes with his saliva a tinge of bitter and the aroma of the sea comes out. He looks at Lex and sees her expression of surprise too. His next bite is mostly the stuff that looks like wild rice to him (the seeds). The sauce on them is thick and transparent. It has a slightly salty spicy flavor to Jay. As he chews it he feels a strange warmth growing in his mouth then a savory flavor peeks through when the seeds are all mashed by his teeth. He chews some more and the warmth continues to grow sensitizing his mouth. He uses his tongue to get every last bit of it swallowed and looks at Drowin and Lex focusing on their own experiences with the flavor. "Wow, this is good." Jay takes another forkful of both seeds and fish this time. The flavors start and mix but he can't discern them as well. The next bite is just seeds and the clear sauce, a drink of sour to clear his pallet and then the fish again; a sip of wine, and then the seeds, wine, fish, sour, and the mix. Jay slowly chewing looking at his Lex, he feels his heart pulling to her as he watches her chewing and looking back at him. He sees her nod at Drowin and wink at him. Jay looks at Drowin and winks at Lex then remembers why they invited him to sit with them for and smiles and nods. "Drowin," he takes a sip of wine, "we are wondering if you would help us with something after dinner?"

Drowin continues chewing and nods, swallows, looks at Jay in the eyes "what?"

"We are going to have a family and we would like you to be our Juice."

Drowin looks at Jay for a second then at Lex and has a big drink of his sour. "I would be glad to"

Lex looks at Jay then at Drowin and realizes that she will soon be naked with a male she has no feelings for, that she will have him ejaculating into her and then the male that she totally loves will be there watching and then he will be with her too.

Jay sees the fear on her face as she starts looking at Drowin, and he sees Drowin starting to turn his head towards her, "Drowin, we haven't been on Ramga for a long time, we haven't had relations with others before and we are a little nervous about it. We like you and we want to do this tonight. Are you busy just after dinner?"

Drowin looking at Jay, "No, I didn't even get a room yet" I just got here an hour ago and don't know anyone on the station."

Jay lifts his wine, smiling, "what do you think of this amburst food?"

Lex takes a big drink of wine and then another bite of the seeds.

Drowin nods his head, "it is really good. I think it is intoxicating though." he drinks the rest of his sour, the last few drops, and then puts another bite of the fish into his mouth, points down at his plate and smiles, chews and nods all at the same time. Then turns to wave at the server, seeing that he has his attention he points at his empty glass and nods. Then swallows and looks back at Jay.

"We have a room, you can come stay with us" Jay offers and looks at Lex realizing that he should have asked. He sees her smile and hopes it is ok.

Lex looks at Drowin and then at Jay. She takes a deep breath and looks at Drowin again. She looks at the features of his face closely and at his body. She looks at Jay and has another bite, then a sip of wine. She feels the excitement of what she is going to do, and she feels the fear that it could make a problem for Jay's feelings toward her. Taking another bite and pushing the plate away she finishes her wine and looks at Jay.

Jay sees the look on her face. He finishes his wine too as the server comes with the sour for Drowin. "The meal was delicious, I can honestly say it reminded me of being in the sea. I have never had anything like that before sir, Thank you for such an honor."

The server smiles at Jay. "Would you like anything else?"

Jay looks at Lex. "No, thank you, please put our friends meal and drinks on my bill too." then looking at Drowin, "Lex and I are going up to our room now, enjoy the rest of your meal and the drinks, and come along when you are done here."

Drowin looks at Lex as she starts to stand. Then back at Jay and smiles. "I will take my time, about ten, maybe fifteen minutes?"

Lex looks at Jay as She says, "that is perfect."

Jay tells him how to find the room and what symbols are on the door. He nods and takes Lex's hand as they leave and walk to the room. In the hall Jay says "I am so glad we can do this for you today, I will feel better knowing you had your fantasy. I hope you won't worry about jealous thoughts that gyrekians would have. I want you to know Lex, I have none about this, I never will. I want you to feel free to ask for anything you want and say and do anything that you want or think that you might want. Even if you are scared, if you want it tell us to do it." He listens to her silence as they walk closer to their room. "We will be gentle Lex, we will be doing it for you, not to please ourselves, of course we will enjoy it, but we want you to enjoy it too."

Lex stops in front of the door and looks in Jay's eyes. Then opens the door and goes in, closes the door behind Jay and asks "Jay, if you see him putting his, cock, inside of me and having his orgasm, will you hate me some how every time you are reminded of it?

Happy endings

Jay looks at her. He thinks about it. He walks across the room and sits on a chair and visualizes her with Drowin, and asks himself how he feels about it. He imagines watching them together and he starts to feel excited and notices that in his imagination he is holding her and she is looking at him as she is feeling her arousal building, he starts to smile, and looks at her. "Lex, it is not like that, I will be with you too. The three of us will be together he will be helping us it is our way. It can't happen for most kyranins without the third so we grow up expecting it, wanting that day to come when we will be able to do this. I want it as much or more than you, it's normal. Lets get our clothes off and get into bed so that he will feel comfortable when he arrives."

Lex walks over in front of Jay and starts to undress. Jay stands watching and starting to take off his own clothes. She finishes first then smiles watching him pulling off his shirt. She looks all up and down and smiles then puts out her hand towards his. As he put his into hers and she leads him to the bed. She climbs on and lays back in the middle. Jay climbs on top of her then slowly lowers himself onto her. He can see her excitement and fear. His cock, half hard bumps her vagina as he moves to kiss her and he notices that she is already very wet. He smiles and reaches down and slides it in. Her eyes widen and her smile glows.

"It is really going to be Ok? Are we really going to do this?" she asks.

Jay slowly glides in and out a few times as she spreads wide to give him easy entry with his half hard. "As soon as he gets here, we will. He can feel her heat on his cock, he looks down and her nipples are rigid, pointing and as big as ever. Jay feels warmth in his heart knowing how excited she is. He leans and kisses her. Her mouth meets his with passion and her legs clamp around him as she starts to moan. He feels her throbbing and does his best, as his cock is still getting harder. He feels her grasping at his back and he hears the door open, and close. Slowly thrusting as she finishes and slows down he hears garments hitting the floor and as she loosens her legs and slows her kisses to relax back onto the bed Drowin climbs on the bed beside them. He sees the surprise in Lex's face as she turns to see his smiling face only inches from hers.

"Hi, is there anything that I should know, how do you want me to be?" Drowin asks without actually touching her yet.

Lex looks up at Jay then back at Drowin, "Be gentle"

Jay roles to cuddle Lex on her other side giving Drowin room to be near her. Jay slides a hand slowly up her belly toward her breasts as he says, "start with some caressing and do what feels like she is comfortable with. She is a little nervous we didn't grow up on Ramga so it is not as normal in our minds as for most of us, start slow and follow her lead."

Drowin does the same as Jay, caressing Lex's belly and kissing her face and shoulder. Then fondling her breast.

Lex's heart is pounding, she wants to touch Drowin's cock but doesn't want Jay to think she does. She thinks about Jay's words each time they talked about it but has doubts that he can actually be OK with it. She feels Jay's hand sliding down her belly as Drowin is softly stroking her breast. As she breathes feeling his pressure increases, as she inhales and his fingers swiveling her nipple as she exhales. Jays' hand is moving over her pubic bone and Drowin's is sliding to her other breast. Jay lifts himself to lick her breast closest to Drowin. Drowin's hand on her other breast cupping it with delicate pressure and movement. Turning to look at him, she sees his lips are moving toward hers, they stop only millimeters from her lips. She feels Jay's lips pulling her nipple and then his fingers on and around her clit. Drowin's lips still millimeters from hers. Drowin's leg crossing hers' as Jay's fingers are moving in her folds, such a feeling. Drowin's hand softly squeezing her breast, then sliding down, his fingers pressing on and around her genitals like keys on a piano and his lips still waiting. Jays tongue on her nipple, pushing it side to side slowly and her clit, under his finger, she inhales, feeling the pressure on her breasts and smelling Drowin's breath, so sweet. Her lips open as she looks at Jay's eye watching her with her nipple in his lips and his tongue sliding across the end of it softly, She sees him smile, as she exhales her lips touch Drowin's. Jay's finger slides smoothly into her vagina, her reaction presses her lip slightly onto Drowin's. She feels his kiss, looking in Jay's eye and seeing his smile her arousal starts to build and she starts kissing Drowin. Worried that Jay won't like it she slides her hand to Jay's cock and softly grips it. The feel of his cock distracts her from the stimulation of her vagina as Jay's finger slides about in side. The kissing with Drowin starts to feel real and she looks into his eyes. Seeing him as a male, a real living male that is holding her breast again and looking into her eye with kindness and caring. Her kiss, tastes him, feels him. His hand on her breast responding to the kiss; and her gripping Jay's cock and feeling his lips pulling her nipple, just the way she likes it; and his finger found the spot inside. The warm pressure building as her other hand slides down, his belly, touching his cock her tongue on his lips and feeling Jay's cock in one hand and gripping Drowin's with her other. Drown's hand leaving her breast and sliding down onto her belly, over her naval as Jay's kisses across her chest to the other breast as the warmth starts to glow and Drowin's kisses retreat. Lex looks down at Jay starting to lick her other nipple and Drowin kissing his way onto her breast that Jay just left. Putting her head back down and trying to relax as she holds their hard cocks in her hands and Jays hand is so sweetly working inside her, and now Drowin's fingers are in her folds, she tries to relax as the pulsing starts her heart is pounding and she squirms from the hot orgasm filling her body with bliss. Drown and Jay both feel her quaking and stop moving their hands in her genitals and mouths on her breasts, snuggling against her sides, and softly kissing her face, each from his side.

Lex takes a few breaths and a few more, enjoying the kisses on her face and the hard cocks in her hands. Realizing that Jay is OK with this and wanting to live her fantasy "Guys, I want to do something now"

"Anything you want Lex" Jay says between soft kisses.

Lex thinks for a few seconds, "Ok" siting up and looking at Drown's leg over hers and their cocks in her hands. She wants them both, but how, which one where, "um, first, I, I will suck on you Jay and Drowin can you slowly put it in from behind?" She looks at Jay's eyes for approval.

Jay sees the worry in her look, "sounds good, I'll slide this way to make more room for Drowin over there". Jay slides close to the side of the bed thinking that Lex will go down on him with her but up and Drowin behind her on the bed.

Lex lets go of their cocks and gets off the bed. She walks around the room and looks at them both there naked with rock hard dicks and their eyes fixed on her. She smiles, "ok" she walks over to beside the bed where Jay is and bends down putting one hand on Jay's Belly and one on his thigh. "Drown can you make it from behind me?" watching him walking around behind her she steps so that her feet are about shoulder width apart and slowly lowers her mouth to Jay's dick. Moving her hand from his thigh to his testicles and gripping them softly as she feels Drowin stepping against her from behind and changing his stance to get his cock between her legs. She looks at Jay and feels a tear coming to her eye. She can feel Drowin's cock on one thigh then the other as he shifts his hips and slides his hands on her butt and thighs and back. She looks over at Jay and sees him Smile and wink at her. Drowin still isn't trying to put it in, but she can feel it slipping around and she does feel like she wants it. Her heart pounding and her cunt aroused she puts Jay's cock in her mouth, holding his balls in her hand, with her other hand taking a little of her weight. She starts working her tongue on his cock in her mouth. Sucking and looking at him smiling at her, and still not sure if she can let Drowin do it. Slowly sucking on Jay's cock, long strokes with her mouth as she feels Drowin's cock pressing up on her belly then sliding over her folds and his hands massaging her ass and back and thighs. Jay's Cock all the way in to her throat, and then her lips around his head and his balls between her fingers, she can feel his hard abdomen muscles with her other hand as it takes the weight. Drowin's hands on her knees and his teeth on her ass, Jay's cock in her throat. His nose in her ass, and sucking on her cheeks, Jay's balls in her hand as Drowin's tongue slides across her anus. Her knees lock, she sucks harder and his tongue strokes it again, the sensation of it sending a tingle through her mind. Slurping on Jay's rigid cock as she feels Drowin's tongue plunge slightly into her vagina, and up to her anus and over it and up over her sacrum, and the teeth sliding down her buttocks and under to her hot vagina again with that tongue. Jay's cock in the back of her throat, and her suckling on it as his tongue tries to slid into her anus, clenching and wanting to let it in too. Lex feels her heart pounding hard. She feels her cunt getting hot, she wants to feel a cock in it. Jay's cock feels good in her mouth and she massages his balls as she slides her mouth over it lets it out, "fuck me". Hearing her own words surprises her. She looks at Jay smiling nodding at her as she feels the worry on her face and then the cock pushing into her dripping wet slippery vagina. It goes so far in, smoothly, in one slow thrust. Feeling Jay's balls in her hand and his hard belly in the other, his cock starting to pulse in her mouth, and the cock sliding around in her vagina, the hands on her hips and the penetration at this angle. The pressure up inside her as her cunt feels hot and tingly, and Jay's cock is so hard and his balls feel so good in her hand. Jay's belly holding her up feels good in her other hand as her orgasm starts again. Lex – trying to suck Jay to come the same time as her and feeling the throbbing of her orgasm more than the thrusting of Drowin and hearing Jay moan and gripping his belly as her orgasm shoots through her. Loosening her mouth to breath past it and realizing that her grip on Jay's balls might be too tight, and feeling Drowin's grip on her hips. But he stopped thrusting, and She is breathing hard. "Let me lay down"

Drowin lets go of her and withdraws his rock hard cock slowly, it strokes up over her anus as it exits surprising Lex at the sensation of it as she is still super sensitive from her climax. Climbing across Jay and onto the bed and cuddling up to him. Looking into his eyes and kissing his face and lips, then holding her breast, "my nipples are sensitive like never before."

Drowin climbs on the bed behind Lex and cuddles them both. "I think it was the food" he says. "I have a body awareness that is more intense than usual."

Jay adds, "interestingly not for pain, I could feel your fingers on my balls tightly but it didn't actually hurt"

Lex looks at Jay, hesitates as she remembers, "sorry"

Jay laughs and kisses her. "Ok what's next" Jay waits a few seconds. How about I lean on a stack of pillows and you lean back on me and Drowin slowly fucks you until he juices as I cuddle you from behind, you can kiss us both?"

Lex looks at Jay then at Drowin, "ok"

Jay moves all the pillows into a pile against the wall at the end of the bed and leans back on to it, stuffs a few of them a little and says "ok"

Lex slides back into him and pulls his arms around her. Under her breasts, feeling Jays cock on her back and pulls her knees up and apart, "no wait" She moves Jay's hands and says, "push the pillows back a little and slid down a bit" she slides to follow him then lifts herself onto him so that his cock is between her legs and under her. Jay can you hold me like this?" as she reaches behind herself putting her hands on his hips and lifting her knees again and spreading them. Her back on Jays front and the pillows starting at Jays ribs lifting their shoulders and heads. "Drowin, are you ready?" as she looks at him still pretty hard and smiling.

"I am ready, are you two ready?" as he crawls towards them.

"'I'm ready" says Jay as he slides his wrists down to the sides of Lex's hips so that his arms are at her sides and grips her thighs firmly with his hands.

Drowin gets into position, his cock at her crotch and his face by her's and Jay's, his legs between Jay's, and her legs up hugging his hips, his arms into the pillows taking the weight.

"I'm ready" Lex says.

Drowin maneuvers his hips several times so that his cock slides over and across her genitals and Jay's too then Jay moves one hand to grab Drowin's dick and guides it into his Lex's vagina. Jay's fingers feeling it slid into her and him feeling her body react to the sensation of another male moving inside of her. Jay's fingers still on her vagina he fondles and massages her folds as Drowin starts his sliding thrusting movements, Jay feels Lex's head snuggling into his and her grip on his hips increasing as Drowin's movements press her into him. Jay sees Lex turn to look for his approval a few times as he watches Drowin's face show the expressions of increasing pleasure. Jay still with his fingers stimulating Lex's clitoris start to pull his hand out, and hears Lex whisper, "no Jay, keep it there, keep doing it" and then feels her clenching her shoulders and puling her hips wider he realizes that she is trying to hold back her orgasm until Drowin has his, looking into Drowin's eye's, half closed, Jay knows he is close, and smiles and winks at Drowin, and keeps the same slow full pressured motion on Lex's clitoris. Lex lifts one leg onto Drowin's back then the other and starts making soft grunting sounds. Drowin is sweating hard and breathing harder, slowly extending his deep sliding thrusts and grinding slightly side to side as he enters each time. Lex's hands gripping Jay's sides tightly and whining as she starts to pant. Drowin groaning and his eyes squinting and he starts to make a strange grunting with his exhale and starts going faster and less controlled, and faster then almost like having a seizure, Drowin crunches and moans and breaths and moans again and relaxes limp onto them.

Lex reaches down and pulls Drowin's cock out and reaches to grab Jay's and pops it into her and starts gyrating and grunting and whining as she rides Jay as best she can from between them. Drowin lifts his weight to slide down off of her and stops so his mouth is at her vagina. Lex sits forward some so she has more control and a better angle on Jay. Looking down to see Drowin turning his head up to try and put his tongue into her groves. She slows her movements, distracted from her near orgasm by seeing him try to lick her. Lex steadies her position and movements so that he can. Jay seeing Lex feeling free to please herself feels happy and relaxes into the pleasure then notices that there are a lot of fingers playing with his balls as Lex is riding him. Jay feels the juice on his cock and the tingle in his balls from the massage and the inside of his mate bumping her contours over the shape of his hard cock. He starts to notice the heat and the throbbing from his perineum growing all though his guts. The pressure of the massage on his balls increases and the feeling of Lex holding his hips and grinding on him with the juice soaking into his skin; draws him out of his thoughts and captures him in his experience of physical sensations. His heart slows and pounds harder, his balls hurt and feel sweet, his cock feels the zing and the hot fluid shoots out of him into the juice and he feels the sensation of friction with her and hears her crying his name and throbbing with him.

Lex feeling Jay hard, deep, pressing and throbbing into her as that tongue is sliding and slapping just right on her clit. Feeling her orgasm pressing up against her heart. Throbbing up her back as she stretches it and then leans back against her bonded mate. The tongue is gone and the sticky glue like feeling in her and all over her crotch. It is tingly and warm. Like a spicy sauce in the mouth, but in there, spreading deeper. "ooohhh. Jay" Still feeling it getting warmer and deeper and stickier. Looking down to see Drowin smiling and climbing up to her. Then feeling him cuddling them both and putting his head on her shoulder and his arm on Jays shoulder, she feels his soft cock on her leg and his weight on her. Them his hand on her breast and his breath blows across her ribs and belly. She can feel Jay's heart beating beneath her and his hands on her sides still and his cock softening but still in. She waits and feels everything again, Drowin, Jay herself, and the feeling of the juice and the seed in herself, Jay's heart beat, the hand on her breast, her heart beating. She takes a deep breath. "How are you doing Jay?"

"mmmmm, I am good, how are you?" Jay replies. Sliding one hand up and onto Drowin's back, "How you doing Drowin?"

"I'm good, If you want more I'll be ready in a minute" and he takes a slow deep breath.

Lex feels the warm exhale from Drowin's nostrils across her ribs. It feels good. She feels the heat from him and his sweat sliding down her sides and she starts to feel horny as the drips of sweat tickle between her sides and Jay's arms holding her. "Jay do you want to go again?"

Jay thinks about her question. 'If she asks she probably wants to' he thinks to himself. "If we are going to do more, how, what type of position, who does what, what would you like to do this time Lex, I chose last time, you choose."

Lex hesitates. "I have never had two cocks in me at once".

Drowin says, "Just a minute ago, one in your mouth and one in your vagina."

"I mean, two down there" Lex says.

Jay kisses her on the side of the head, "ok, both in the vagina or one in the anus?"

Drowin offers, "either way is good by me"

Lex hesitates, moves her hands, one to each of them giving a soft but intentional touch "can we try both?"

Jay thinks for a minute about the positions that might work. "Well," He feels Lex's body tighten, realizing she might be worried about a judgment from him. "I and happy with both, it is the positions that could work best that I am not certain of."

"Oh, that's easy Jay," Drowin says. "One of us on the bottom with our feet off the bed on the floor, her next and the other standing and leaning on the top of the other two. The top is tricky, but not difficult."

"Ok", Jay says. "So both in the vagina first then?"

"I,,, you're both so big,, I'm worried it might not fit" Lex says.

Drowin says, "it will be ok, but if you like we can go the other way, You will have to relax a lot for one of us to get into your anus though."

"Ok" Jay says, "do you have a preference of who goes where?"

Lex hesitates, "I hadn't thought about it"

Jay says "Maybe if we use some oil or something slippery on your anus to help entry"

"Some saliva usually works" Drowin says.

Lex offers, I can go to the body function room and make sure I'm ready. Drowin rolls off and Lex gets up and walks to the other room.

Jay sits up on the bed, looks at Drowin. "Thank you for this."

"I thought about what you said at dinner about the bribes, I think I will go back and ask those guys about it. Maybe I can make it there. I liked that planet a lot."

Jay looks at him. "I hope it goes well there then". Jay looks at the door to the room Lex is in. "Do you have a preference which one of us is on top?"

Drowin looks at Jay. "Lets take turns, if she is ok with it" Then he shrugs, "and after we can try both in the vagina at the same time is she wants, are you ok with that?"

Jay thinks about it for a few seconds, "if she wants, yeah, why not" He smiles at Drowin, "if the bribe works how long will you stay on that planet?"

Drowin looks at Jay, and says softly. "If the bribe works I am going to settle down there. I have an amburst female that wants to spend her life with me. Things are different there. We can have a family and no one will say a word, not to us and not to our children. That is why we went there."

Jay smiles, "I hope it works."

"Jay, you should go on the bottom and have her face you, it will be better I think, she seems a little shy with me."

"Thanks, that is a good idea". Jay smiles at Drowin and nods. Then he looks at the bed. Drowin takes some pillows and puts them near the edge, "lay down here face up. With you legs here, then slide so your butt is at the edge of the pillow"

Jay does it and gets in the position Drowin says as Lex come back into the room.

Drowin looks at Lex and smiles. "Ok? You ready?" seeing her nod and smile he points at the bed as he says, "so you go on top of Jay with your knees beside him and align yourself up so you will be comfortable, then I'll lick your anus until it is slippery enough and I will slide it in."

"Ok" Lex says and gets on top of Jay. She gets into the position and starts kissing him. Jay starts kissing back and is liking it, as he is feeling her back with his hands, and is feeling a little intoxicated and happy to be kissing with Lex. He notices that there are some hands on his cock and balls as he is kissing her. Then he notices that Lex is kissing passionately but slightly distracted, and that his cock is getting hard from being played with too. Then he feels Lex lift and the hand help his cock find it's way into her.

Lex feels Jay's cock in her and likes it she keeps kissing him and pressing her breasts into his chest and holding his shoulders. She is trusting all that is happening at the bottom of her, the hands on her ass and the tongue that was in her pussy and now in her anus with Jays cock so hard and in her, and her knees at his sides and her anus feeling that tongue poking into it again and again, it is feeling pretty relaxed and opening pretty good. Lex feels the anticipation and the excitement and the sensation of the tongue poking and sliding in more easily as she relaxes it more. Then the cock rubbing on it, and Jay in her and kissing her and she focuses to relax and the cock slides in a few centimeters. Lex clenches, kissing Jay and feeling the pressure, the gentle good soft pressure she relaxes and the cock goes and the tongue is back, then as she feels the tongue finding itself deeper and the sensation making a hunger there for more. It is gone and that cock comes back slipping around and in further. She is clenching and relaxing, and further in it goes. "ohhhhhwwwooo" the pressure feeling sweet to her and as she relaxes a little more. It goes deeper, and deeper, and Jay's cock moving in and out feels so much more with the other one there too she is thinking. Relaxing her whole body and focusing on how the kisses with Jay and her love for him as her vagina is full of his cock and her ass has that pressure, the slow sliding of it and Jay beneath her. Staying still as Jay slowly crunches under her and that cock in her ass filling her with that hot growing pressure, against her sacrum and against her cunt and she can feel the juice pumping into her as her heat from Jay's cock starts to feel like a glow and she hears Drowin moaning and pumping slowly sliding in his own juice zinging sweet waves of throbbing delight as Jay starts to twitch and suck and slip with his kisses and her heat in her vagina with the zing in her anus and the ringing of her clit as Jay's pubic bone squashes it when he thrusts. 'He is panting', she thinks as she feels the glow spreading from both of them in her. Forgetting to breath she feels it like a convolution in her guts and the throbbing of joy between her pubic bone and sacrum, closing her eyes she can't move. Clinging to Jay and squeezing him with her knees and arms and feeling the smooth ripping glow in her ass throbbing like hot honey, then he slides out. She looks at Jay, then back at Drowin, then kisses Jay again and whispers in his ear "I love you Jay, lets go home". Focusing on Jay, still half hard inside of her, seeing his smile, she feels the ripples of joy from her heart as she notices the satisfaction of having done her fantasy filtering through her mind and body.

Jay says, "Drowin, the room is yours, we are going to go home now."

Drowin smiles at Jay looking into his one visible eye as he lay under Lex. Drowin nods and walks into the other room and starts the shower.

After another minute they get up, get dress and leave the room, walking hand in hand back to the loading bay to find their ship. Jay feels the smile on his face but his mind is empty, he feels Lex's hand in his and walking beside her without a though. Lex remembers how to find the loading bay. She is still feeling the lingering sensations in her vagina and anus. Her entire abdomen is retaining some after feeling, some sweet sensation that hasn't faded yet. She thinks about Jay, and how he was, and how Drowin was, and glances over at Jay. Feeling different in her body somehow and comfortable with herself. She sees the docking bay entrance. They stop in front of it, it opens, they, go in and walk to the shuttle. A guy comes over with a tablet and says "it has been fuelled, and tested and is cleared for travel" as he hands the tablet toward them. Jay looks at it and Lex takes it, looks it over and asks Jay if he wants to pay for the fuel now. He takes out his tablet and tells it to transfer the amount for the fuel and services. Then puts his tablet back into his pouch. The guy smiles and turns and goes.

Jay looks at the small ship, "lets get in". Inside he sits in the seat and watches Lex work the controls to bring the ship back to the Gyrekian freighter, then they go to their other ship and Jay lays down in the lounge while they start traveling back to the moon. He is soon asleep.

Lex sees Jay sleeping and makes herself a pot of tea, she sits across the room and sips it and watches Jay sleep. As the tea finishes the ship tells her she is approaching the moon. She tells it to coordinate a landing back in the bay that they took it from and makes a tea for Jay. Lex sits with him, jiggling him, "Jay, Jay, I have a tea for you"

He opens his eyes and looks at her. Jay remembers he is on a ship, he remembers what they did at the station. He sits up and takes the tea, "Thank you Lex. How are you doing?" He looks at her looking back at him with a blank look. He leans over and kisses her, and again on the lips. He smiles. "We did it Lex. Are you ok?"

Lex smiles, "I can still feel it Jay" she looks into his eyes and realizes he is not sure what she means. "My ass is still throbbing in a good way" she looks down at herself. "My vagina feels it too, it is still tingly and warm feeling inside." She looks at him smiling back at her, smiles hard as he reaches to embrace her.

"Lex, I am glad you went through with it. I was worried you would get scared and change your mind at the last minute. Then we would have to talk about it again and again until we finally did it or you felt it was to late for us to do it. It was an adventure, I was a little scared too."

The ship announces that they have arrived in the moon. Jay gets up and finishes the tea. "Do we wash the cups?"

"No leave them, there are service workers that enjoy cleaning the ships" Lex starts walking toward the stairs "let's go home Jay".

As they are walking through the corridors back to their home Jay realizes that he has no idea if it is day or night. He tries to estimate how long they were away and still is not sure, he checks his tablet and sees that it is the middle of what would be night in his estimation of time but sees that a similar pace of activity is happening in the corridors as during the day. "Lex, do Gyrekians follow days and nights like beings do on the planets?"

She looks at him. "What do you mean Jay?"

Jay thinks, "on planets the light hours are day and the dark hours are knight. Here on the moon the situation is different both because the orbit of the moon is around a planet and the spin is at a different rate than on most planets. How is it decided when things will be done? Um, when does the time for work start for most gyrekians?"

She looks at him. "We aren't as regimented as most places in the alliance Jay. We have adapted to an ebb and flow of commerce to accommodate our visitors but we basically work when we want." She looks at him as they approach their door and stops short of it. "Is it uncomfortable for you?"

"No, I hadn't thought about it. It is different. So the shops and businesses will be open day and knight?"

"Some". Then stepping toward their door. But most follow the rhythm of the city that they are in. We follow a Ramga day here but in several cities they follow a Ryberian day, much longer with longer work hours and longer rest times. A few cities follow traditional Gyrekian time, everything is open random hours. If you like we can move to another city." Lex opens the door and steps inside. "Jay do you want some tea?"

Jay looks down the corridor. Then steps in and closes the door behind him. "Yes, tea sounds good." he looks around, "I'm going to have a shower".

Lex says, "I'll bring the tea and join you"

Jay is enjoying the shower when he feels Lex's hands on his back then sliding around him and her hugging snugly on his back. "I like that Lex"

"The tea is on the ledge Jay" as she shifts her hugging, "Jay your tablet said you have a message from Herfermks. Can we sleep for a while after our shower? I want to sleep after today, I want to remember this day without adding more to it."

Jay slides around in her hug to hug her back under the warm shower. "Me too, let's sleep for a long time." After a few slow breaths, feeling her embrace he starts scrubbing her back and notice her doing the same to him. They lovingly scrub each other well and dry off, then go to bed and fall asleep in each other's arms, spooning, her in his arms, and her arms holding onto his. After some time Jay wakes up to go to the toilet and remembers Herfermks message, he goes to check it. It asks him to meet Herfermks at his place in the moon. Jay goes back to their bedroom and looks at Lex. He softly tells the room to inform her if she wakes before his return that he went to meet Herfermks and will be back soon. He dresses and goes to the door of Herfermks place in the corridor near the bar. He stands outside for a few seconds then knocks. He waits and checks his message then asks his tablet if there is a specific time that he is to meet with Herfermks. The tablet doesn't respond. Then the door opens.

"Jay" Herfermks looks both ways down the corridor, "come in my good friend. It is good to see you."

Jay smiles and walks into the room seeming well lit, and with furniture, and two other Ryberians sitting at the table looking his way and smiling at him. "It is good to see you too Herfermks, and an honor to see you Berkjets, and to meet you sir," as he nods the Ryberian that he hadn't seen before.

Berkjets stands and turns to the other Ryberian at the table then looks at Jay. "Jay this is Twrelark, He is a long time friend and colleague of ours. He is working on a project that we hope you can help us with."

Jay steps closer as Twrelark stands and faces him.

"Hello Jay," bowing slightly and extending both hands open palms up to him, "thank you for the assistance with the war, your help will be remembered for many lifetimes by my family."

Jay feels a little surprised and puts his hands in Twrelarks, "Thank you, the honor is mine sir, I am glad that I could help."

Twrelark holds his hands for a few seconds as he nods and looks into Jay's eyes then steps back to the side and gestures with one hand towards a chair while saying "please have a seat with us Jay."

Herfermks comes with a cup in his hand and places it on the table where Jay is expected to sit. "I brought a coffee from Earth, Reggie said that he asked for what you wanted and the man called it a flat white." The others both look at the cup with interest. "I tried one Jay, I couldn't drink it. It is not palatable. But I remembered you mentioning it several times so I thought I would get you one for this meeting."

Jay sits and sips the coffee. He looks at them looking at him and realizes that they are going to ask him something. Jay thinks that since they are all so polite it that it must be something big. He takes a drink. It is a good latte, bold and smooth. "mmm, thank you, it is a good coffee. How are you all doing?" he looks at Herfermks, "I hope your family is well," then looks at Berkjets eyes.

"I didn't taste it Jay but the smell, it is not comfortable to me, If you like it though, I guess you can choose what you like" Berkjets says then looks at the drink.

The three of them take their seats, Berkjets on one side, Twrelark on the other and Herfermks across from him. The ryberians look at each other back and forth then they all look at Jay. Herfermks sits back in his chair then looks at the others again. "Jay," He asks "we want to clone you so that you can be here while we take you to work with us on other worlds."

Jay looks at him. "Is that a good idea?"

Berkjets looks at Herfermks than at Jay and admits, "We are not sure Jay that is why we all came to ask you about it. There are issues with cloning that are complicated and uncertain. How do you feel about being cloned?"

Jay looks at him, "I haven't ever thought about it. Would my clone know that it is a clone, would it know anything, would it be physically better than me having not gone through the trauma and injuries that I have, or would it be weak and unskilled in motor functions like an infant, and with no understanding of what it is?"

Twrelark says "it is true, but we can record your memories and imbed them into the clone so it will have your experiences to draw from. The motor skills will develop faster that way and the personality will be easy to coach to become like yours."

"Are there ethical issues with cloning in the alliance?" Jay asks.

Berkjets interject "many Jay, but you are not recorded as being in the alliance so we could do it without braking any laws. I don't endorse this procedure, but I have been asked if we can so we are here asking you."

Jay looks at Herfermks and sees nothing in his face, then looks at Twrelark urgent expression. "Well?"

"Jay," Twrelark starts, "we know how well you performed in the past with the gowrlacks and we would like to be able to use you in other situations as well. If we have clones of you, you could live your life without having any risks to your self or your life that you want to continue on earth after your time with us."

Herfermks' face hasn't changed when Jay looks at it. He looks at Berkjets also and sees no hint at what he should say. Taking a sip of his coffe he remembers the words of Herfermks and his father, 'bad taste, bad smell'. "I am not sure that I want to be cloned" Jay says. "Will you do it anyway if I say no?"

Twrelark leans on the table and turns his head toward Jay. According to our law on Ryberia you are the possession of the department that Herfermks works with. You have no autonomous rights as an alien of a non-aliened planet that is without treaty with any alliance planet. If I ask the chain of command in my department I could have you borrowed from their branch to have this done. This meeting is a courtesy that they have asked for personally and out of respect for them, and that our cultural demands that such a request is appeased I am going through this process."

Jay looks at Herfermks then he looks at Berkjets. He remembers that the Pixies have an agreement with the Ryberians concerning his planet. Jay deducts that they must have kept this information from Twrelark. Jay thinks about how his two friends are staying silent while this ryberian is pressuring him to do something that is not ethical according to their rules. "Well," Jay looks at each of them. "I can't let you take such a risk. It would not be fair to jeopardize your careers when I am available for what ever Herfermks want me to do as I am."

Twelark says, "what risk? You will be left intact after the cloning process and know one will ever know except those involved, it is not a crime as you are not a member of a species with any possible legal recourse."

Jay looks at him and hesitates as he looks into his eyes. "I have been bonded as mate to a Gyrekian female here on the moon, we are having a family. I have been recorded as her bonded mate and thus accepted in their law as a Gyrekian. In their law I am one of them, so it would be against them that the crime would be committed. Do they permit cloning of their species? Would the alliance be willing to hide such a matter if it was found out? And, if they found out that the Ryberians had planted a human in their midst to breed with one of their females, disguised as a Kyranin, what would be said about it on Ramga?" He looks at Herfermks and sees a slight sparkle in his eye. "I can't let you take the risk. It would be too devastating for your alliance if any of the clones got caught, or found out, or got away and did something terrible. We humans are so unpredictable, that is why you want my clone isn't it?" he looks at Twrelark, "why do you want my clone?" There must be a good reason? I can't think what it could be though."

Twelark sits back in his chair and looks at Jay, then the others. "When did you bond with a Gyrekian?"

Jay smiles and looks at Herfermks. "Herfermks, remember that server at the bar, she flirted with me and it went forward so fast, we are on our bonding holiday now. Her father says I should take at least two weeks from work to assure a good bonding. I didn't have time to research it but I think I am doing well. We are becoming very close. I actually want to take some time from my work with you too, to spend here with her. I want to live the life of a Gyrekian with her here in the moon. Can I do that?"

Herfermks looks at Jay with a perplexed look, "what do you mean?"

Jay looks at Birkjets and gives him a soft kick under the table. Then looks at Twrelark, then back at Herfermks. "Well I understand that on your world it is a custom to bond for life and that the family is the top priority. I believe it is the same here in the moon. Now that I am a mate and thus a member of the moon I want to live my life with my mate, at least for the short time that I am agreed to have here. I want to be able to stay here on this moon and live my life with my mate as one of them."

Twrelark looks at Herfermks then Berkjets, then at Jay, "it was interesting, and it is an honor to meet you Jay." then he looks down at his tablet and moves his fingers on the screen and fades out of view.

Birkjets smiles and nods at Jay then turns to Herfermks "I'll go and be sure all is well on our side" and fades out as well.

Herfermks smiles and nods, "Thank you Jay, for not mentioning the Pixies. It is best that we don't share their treaty until they are ready to become full members with the alliance. I am glad that you said it so gracefully. He is a pushy ryberian and likes to get what he wants. I didn't like the clone idea. But he has got influence and could have made things difficult for us all." Herfermks smiles, I brought you a machine to make that drink you like from earth and the other ingredients too, they are in the next room. I don't know how you will power it here though, I am sure there is a way."

"How are you doing?" Jay asks

"It is always interesting Jay." Herfemks looks around the room. "I fixed it up a little for you. If we have to meet we can meet here and if Lex comes with you we won't have to explain anything." Then looking directly at Jay "I was spending a few months at home with my children when Twrelark had me called into a meeting. None of us liked his idea but he pushed so we had to ask you. I will be glad that I can go back to my children. My father is thorough, it will be closed and there is no possibility of you being cloned without us knowing about it."

Jay smiles and takes a drink of the latte, licks his lips and says, "I found something that you might want to look into. It is about the origin of the pyramids here."

Herfermks looks at Him. "What do you know of the pyramids Jay?"

I am one of them now Herfermks, so I have free access to all security here, I know it all, I think?" I went back and recorded what happened to the being from the pyramids" taking out his tablet and handing to Herfermks. "I would like to share it with the gyrekians but they don't know about the time tool, so I can't." sitting the tablet on the table then pointing to it, Look at the files I recorded, I am sure you will find some helpful data about the workings of the pyramids and the being's demise who brought them here."

Herfermks looks at the tablet and asks Jay to use his new security status to hide the files in his tablet. "Jay things are getting more complicated in Ryberia. The various departments are spying on each other.

What I wanted from you here is likely in there but I can't look into it now. I know where to find it and I will when I get a clean chance. For now I will only be here to visit you and your family. It won't be often. Your identity will be as was created by the Gyrekians when they accepted you as a kyranin bonded mate to a gyrekian female. We will prevent further traces from your work in the war and assure your request to live your years here is secured." Herfermks smiles and winks at Jay" Home, grant Jay full and total access to his level of security here both as my subordinate and ryberian diplomat, and also as a member of the moon." He looks at Jay, "my family is well, and yours will be too." He smiles and fades out of view.

Jay looks around the room, finishes his coffee and goes home to his bed, cuddles up with Lex, feeling a little jittery from the coffee and goes to sleep.

Herfermks fades in behind his father and watches his father watching Twrelark's meeting with his colleagues. Herfermks slides backwards and forwards in time watching to be sure that his father is undetected in his surveillance of Twrelark and his team. Then he fades into a meeting with Berkjets. "They don't know you attended their meeting. I couldn't detect anyone else there. My other scans showed that no one was watching us on the moon. I have seen that Twrelark's team have all started other projects, but still I worry about them cloning Jay without his consent."

Berkjets leans forward, "I left some probes from the future to watch him and alert us if he does anything with Jay or data that was taken of Jay."

"Lets go back to a time when we can be sure we are not followed." Herfermks says, "I want to go fishing on the ruysec world before the calamity" and he looks at his father with a serious look.

"Just before or a long time before." Berkjets asks.

Herfermks makes some hand signals on the table as he looks around the room. "I am going to go back and see my family, lets talk again in a few weeks."

Brekjets smiles, I want to go to the city, Vbransto, to the market for some fruit to go with the birds Yintenshix said she acquired for our evening meal tonight. See you at dinner!" Berkjets smiles and fades out of view.

Herfermks fades out of view and into his family home's front entrance. He looks around and sees his children out in the yard basking in the sun. He looks inside and sees the vast entrance hall and sees up two levels Kadjieken swinging out and then coming down a ladder. "Hello, have you seen my mother around today?"

"Herfermks, hi, no, I think she is in her room sleeping, we went to hunt in the forest yesterday and she ate a lot." he jumps down the last 6 feet and runs over stopping in front of Herfermks. Do you want to go hunting with us next time?"

Herfermks smiles, "Yes, actually I would like that. Be sure to tell me when you will be going next, the day before, so I can be there." Herfermks puts his hand on Kadjieken shoulder as they walk past each other. Herfermks walks into the next room. "Home, security, full security sweep and report."

Seconds pass then the home responds. "Two time surveillance probes watching the house form outside, one event recorder in the kitchen, a visual record and transmitter device in the entrance."

Herfermks says, "house, top security sweep for this room" and waits for the all clear tone and detailed response. Then he pulls out his tablet and asks to travel back 30 years. As he is fading he starts working the screen and changes the 30 years to 3000 and changes the location too. He unfades in a grassy field with a fence around it. Then working the tablet with his fingers he fades again and appears on Ruysec world during the calamity. As Herfermks starts to fade in he is working his screen and a shield appears before that, and he un-fades inside of it. There are several small explosions in close proximity to him. Then him and the shield fade again back in time a few days. He looks at the data on his tablet and scrolls through several screens then asks his tablet to scan for technology in the area.

His tablet responds "water driven electrical generator 3 kilometers to the north, many variable wave communication devices in the area of the generator, two surface vehicles with similar communication equipment and projectile weapons .6 kilometers to the east, a small city 5 kilometers to the southwest with various similar technologies in it. Nothing to detect your presence if uncloaked an in this faze and time."

Herfermks moves his fingers on the screen of the tablet and hears his fathers voice beside him, and turns. "Hello, were you followed?"

Birkjets nods, "only to the calamity" then looks around, they will be here looking for us soon.

Herfermks looks at him and hesitates then reaches out and touches his arm "earth" and they both fade and fade into a room. A small room, that smells bad, "sorry father, I thought of it as the least likely place that we would be looked for. We can relocate from here to an out door location."

"Where are we?" Birkjets asks.

"It is a toilet room", Herfermks says.

"I can see that but where?" Birkjets asks.

As they start to fade Herfermks says "it is where I met Jay once when I had to send him back to earth during his training to get him to think about his situation. It is on Earth, Jay's home planet. We have an alliance with the Pixies here so we will go to where we can meet with them."

"Why", Berkjets asks.

"In case we are ever asked what we were doing here" Herfermks asks. "Do you have any idea who authorized it and why we are under surveillance?"

Berkjets looks at him as the forest starts to appear around them. "No" he takes out his own tablet and starts working the screen. He looks at Herfermks doing the same as he searches the scans and information about the probes at their home and the ones that exploded an the ruysec world as he arrived during the calamity. "It looks like it is our own department, except these two probes." tilting his tablet to show it to Herfermks.

"Those are not ryberian probes," Herfermks says. Then he taps his screen to his fathers tablet, works the screen with his fingers, and asks his tablet to do reconnaissance and return. He watches as his tablet half fades out of view for a split second. Then has a new screen of data on it.

Berkjets looks at it, "that is good son, what did you do?"

Herfermks smiles, "I wrote a program to get it to travel without me to scan things and return in the same second in time to where it leaves form. It works petty good. I lost one though. I had to go back to see what happened to it. It was melted by a weapons blast, I was researching a battle in the war with the gworlacks."

"Did you watch to see that it is all that happened to it?" Berkjets asks.

"I did" Herfermks says, and then I checked again more thoroughly after I noticed the discrepancies.

"What did it find" Berkjets asks as they both start looking at the screen, after a second Berkjets taps his screen to it and starts working his screen with his fingers as Herfermks does the same with his. "It is an older variation of one of our time probes, it was only used by the genetic development science

teams for their results research" Berkjets says. Then he
looks at Herfermks, Why would they want to watch us?"

Herfermks looks up then back at his screen, "lets go see, it was
sent from three days before we went to meet with Jay on the
moon", as he works the screen and then reaches for his fathers
arm. Looking up at him as he touches his arm he says "we will
stay out of faze and cloaked to watch, I will let go of you and I
will slide past the event to see that we are not detected as you
scan the event."

Berkjets smiles, "ok" and they fade. Berkjet starts to see the
meeting with four ryberians that he knows talking about him
and Herfermks as he feels his son let go of his arm. He starts
scanning as he is listening to what they are saying then moves
to the next room and scans form there then the rest of the area
and adjoining rooms in the building that the meeting is in.
Then he stays in the room and listens for a while as the
meeting continues. One of the ryberians in the meetings raises
several questions about him and his son's activities and asks
why are their no records of so many uses of the time travel
technology. The other says some things are best not recorded.
Another asks who gets to determine that. The other say we do,
all of us who do past or future research get to determine what
we should have records of and who gets to see the records.
The first one says I want to see the records of all of Herfermks
time travels. The one that had not yet spoken starts to laugh. I
have worked with him, once, a long time ago. It would take
you all of your life to look at all of his time travel records, if he
kept any. "I want to know what he is doing" The first one says,
the others say nothing. "We can put some probes on them and
watch their activities to see what they are doing, but I suspect

we won't learn much" the other says. The first says, "lets do it" and looks at the other two, "get it done".

Berkjets takes a scan of each of them then a second scan of the first one. "He is a clone!" he says.

Herfermks appears beside Berkjets. "I watched from two days before until a day after the meeting. We were not detected. So you say it is a clone, who did it?"

Berkjets looks at him "I don't know, lets see what Twrelark's connection to this clone is."

Herfemks asks, "Where is the real ryberian that this was cloned from?" They both start to fade.

Herfermks travels back in time out of faze following the movements of the clone as his father searches for the real ryberian that the clone was made from. Herfemks follows the clone back for three days until he is in a lab on a table hooked up to a machine. He stops and watches and sees that Twrelark is at the controls of the machine and watches as the clone is programed and then tested with activities and conversations with lab staff after being unhooked from the machine. Herfemks watches back several more days and finds out that Twrelark has several clones working for him discreetly. Then he goes back to the second he left his father.

Berkjets traced the ryberian that had been cloned to a month earlier when he had traveled to a world outside of the alliance and had been missing for a day. But he could not find proof that he had traveled back to ryberia. So Berkjets returned to one second after he left to appear at the same time as Herfermks.

"I think the original may be gone. I can't find him."

Herfermks says "Twrelark is programing these clones, I don't know why though. Can you think of a reason?"

Berkjets looks at Herfermks "I don't know where to look. It doesn't make any sense to me. We are no threat, and why the clones, what does he want to have clones, what for?"

Herfermks shrugs, "in the scans of him was there anything irregular? What about wanting to clone Jay, any reason given?"

Berkjets works his tablet, "he had a very low security for a long time, and then it was upgraded a lot last year, and just a few months ago to near our levels. Usually it would take gradual upgrades for a century, I wonder if a clone did it for him?"

"I will watch to see if he tries to access Jay some how." Herfermks works his tablet and sends it off. It shifts in his hand with a new screen showing. Herfermks grabs his father arm, "take me with you" then starts reading his tablet and reading information on the screen.

They fade and appear in a ship with transparent floors ceilings and walls with a lot of ryberians working at consoles and desks that are also transparent. A few of them look up and give them a nod as they appear and start walking through the room to the next room. Berkjets says "lets sit there" gesturing to a console with a chair on either side.

Herfermks looks up from his tablet and nods then seats himself and works his tablet again. "No Jay seems Ok until his time is up on the moon".

Berkjets taps his tablet to the console and asks "full security history of Twrelark." The console screen shows three sections, one of a list of infractions to security, one a graph of his security over time and one of the details of his present security codes and clearances. "Look, he had his security held back for good reason, he has suspicious ambition syndrome."

"That is rare" Herfermks says. He looks up to see a few other ryberians coming from the other room. "Console, top most security, research the activities of Twrelark, regarding actual cloning of ryberians and locations of the original ryberians cloned."

The three other ryberians stand around the console and watch the search results appear. Berkjets reads the results aloud as it starts to appear on the screen saying "He has cloned three ryberians that are no longer with us and these five that are now stationed on informal duty in distant colonies. He looks up at the other three agents. "He has had probes watching us for several days that we know about but we don't know why."

Herfermks looks at the screen, "I can't see a reason either". Then looks up at their colleagues "Can any of you?"

The largest one looks at the others and shrugs. The other two start working on their tablets and fade out and back again. One is shaking his head from side to side and the other says can't make any sense of it either, should we have him collected?"

Birkjets says "if he does have a reason I want to be told what it was."

Herfermks says "are there others making clones? Is he one himself? Or is he simply a sick ryberian?"

The tall one says, "ship, analyze situation with Twrelark, collect him and the clones and the originals and bring them securely into my meeting room now." then he looks at them all, "puts his hands on the other two's backs, "Should we have something to eat first?"

Herfermks says, "I'm going to have dinner with my family" and looks at Berkjets.

Berkjets turns and looks at the three of them smiling at him arm in arm, "not this time, I'm going to eat with my family too, and could you not mention to him that we found out, we have several associates in common with him and it could cause riffs in our working relationships if he mentions it." He watches as the three start to fade, then one is covered in blood. Berkjets leans back and sees Herfermks jump in his seat to look too. "What happened?"

The other two stepping back from him, "it didn't look so big until I got to it, it was more than I could handle so I had to use a weapon, sorry, I should have stopped to clean up before coming back, I didn't look at myself."

They all burst into laughter, "well we better get you cleaned up before we let you interview Twrelark" Herfermks says, and they all laugh harder.

Herfermks looks at Berkjets. The three turn and start walking and laughing then splitting up in different direction across the room. "Well dad" he smiles, Should we go to dinner? Or do you want to look at what Jay learned for us first?"

Berkjets looks with curiosity "dinner first, let me enjoy the mystery for a while."

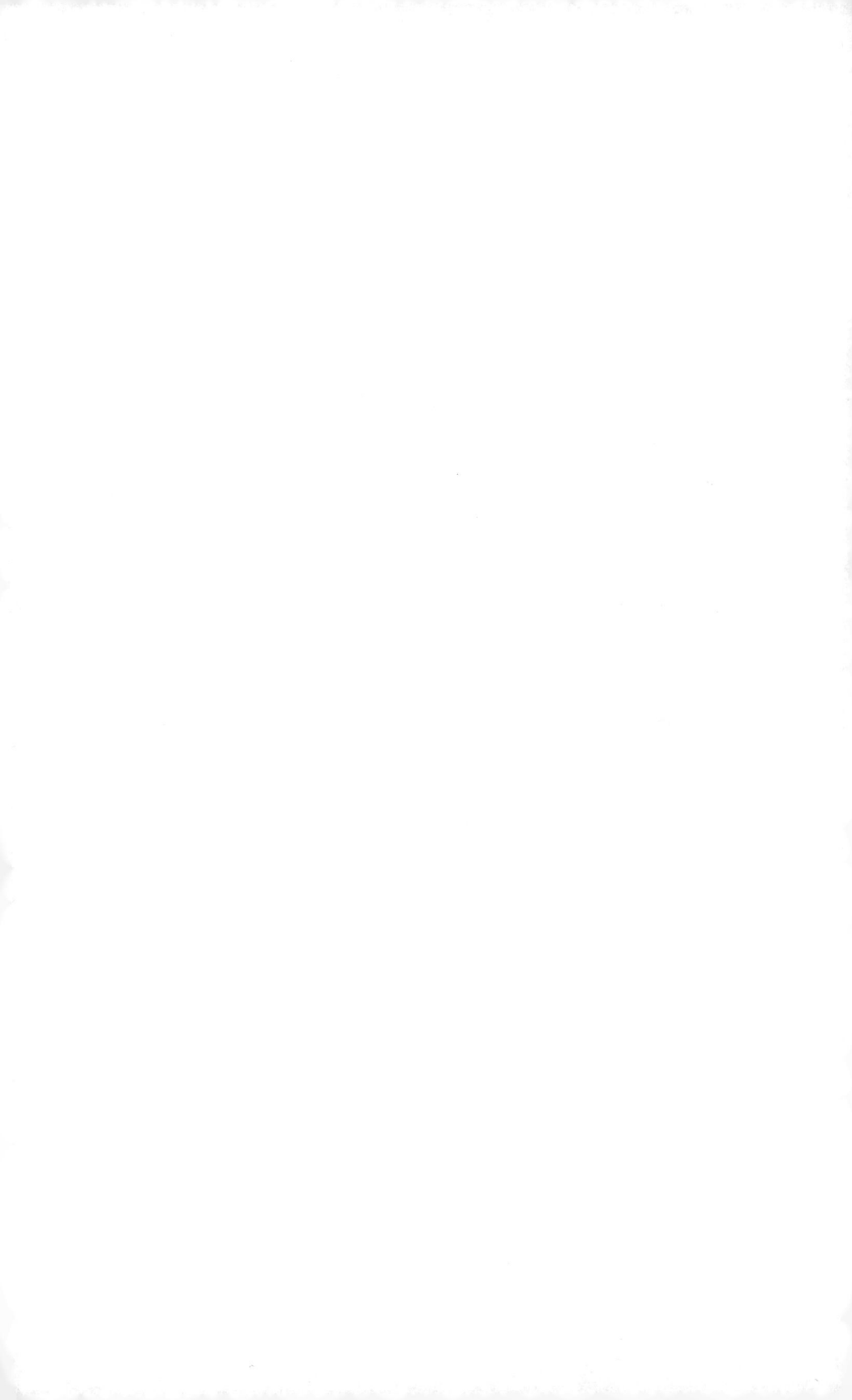

Made in the USA
San Bernardino, CA
31 August 2017